MW00709491

Bone-setting Skills in Traditional Chinese Medicine

Written by Zhang Zhigang
Translated by Wang Baoqin
                Zhang Yuxi
                Liang Suqian
                Zhao Huaying

Shandong Science and Technology Press

First Edition 1996

**Bone-setting Skills in Traditional
Chinese Medicine**
Written by Zhang Zhigang
Translated by Wang Baoqin   Zhang Yuxi
Liang Suqian   Zhao Huaying
Published by Shandong Science and Technology Press
Printed by Shandong Dezhou Xinhua Printing House
Distributed by China International Book Trading Corporation
35 Chegongzhuang Xilu, Beijing 100044, China
P. O. Box 399, Beijing, China
ISBS 7−5331−1797−2
Printed in the People's Republic of China

Preface

Orthopedics and traumatology of Traditional Chinese Medicine (TCM) date back to ancient times, and have long been an integrate part of the great TCM treasure house. In the prolonged struggle against diseases, injuries and wounds, and through ages of uninterrupted explorations and summarization by doctors of past generations and scientists of modern times, the Chinese nation has accumulated a wealth of experience in medical theories and practice, some of which can be rated as the earliest in the world.

This book is aimed at promoting further progress in the field of orthopedics and traumatology through academic exchanges and joint explorations among the Chinese and foreign medical scientists. It introduces and explains TCM orthopedics and traumatology, focusing on common fractures and dislocations, to our fellow practitioners and friends abroad, with the hope of finding better cures for these diseases.

The first two chapters of the book present a brief introduction of the history of the development of TCM orthopedics and traumatology and some general principles of the diagnosis, manual reduction, fixation with splints and bandages, functional exercises and herbal therapy. Other chapters expound on the diagnosis and treatment of various individual fractures and dislocations and, with the aid of illustrations, describes the characteristics of the synopses and treatment mentioned above. An index is appended with the book which may help the readers learn how to use traditional Chinese medicinal materials.

This book will benefit our fellow practitioners abroad in applying the Chinese medical skills, and through imparting an understanding of the features of TCM orthopedics and traumatology in combination with their own knowledge, enable them to improve therapeutic efficacy, relieve pain of the patients and hence benefit mankind with better and more effective remedies. It is also helpful for domestic readers to learn medical English.

We are sure there is still much room for improvement with the content and English translation of the book due to our limited knowledge, pressing time and especially the great difficulty in putting the profound terminology of TCM and the complicated descriptions of the manual maneuvers into English. We hope the readers will not hesitate to let us know their kind advice and suggestions, if any, for further improvement.

Acknowledgments are hereby made to Song Ligang of the Anatomy Department of Shandong College of Traditional Chinese Medicine, who has carefully prepared the illustrations for the book.

Zhang Zhigang
Professor of Department of Orthopedics and Traumatology
Shandong College of TCM
April, 1996

Contents

1

Chapter 1

A Short History of the Development of Orthopedics and Traumatology of Traditional Chinese Medicine

The orthopedics and traumatology of Traditional Chinese Medicine (TCM), an important branch of TCM, has a long history and has made great contributions to the existence, development, reproduction and prosperity of the Chinese nation. Early in the primitive stage of clan society, our ancestors tried to conquer the harsh environment in their life. They suffered diseases and traumatic injuries in their fight against poisonous snakes or wild beasts, and in their labor and wars, so they kept exploring and searching for various ways of conquering nature and relieving the suffering of diseases. They experienced a course from unconsciousness to consciousness in learning and summing up a vast amount of medicinal knowledge and practical experience such as massage for treating injury, external application of herbs and hot compress therapy, etc. Stone knives, axes, spades, etc. which were both productive and medical tools were found in the ruins of Banpo Village of the matrilineal clan society dating back to 6 000 years ago. The stone and bone needles show that people may have treated diseases with them.

Among the unearthed relics of the Shang Dynasty (16th century B. C. — 1066B. C.), there are bronzeware such as needles, knives, axes and arrows which are more advanced than stone needles.

According to the records of Western Zhou Dynasty (1066 B. C. — 770 B. C.), *Zhou Li (Volume 9)* , the doctors were divided into

1

four kinds, that is, food doctors, doctors treating diseases, doctors treating sores, and veterinarians. The doctors treating sores might treat sores, abscesses, ulcers, fractures, metal-induced wounds, etc. In the Spring and Autumn period, Warring States period and Han Dynasty (722 B. C. − 220 A. D.), with the economical development, traumatology of TCM has made rapid progresses. First, the publishing of *Internal Classic*, *Classic on Medical Problems*, *Shen Nong's Herbal Classic* and *Treatise on Febrile and Miscellaneous Diseases* laid the theoretical basis for the development of traditional Chinese medicine. The *Internal Classic* with rich content made comprehensive exposition on the basic theories of anatomy, pathology, physiology, diagnostics, pathogenesis and therapeutic principles. Based on the anatomic observations of corpses, the shape, size and length of the skeleton of the skull, trunk and limbs were described. The theories that the kidney is in charge of the bone, the liver is in charge of the tendons, the spleen has the function to nourish the muscles and skin, pain is caused by *qi* disturbance, swelling is due to injury to the tissues, etc. were elucidated. The pathology, pathogenesis, clinical manifestations, and diagnostics and treatment based on differentiation of symptoms and signs of hematogenous pyogenic infections of soft tissues, ostarthritis and the whole body were recorded. Acupuncture, hot compress, massage, as well as medication were adopted in treatment and timely incision and drainage of pyogenic infection were also introduced in the book. In one of the unearthed relics from the tomb of the Han Dynasty at Mawangdui, *Fifty-two Diseases and Prescriptions* written on silk fabrics in the Qin or Han Dynasty, the therapeutical methods and recipes for many kinds of traumatic diseases such as wounds by knives, metal tools and traumatic bleeding, and many ways of analgesia, hemostasis, prevention of cicatrices after healing, and cleaning of infected traumatic wound were recorded. The famous doctor in traumatology in the Han Dynasty, Hua Tuo, was not only good at treatment of diseases with acupuncture and herbal drugs but also good at surgery. He performed such operations as sequestrectomy and la-

2

parotomy under the anesthesia with *Mafu Tang*. He also developed an exercise named "Exercise Imitating the Movements of Five Kinds of Animals" as a physical therapy. From the Wei and Jin Dynasties to the Sui and Tang Dynasties (A. D. 220—960), there was great improvement in the diagnosis and treatment of traumatic diseases and traumatology became a separated branch of medical science. The intraoral reduction for dislocations of temporomandibular joint recorded in *A Handbook of Prescriptions for Emergencies* written by Ge Hong is the earliest reduction method in the world used for dislocation of this joint and is still in use now. Thirty-four recipes for traumatic injuries were recorded in *Liu Juanzi's Remedies Left Over by Ghosts* written by Gong Qingxuan of the Southern Qi Dynasty.

The book *General Treatise on the Causes and Symptoms of Diseases* compiled by Chao Yuanfang of the Sui Dynasty is the first book on etiopathology, which sets aside a special chapter for traumatological diseases and discusses the causes and symptoms of 32 kinds of fractures and their complications. Reduction, debridement and suturing are suggested to be taken for open fracture and the broken ends of bone should be sutured and fixed, which is the earliest record of internal fixation of fracture.

It was recorded in *Prescriptions Worth a Thousand Gold for Emergencies* compiled by Sun Simiao of the Tang Dynasty that kerotherapy and hot compress were used after reduction of the dislocation of temporomandibular joint to help restore articular functions. It was recorded that hot wet felt compress could relieve the pain after injury in *The Medical Secrets of an Official* compiled by Wang Tao. *Secret Recipes of Treating Wounds and Bone-setting Taught by Celestials* written by Lin, a Taoist, is the first monograph on traumatology and orthopedics in China. Four therapeutic principles for managing fractures, i. e. reduction, splintage, dirigation and herbal therapy were initiated in the book and their manipulative steps and precautions were also recorded, such as "reduction with the aid of chair-back" for setting dislocatioin of shoulder joint, which is based on "lever principle", were recorded. The

3

book also recorded 40 prescriptions. Taoist Lin is a famous ancient traumatologist in China.

The orthopedics and traumatology made further advances in the Song and Yuan Dynasties (A. D. 960—1368). In the Song Dynasty medicine was divided into nine specialties, two of which were specialty of sore and traumatology and specialty of war wounds and incantation. Four therapies for fractures, i. e. reduction, fixation, medication and massage, were recorded in *General Collection for Holy Relief*, which collected 160 prescriptions for treating traumatic injuries. In *On Medicine* by Zhang Gao, the method of rolling muscles and tendons with bamboo-tube for relaxation was introduced to treat functional disturbances of traumatic injuries in the ankle and knee joints, and open reduction was described for treating polysegment fracture of tibia.

In the Yuan Dynasty there were many wounds caused by frequent wars, so the development and improvement of traumatology in theory and practice were promoted. There were 13 departments in the imperial hospital, one of which is for bone-setting and war wounds equivalent to the specialty of orthopedics and traumatology of the modern times. *The Effective Formulas Handed Down for Generations* written by Wei Yilin recorded the great achievements in traumatology achieved before Yuan Dynasty and summarized the main fractures and articular dislocations in the four extremities as "Six types of dislocations and four types of fractures", which perfected the diagnosis and treatment in orthopedics and traumatology. The method of "Suspending reposition" used to treat the flexion type of spinal fractures was recorded in the book. He was the first doctor in the world who applied suspending reposition to treat spinal fracture. He divided the fracture and dislocation of ankle joints into inversion type and eversion type and applied different reduction methods accordingly. He also pointed out that after fixation of fractures of elbow joints, proper exercises should be practiced, otherwise "in the future it would be difficult to extend and flex the elbow".

From Ming to Qing Dynasties (A. D. 1368—1911), with the

4

further development of economy, culture and medicine, including orthopedics and traumatology, stepped into a thriving period. Large number of treatises and books on orthopedics and traumatology were published. There was greater development in basic theories and practical skills of bone-setting. Department of bone-knitting and department of war wounds were set up in the imperial hospital of Ming Dynasty, and later the department of bone-knitting was changed to department of bone-setting. Bone-setting maneuvers, splint fixation and 1256 formulae for treating traumas were recorded in the *Universal Prescriptions* compiled by Zhu Su, etc. For example, backward and forward types of dislocations of the hip joints are distinguished with inversion or eversion of the knee joint involved as the diagnostic reference, and for the forward and backward angled displacements in fracture of the surgical neck of the humerus, flexing the upper arm forwards and extending it backwards are recommended for treatment respectively; for extension type of fracture of the distal end of the radius, the wrist should be fixed in flexion after reduction was described; traction with a towel pulling the mandible is adopted to treat fracture and dislocation of the cervical spine. The reduction followed by knee-crown fixation can be used to treat fracture of the patella. In *Classification and Treatment of Traumatic Diseases* compiled by Xue Ji, sixty-five proven cases are recorded. It was put forward in the preface of the monograph that "when an injury happens to the limbs outside, *qi* and blood are hurt inside, *ying* and *wei* cannot circulate smoothly and disharmony between *zang* and *fu* takes place." The statement indicates the close relationship between local injuries and the whole body. In *Golden Mirror of Medicine* compiled by Wu Qian of Qing Dynasty, the experience of treating wounds before the Qing Dynasty was summed up and the skills of bone-setting were summed up as eight maneuvers, i. e. touching, uniting, lifting, pulling, pressing, pushing, pinching and kneading. The method of "hanging on ropes and standing on brick piles" was described for the first time for reduction of fracture and dislocation of thoracolumbar vetebrae (Fig. 1—1), then pillows are

5

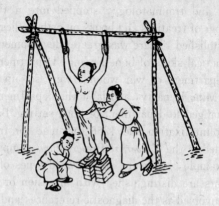

Fig. 1—1　Hanging on ropes and standing on brick piles

put under the lumbus so as to hyperextend the spinal column. The method is suitable for the flexion type of fracture and dislocation. Various fixation devices were invented such as bamboo curtain and China fir fence to carry out fixation for the fractures of limbs. Wooden supporter and lumbar splint were used for fixation of the fracture with dislocation in thoracolumbar vertebrae. In another book, *Compilation of Traumatology* written by Hu Tingguang, there are over a thousand recipes together with 14 drawings illustrating the reduction of fractures. Small splints together with supporting boards were used for fixation of the supracondylar fracture of the humerus, embodying the principle of combination of activity and inertia. *Supplement to Traumatology* written by Qian Xiuchang dealt with 10 kinds of fixation of fractures and dislocations, 17 kinds of traumatic injuries and recorded 92 recipes, which were put into rhyme for the sake of easy memory. Other monographs published in the period, such as *Encyclopedia of Traumatology* written by Zhao Zhuquan, *Jiang's Traumatology* written by Jiang Kaoqing, etc. have made great contributions to the development of traumatology. In a word, the orthopedics and traumatology of TCM with a history of thousands of years reflex the precious and rich theories and experience of the Chinese working people accumulated in their long struggle against traumatic injuries and bone and joint diseases. Some of the theories and methods are the earliest inventions in the world and represented the advanced level of the world at the time.

In the years of the late Qing Dynasty and the Republic of China, because the Northern Warlords and the Kuo Mintang reactionaries took the reactionary policy of banning traditional medicine, the development of TCM was seriously hindered, almost resulting in its extinction and the traumatology of TCM was also in an extremely difficult situation. Some of the theories and skills were handed down from the older generations of the family or secret teachers while others such as open reduction of fracture and internal fixation which were at their embryonic stage did not develop but were lost.

After the founding of the People's Republic of China, thanks to the correct TCM policy adopted by the people's government, the TCM orthopedics and traumatology, just like the withered trees in the spring, were revived and have been thriving. Many colleges and schools of TCM have been set up with departments of orthopedics and traumatology. Large numbers of doctors specialized in orthopedics and traumatology have been trained and brought up. Lots of hospitals and research institutes specialized in orthopedics and traumatology have been established all over China. Great achievements in medicine, medical education and scientific research have been made. The development and systematization of TCM orthopedics and traumatology have been accelerated. Monographs on orthopedics and traumatology have been published like bamboo shoots after a spring rain, of which those with tremendous influences include *Shi's Bone-setting*, *Wang's Bone-setting* and *Wei's Bone-Setting* in Shanghai, *Guo's Bone-Setting* in Henan and Su's Bone-setting in Tianjin. Liu Shoushan and Du Ziming of Beijing, Liang Tiemin of Shandong, Chen Zhankui of Hei Longjiang, Lin Rugao of Fujian, etc. published their books on TCM orthopedics and traumatology one after another. Fang Xianzhi and Shang

Tianyu compiled *Treatment of Fractures by Combining Traditional Chinese Medicine with Western Medicine* in 1966, in which they put forward the four principles of treating fractures, i. e. activity combined with inertia, stress on the treatment of both fracture and soft tissues, simultaneous treatment of both internal and external injuries and harmonious doctor-patient cooperation. In the treatment of fractures and dislocations, guided by these principles, the healing time is usually shortened and complications reduced. In all localities the clinical experience of expert doctors of TCM were summed up and proved folk recipes for treating traumatic injuries were collected. Scientific research on such topics as "the relationship between kidney and bones", "promoting blood circulation to remove blood stasis", "mechanics of splinting materials" and "effects of Chinese traditional drugs in the promotion of fracture healing" have been conducted and great achievements have been scored. In clinical practice, the therapeutic effectiveness for intra-articular fractures was improved. Doctors succeeded in treating malunion of fractures by manual osteoclasis. For open fractures with skin defect, treatment of external application of Chinese herbal medicine on the surface of the wound was given and after the union of fracture, the scar left is small and soft and the functions of the fractured member are desirable. And great achievements in summing up and improving the manipulations of reduction, splint fixation, devices for traction fixation and dirigation have been procured.

In recent years, a dynamic academic atmosphere has prevailed the field of TCM orthopedics and traumatology in China. There have been rapid advances and more and more academic exchanges and cooperation in the field between China and other countries day by day. Chinese doctors and researchers and their international partners are learning from each other. Related international organizations have been set up to promote the development of the whole undertaking of orthopedics and traumatology in the world. With the rapid development of China's economy and the increase of international cooperation, Chinese doctors and researchers in the

field are making full use of the advanced science and technology,
carrying on TCM as well as the orthopedics and traumatology of
TCM forward and making even greater contributions to the rejuve-
nation and development of China and the health of mankind.

Chapter 2

A Brief Introduction of Diagnosis and Treatment in Orthopedics and Traumatology of TCM

Section I   Diagnostic Methods

A clinical diagnosis is made by differentiating symptoms and signs in line with the dialectical viewpoints of TCM theories, through four diagnostic methods, i. e. inspection, auscultation-olfaction, interrogation, and pulse feeling and palpation, with the help of special traumatological examination, necessary x-ray and laboratory examinations, and on the basis of overall analysis of the clinical data.

● **Inspection**

Inspection includes not only the general observations of the patient's expression, look, carriage, picture of tongue but also contrast and dynamic observation of the trauma.

1. Posture and gait

According to observations of the body posture and patient's gait, a rough judgment about the location and severity of the injury may be made. If the patient is quick in action, the injury is usually not serious. If the patient can't sit, stand or walk, it is meant that the location of the patient's wound lies below the loin. If the patient can't stand up and move about by himself or is forced to take a certain posture, it is indicated that there is osteoarticular injury and the condition is severe. Some fractures or dislocations are characterized by particular postures. The gait of the patient is very helpful to the diagnosis of injuries in spine and lower limbs.

2. Expression and look

Rough judgment of the injury may be formed by the expression and look of the patient. The normal expression and calm appearance show that it is a mild injury or an old one. Absent-mindedness, pallor, apathy, dysphoria, cold sweat on the frontal part, short breath and asthma usually indicate that the injury is severe.

3. Inspection of contour, color and luster

Inspection of contour, color and luster of the local skin can help to understand the severity of the injury. Cyanosis of local skin with blisters and localized swelling is caused by the bleeding of fresh injury. If the color of the local skin turns yellowish and the swelling is rather extensive, the injury is an old one. If the local cyanosis darkens progressively and the area expands gradually, it is indicated that there is still bleeding from the injured blood vessels. If the skin is red and hot, it is possible that the stagnated evil factors have been converted into pathogenic fire leading to infection. The dark blue skin may be the manifestation of tissue necrosis.

4. Inspection of deformity

Deformity is mostly caused by fractures or dislocations. Judgment can be formed by observing marker lines or points on the body or limbs. The length, thickness, angulation, bend, high projection, collapse, rotation, inclination or deformity of peculiar shape should be observed. Different kinds of deformities and their changes are of help in the diagnosis of injury and judgment of prognosis.

5. Inspection of wound

If there is open wound, it should be inspected to determine:

(1) the wound is deep or superficial, large or small;

(2) the edge of the wound is regular or not;

(3) whether there is contamination and the degree, if any;

11

(4) whether there are exposed fractured ends;

(5) whether there are damage and fragmentation of nerves, blood vessels, muscles and tendons;

(6) whether there is any change in the pupils and what the tongue looks like.

6. Measurement

The length, thickness of the injured member and angles of articular activity may be measured with a tape measure or a protractor and compared with those of the normal side and analysis of the comparison can be made.

● Auscultation-olfaction

1. General auscultation-olfaction

Attention should be paid to the patient's language, respiration, and cough, and auscultation of the chest and abdomen should be made to find out the condition of the disease, e.g. mild or severe, deficiency type or excess type, any complications, etc.

2. Bony crepitus

Whenever crepitus is felt at the fractured part, complete fracture is proved. Take the fracture of the ribs for example. Sometimes the fracture can't be found on x-ray films but if bony crepitus can be felt when the doctor presses and squeezes the fractured part or when the patient coughs, it can be diagnosed as fracture of ribs. However, after a definite diagnosis is made, repeated examinations for crepitus should be avoided so as not to exacerbate injury.

3. Baby's cry

Because babies can't complain of their injury conditions, their cry is of significance to the diagnosis. When the injured part is pressed, the baby's cry sharpens suddenly, fracture is often indicated at the part pressed. When a parent or someone else carries the baby with hands supporting the baby's armpits, the cry becomes louder, it is usually suggested that there is fracture in the clavicle. .

12

4. Osteophony

Listening to the osteophony is a method of examination combining auscultation with percussion. During examination, the doctor puts the auditory end of the stethoscope on the proper part of the proximal end of the injured limb (such as bony projection) and percusses the bony projection of the distal end of the injured limb with fingers or a plesxor. In a normal person, clear and melodious steophony may be heard. If severe fracture or separated displacement occurs, the osteophy weakens or disappears. A contrast examination with the healthy part should be made.

5. Snap

If there is pathologic change in the joint or tendon, snapping sounds may be heard on moving the joints. After the injury of semilunar plate, for example, when the patient does rotation, extension or flexion movements of knee joints, a snap may be heard.

6. Crepitant rales

When the fractured ends of the ribs stab the lung forming pheumato-thorax and air penetrates into the subcutaneous tissue to form aeroceles, crepitant rales can be heard by pressing there.

● **Interrogation**

Interrogation is especially important in the diagnosis of diseases in orthopedics and traumatology. All patients except the comatose due to severe injury should be questioned. During the interrogation, apart from general questions concerning age, occupation, type of work in production, cold and heat, sweating, diet, stool, urination, etc., questions must be asked with regard to the following:

1. Time and circumstances of injury

The exact time of injury, falling height, position and posture, surroundings and conditions when injury occurs should be known.

2. Causes

The nature, greatness, direction and acting site of external force and anamnesis related to the cause of disease should be inquired to exclude pathological fracture.

3. Course of treatment

Questions like whether the injury has been diagnosed and treated, when and by which method the injury is diagnosed and treated, and what is the result, should be asked.

4. Present conditions of injury

What are the generalized symptoms at present? What are the nature, extent and degree of swelling and pain of local injury? Are there complications or functional disturbances in the limb involved?

● **Pulse-feeling and Palpation**

1. Pulse-feeling

In the course of making a diagnosis, apart from symptoms and signs, the pulse condition should be felt to help judge the severity, deficiency or excess type, cold or heat, of a disease and be used as one of the bases to go by in prescribing drugs and other therapies. Pulse examination mainly involves observation of pulse condition, its frequency, rhythm, fullness, strength, evenness, amplitude, etc. For example, floating pulse suggests that the disease belongs to the exterior syndrome while deep pulse, the interior syndrome. String pulse often suggests there is pain and blood stasis. Accordingly, when a mild injury occurs on the body surface, floating, string pulse can be felt while deep pulse can be felt in patients with impairment of internal organs, blood and qi, or injuries of the lumbus or spine. Because rapid pulse suggests a heat syndrome and full pulse hints exuberant heat. Rapid and full pulse may be felt in patients with fever and infection. Hollow pulse which is floating, large, soft and hollow to the feeling is often seen in cases of severe hemorrhage. Intermittent pulse is temporarily felt in cases of severe traumatic injuries with unbearable pain. For patients with severe traumatic injury but moderate pulse, the prognosis is often good. Thready and weak pulse is mostly seen in weak patients with chronic diseases. In making a diagnosis, both the pulse condition and symptoms and signs should be taken into consideration to make an overall analysis of the patient's condition.

2. Examination of the blood supply of the affected limb

The pulsation of the artery at the distal end of the injured limb should be examined. The sites for examination are usually the brachial artery at the antecubital region, the radial and ulnar arteries at the wrist, the popliteal artery at the popliteal fossa, the posterior tibial artery at the back of the medial malleolus, and the dorsal artery of foot. Sometimes finger nails or toe nails are pressed to observe whether the recovery time of blood supply is normal. On examination, special attention should be paid to whether there is disturbance of blood supply after injury. For example, breaking or contusion of the artery, compression of the artery by displaced broken ends or large hematoma, artery spasm due to irritation of the injury, compression of blood vessels by tight external fixation materials such as splints, compression pads, plaster, etc. may all lead to weak or even no pulsation of the artery at the injured distal end. The causes should be found out without delay and effective measures be taken.

3. Palpation

Doctor's careful palpation of the injured area is of help in obtaining related information about the injury, e. g. fracture, dislocation, severity of injury, displacement, etc. The methods of palpation include touching the injured region by the fingers, squeezing and pressing the periphery of the affected site with both hands, doing percussion along the longitudinal axis of the skeleton, or holding the lower end of the injured limb to rotate, extend and flex gently.

(1) Palpation of the pressure pain point

The nature and type of the injury may be judged by the location, extent and degree of the pressure pain point. If there is tenderness at the affected part, there may be bone fracture or muscle and tendon injury. If there is indirect tenderness (i. e. longitudinal per-

15

cussion pain), a fracture is often suggested. The cricotenderness at the fractured region usually accompanies complete fracture of the long diaphysis.

(2) Palpation of the deformity

Based on the palpation of conditions of bone projection of the body surface, the nature, position, displacement direction, overriding, angulation or rotatory deformity of a fracture, dislocation may be judged.

(3) Palpation of abnormal movement

Abnormal movements refer to those similar to articular movements and occurring at a location without joint in the limb or those movements appearing in the direction in which the joint is unable to move under normal condition. Abnormal movements are mostly seen when there is fracture.

(4) Palpation of elastic fixation

The dislocated joint usually remains at certain abnormal position, and an elastic feeling may be felt on palpation. Since the abnormal position is uneasy to change, it is known as elastic fixation, which is one of the characteristic manifestations of articular dislocation.

(5) Palpation of the skin temperature

If on palpation the skin of the distal end of the injured limb feels cold, and there is numbness, disappearance or weakening of the pulse, it is indicated that there is disturbance of the blood supply.

Section Ⅱ Manual Reduction

🔴 Common Anesthesia

In order to effectively relieve the pain caused by the injury itself and reduction, relax the muscles to make the reduction of fracture and dislocation easier, and ensure that the patient can undergo manual reduction smoothly, anesthesia is often applied before the

16

reduction.

The common ways of inducing anesthesia are local infiltration anesthesia, intrahematoma anesthesia, nerve block (such as brachial plexus block, sciatic nerve block, etc.), epidural anesthesia, etc.

If the injury is mild and easy to reduce, the patient has a good constitution and comes to see the doctor shortly after injury, anesthesia may be unnecessary.

● **Requirements of Fracture Reduction**

The manual reduction requires that it should be done properly, accurately, safely, gently, successfully and by only one reduction without adding to new injury. In the treatment of fracture, anatomic apposition is the most ideal reduction standard, i. e. all the displacements are corrected and the anatomic forms of the bones are completely restored. The better the apposition, the firmer the supporting function of the bone, and the more quickly the fracture is knitted, the better the limb will restore its functions.

But for some fractures, such as fracture of the femoral shaft, ulnar and radial fractures, comminuted fracture, etc., sometimes even if the doctor has made every effort to perform the reduction, the displacements cannot be corrected completely; however, when the bone is knitted, there is no apparent impediment to the functions of the limb. This is referred to as functional reduction, during which the rotated displacement of the fracture should be completely corrected and generally the angulation displacement should not exceed 15 degrees in children, and 10 degrees in adults. The apposition of long diaphysis should at least amount to more than one third. For fractures at the epiphyseal end, the apposition should at least come to three fourths or so. For children with fracture in a lower limb, if the limb involved is shortened by 2 cm and there is no injury of epiphysis, the mismatch may be corrected by itself in the course of development. The shortening of a lower limb

17

is not allowed to exceed 1cm, otherwise, there will be apparent lameness.

If the patient's general condition permits, the earlier the reduction of fracture or dislocation is done, the better the result will be. It would be the best that the reduction be done within 1 to 4 hours after the injury, for the local swelling is not serious then and it is easy to perform the reduction, and early reduction also benefits union of the fracture and the soft tissues in the vicinity. The fracture or dislocation with a history of over 2 weeks after injury is called an old fracture (or dislocation), manual reduction of which is generally difficult to perform. In the case of fracture of long tube-like bones which is sustained within 2 or 3 months with deformed union, osteoclasis may be tried to break the fractured ends before manual reduction and fixation are performed.

● **Manipulative Maneuvers for Reduction**

Repositioning of fracture or dislocation with maneuvers is known as manual reduction. In most cases, fracture and dislocation can be manually reduced with satisfactory results. But manual reduction should be performed with prudence if the patient is weak or suffering from other serious diseases. Clinically, the basic manipulative maneuvers commonly used in reduction are listed below.

1. Palpating and feeling

Palpating and feeling is the maneuver of first choice in bone-setting and repositioning. The operator may press the injury slightly with the thumb, the thumb together with the index and middle fingers and palpate carefully to find out the location, degree and direction of the displacement in a fracture or dislocation. With reference to the x-ray films, a stereo-scopic image of the displacement can be formed in the operator's mind so that the operator may do the reduction with a clear picture in mind.

2. Counter-pulling

The gist of this maneuver is that bone reunion follows remedial separation and remedial separation is for the purpose of bone re-

18

union. When a reduction is done in this way, an assistant and the operator hold the proximal and distal ends of the injured limb respectively to perform countertraction. At the beginning, the traction is done in the same direction of the fractured position of the limb. Then the rotatory deformity will be corrected gradually and countertraction along the physiological vertical axis should be done. The force applied should be increased progressively, firmly and continually. Generally, it takes several minutes to separate the overriding ends by countertraction. Counter-pulling maneuver can correct overriding of fractured ends and rotatory displacement, and it is often a preparation for other maneuvers (Fig. 2—1).

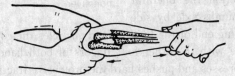

Fig. 2—1 Counter-pulling maneuver

3. Elevating and pressing

Under sustained counter-pulling traction, the operator firmly presses down the distal end of the fracture with two thumbs and elevates the proximal end of the fracture with the other fingers. The maneuver may correct the forward, backward and other lateral displacement so that the concave part can rise up and the protrusive part can lower back to its original position (Fig. 2—2).

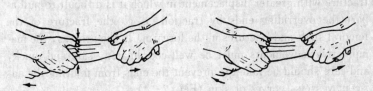

Fig. 2—2 Elevating-pressing maneuver

4. Pushing and pulling

The operator uses his thumbs or palms to push and pull or

squeeze the displaced ends of fracture in opposite directions, i. e. from both anterior and posterior or from the left and the right. The function of this method is similar to that of elevating and pressing method, that is, they both correct the lateral displacements of fracture or dislocation (Fig. 2—3).

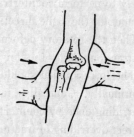

Fig. 2—3 Pushing-pulling maneuver

5. Contra-angular flexing

Under traction the operator presses his thumbs side by side on the projecting end of the fracture and encircles the concave end of the fracture with the other four fingers of both hands. First, the operator presses and pushes hard the protrusive fracture end to increase the degrees of angulation with both thumbs. Then when the operator's thumbs feel that the cortex of the two fracture ends come together, the other fingers encircling the concave end elevate it to make a sudden contra-angular bending and then pull the concave end straight. Meanwhile the operator keeps on pressing downwards the protrusive end with both thumbs to restore the normal axial alignment of the bone, and the reduction of fracture is completed.

This method is mostly applied in the correction of transverse fracture with greater displacement in which it is difficult to pull apart the overriding ends by traction, e. g. the fracture of the femoral shaft and fractures in the forearm. In the process, the manipulative movements must be well-coordinated, safe and quick, and care should be taken to prevent the ends from injuring the adjacent vessels, nerves or skin (Fig. 2—4).

6. Separating parallel bones

This method is applied in reducing fractures in a part where there are two or more parallel bones, for example, the ulna and the radius, the tibia and the fibula, the metacarpal bones, and the

20

metatarsal bones, and where the fractured segments are so close to each other due to a violent force or contraction by the interosseous muscles or interosseous membrane that the gap between the bones are narrowed. During reduction, the operator should put both thumbs on the palmar side and index, middle and ring fingers of both hands on the dorsal aspect to pinch the gap between bones in opposite directions so as to restore their normal gap. In this way the fracture ends are easy to reposit (Fig. 2—5).

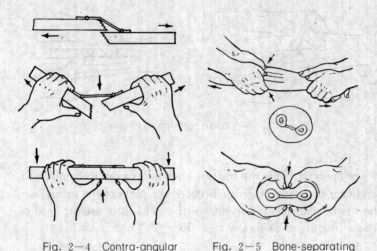

Fig. 2—4 Contra-angular flexing maneuver

Fig. 2—5 Bone-separating maneuver

7. Contra-rotating

When this method is adopted, the traction can be relaxed. The operator holds the proximal fractured fragment in one hand and the distal one in the other and performs back rotation to retrack the rotated fragments to apposition. For the oblique fracture in a back-to-back position, sometimes even forceful traction is inadequate to pull the fractured ends apart and make proper apposition. In such cases, on the basis of a sound judgment of the way in which a back-to-back displacement has rotated, contra-rotating maneuver is employed. So this method is suitable for the correction of an oblique fracture displaced to a back-to-back position, a spiral fracture or a fracture with soft tissues impacted into the broken ends. During the manipulation, the operator should try his best to make both fractured ends come in close contact with each other. If the operator feels that there are soft tissues blocking his attempt, he should change the direction of the contra-rotating from back-to-back to face-to-face and go on to correct other displacements (Fig. 2—6).

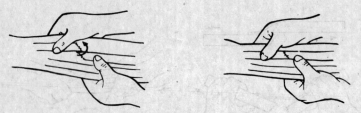

Fig. 2—6   Contra-rotating maneuver

8. Pinching

The operator holds the fracture ends in between a thumb and a forefinger or middle finger or between the parts of the palms near the wrists and squeezes or pinches the ends. It is usually used to reduce fracture of fingers or toes (Fig. 2—7).

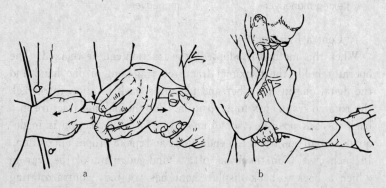

Fig. 2—7   Pinching maneuver

9. Pneumatic supporting

When fractures of ribs with concave or protruding displacements occur, the assistant presses the upper abdomen with both hands and asks the patient to take deep breathing and make strong coughing. At the instant of coughing, the assistant exerts force to press the upper abdomen and the operator presses the highly protrusive fracture end downwards with the thumbs or palms to reposit the displaced fractures of ribs (Fig. 2—8).

10. Shaking

After basic correction of displacement with other maneuvers, the traction should be relaxed a little and the operator holds the fractured ends to keep them steady with one hand and holds the distal end of the injured limb to do gentle shaking for several times. This may make the reposited fracture ends come in closer contact with each other. Shaking maneuver may also be employed in the reduction of intraarticular fracture as it has a "self-remolding" effect to benefit the articular surface in restoring the original shape and smoothness. The maneuver is mostly applied in a transverse fracture or serrated fracture (Fig. 2—9).

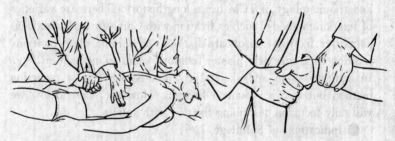

Fig. 2—8 Pneumatic supporting   Fig. 2—9 Shaking maneuver
maneuver

11. Clapping

After reduction and fixation when the broken ends are in apposition, the operator may hold the splints on the fractured part with one hand and gently clap the distal end of the fracture several

23

times to make the ends impacted to each other more closely (Fig. 2—10).

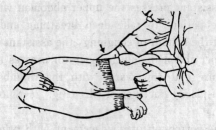

Fig. 2—10　Clapping maneuver

Section Ⅲ　Fixation with Splints and Bandages

Fixation with bandages or splints is also an important treatment for fractures and dislocations because the reduced fracture and dislocation must be fixed effectively and steadily in a good position to enable the fracture to unite and the injured tissues caused by dislocation to recover. Fixation with bandages or splints in orthopedics and traumatology of TCM has a long history. There are varieties of fixation methods, such as fixation with China-fir bark, wooden-supporter fixation, cardboard fixation, aluminum plate fixation, fixation with wire net, plaster fixation, small splint fixation, etc. In addition, skin and skeletal traction is not only a reduction method but also a sustained fixation. However, here below we will only focus on describing fixation with splints.

● **Indications of Splintage**

1. Closed fractures in the four extremities. Splint fixation of the fractures of the femoral shaft may be applied in cooperation with the skeletal traction because there are rich muscles around it.

2. Open fractures in the four extremities with a small wound or healed wound after management.

3. Old fractures suitable for manual reduction.

● **Functions of Splintage**

24

1. To keep the injured limb at a proper position so that the fracture is in a relatively stable state which will provide necessary conditions for healing.

2. To retain the effect of reduction, protect the fracture site from any harmful force, and prevent redisplacement of the ends.

3. To provide favorable conditions for earlier dirigation.

4. To have certain repositing effect for the residual displacement after reduction.

5. To protect the wound and relieve pain.

● **Materials often Employed for Splintage**

1. Materials and preparation of splints

Splints are the main implements of fixation. The materials used to prepare splints must have plasticity (i. e. they are able to be curved into various shapes fit for the physiological radian of the limbs), tenacity (i. e. they are strong enough to maintain their given shape without breaking or cracking), elasticity (i. e. they must be able to accommodate to the change of the internal pressure of the limb during local muscular contraction and relaxation), permeability and absorbability, and they should also be penetrable to x-ray to facilitate x-ray examination.

Splints may be made of local materials, such as willow and poplar board, bamboo, thick cardboard, etc. They should be cut according to the length and thickness of the injured part and then be soaked in hot water, pressed by a board machine or heated dry on an alcohol burner, shaped according to clinical needs and lined with felt pad.

2. Compresses

(1) Property of compresses

Compresses, also called fixation pads, are generally placed between skin and splints. They can exert pressure and lever function which are utilized to maintain the fracture ends at the right position and correct the residual displacement. The materials for compresses must be soft, tenacious, elastic, water-absorbent, and heat-diffusive. The common materials used include cotton, felt, tissue paper and bandage gauze. They should have proper hardness and their shapes, thickness and size all depend upon the location and type of fracture, conditions of the displacement and muscle thickness in the fractured area.

(2) Types of compresses frequently used (Fig. 2—11)

① Plane compresses: They may be square or rectangular and are applicable to flat parts of the limbs (Fig. 2—11—a).

② Pyramid-shaped compresses: These compresses look like a pyramid and are applicable to concave parts near joints (Fig. 2—11—b).

③ Stair-shaped compresses: This kind of compresses are like stairs and are applicable to slope parts of limbs (Fig. 2—11—c).

④ Note-shaped compresses: They are applicable to fracture of the clavicle (Fig. 2—11—d).

⑤ Bone-embracing compresses: The bone-embracing compresses are something like a half moon and can be cut out of felt and are applicable to fracture of the olecranon or patellae (Fig. 2—11—e).

⑥ Spindle-shaped compresses: They are applicable to fracture in the head of the radius (Fig. 2—11—f).

⑦ Transverse compresses: They look like a long strip and are applicable to fracture of the distal end of the radius (Fig. 2—11—g).

⑧ Bone-regathering compresses: They are high on two sides and concave in the middle and are applicable to separation of the lower radioulnar joint. In order to prevent ulna capitulum from being pressed by the compress, a small hole must be cut in the corresponding part of the compress (Fig. 2—11—h).

⑨ Bone-separating compresses: They are made of a piece of iron wire which is 2—3cm long and wrapped with bandage or cotton and rolled into a cylinder-like rod. They are applicable to fracture of radius and ulna (Fig. 2—11—i).

⑩ Mushroom-shaped compresses: One end of a splint is wrapped with cotton and wound up with bandage so that it looks like a mushroom. It is used as the medial splint for fracture of the surgical neck of humerus (Fig. 2—11—j).

⑪ Center-holed compresses: It is a piece of flat compress with a round hole cut in the center, which is used for fixation of fracture in the medial malleolus or lateral malleolus (Fig. 2—11—k).

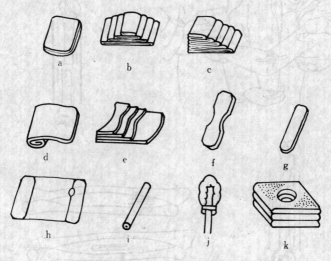

Fig. 2—11 Types of compresses

(3) Placement of compresses

After reduction, a compress is applied to a proper part of the body surface in the affected area and fixed with adhesive tapes. It is then wrapped with bandages or cotton pad before placing splints (usually four splints), which are fastened with cloth strings. Compresses should be placed at a due position. The following are the ways of compress placement commonly used.

① Single-spot compression: Only one compress is applied to avulsion fracture and is placed on the bone fragment.

② Double-spot compression: It is usually used in fracture of long diaphysis with lateral displacement.

③ Triple-spot compression: It is mostly used in fracture of long diaphysis with angulation deformity. The length, size and shape of the compresses should be in conformity with the location of fracture. Attention must be paid to the thickness of compresses. If a compress is too thin, it will not serve the purpose; if it is too thick, skin pressure sore is likely to develop (Fig. 2—12).

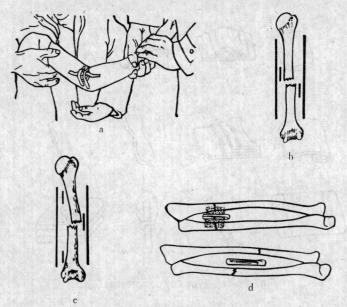

Fig. 2—12 How to lay compresses

● **Methods of Splinting**

After reduction, under sustained traction, the injured part is wrapped with 4 or 5 layers of cotton paddings or bandages. With regard to the fracture type and displaced direction, compresses should be properly and accurately placed and then proper splints are put at the fractured part, and tied with laces. At last, a supporting splint is placed in the light of requirements of different parts or the affected limb is suspended.

Local external splintage is applicable to fractures in long diaphyses, for example, fracture of the humeral shaft, etc. Supra-articular splintage is applicable to fractures near the articular parts or intrarticular fractures. Sometimes, both splintage and skeletal traction should be applied at the same time, e. g. fracture of the femoral shaft.

During splinting, each splint must be placed in good order. The tightness of the laces binding the splints should be most appropriate. It is advisable that the splints are allowed an up and down movement of 1cm. After fixation, the artery pulsation of the distal end of the limb and the skin temperature, color, feeling, etc. must be examined. If disturbance of blood circulation is found, the laces must be relaxed so as to avoid ischemic contracture or necrosis of the limbs.

During splintage, regular x-ray examination should be ordered. If displacement happens, prompt measures should be taken to rectify it. After clinical healing of fracture, splints should be removed because prolonged fixation will affect the restoration of functions.

● **Cardboard Fixation**

Hollow hard paper board of 1mm thick or cardboard of daily packaging boxes, etc. can be used for fixation. It is cut into a definite shape according to the needs. Cardboard fixation is done practically in the same way that splintage is. It is applicable to fixation in the articular region. Though less strong than splints, it is more comfortable to the patient, convenient to obtain and easy to prepare.

Section Ⅳ   Dirigation

Dirigation or functional exercises, known as physical and breathing exercise in ancient times, is one of the key links in the treatment of fractures and dislocations. There were records of treating diseases with physical and breathing exercises in *Internal Classic*. Dirigation therapy for which rich experience has been accumulated in the clinical practice over thousands of years has developed into a characteristic therapy.

● **Effects of Dirigation**

Following the principle of "combination of movement with

rest", functional exercises play an important role in improving the curative effect and reducing sequelae in the treatment of articular injury. It has the following advantages:

1. Promoting blood circulation to remove blood stasis, relaxing muscles and tendons and activating the flow of *qi* and blood in channels and collaterals

An injury is often followed by swelling and pain resulting from stagnation of *qi*, blood stasis and obstruction of channels and collaterals. Being able to promote blood circulation to remove blood stasis, relax muscles and tendons and activate the flow of *qi* and blood in channels and collaterals, dirigation is practiced to promote subsidence of swelling and relief of pain and to ease the movement of joints.

2. Promoting the union of fracture

Since it is able to promote blood circulation to remove blood stasis, and the removal of blood stasis will in turn promote regeneration of new bones to accelerate union of fracture, dirigation during splintage is beneficial to the correction of slight residual displacement, creation of conditions for porosis and restoration of calli at the injured ends and union of fracture.

3. Minimizing myatrophy

Long-term inactivity of the injured limb due to fixation leads to disuse-myatrophy. Proper functional exercises may reduce the negative effect.

4. Preventing articular adhesion

Both articular adhesion and osteoporosis are the results of inactivity of joints. Reasonable functional exercises may minimize or prevent articular adhesion, rigidity of joints and osteoporosis.

5. Improving the patient's general health condition

Doing exercises can enhance the circulation of the blood and *qi*, harmonize the functions of *zang* and *fu*, whet appetite, improve sleeping and promote metabolism, and so it is of great significance in improving a patient's general condition and accelerating recovery after injury.

● **Precautions of Dirigation**

30

1. A plan for exercises must be worked out on the basis of conditions and pathological characteristics of injury, and should vary in individuals.

2. Main points of exercises must be known

The purpose and significance of dirigation should be fully understood. For example, exercises of the upper limb are designed for the purpose of restoring the functions of all the joints of the hands. Exercises of the lower limbs aim at restoring the functions of weight-bearing and walking and at maintaining the stability of relevant joints.

3. Dirigation should consist of more active exercises and less passive exercises and movements must be performed step by step

The patient should increase the number of movements gradually, expand the mobile amplitude little by little and prolong the exercise session day by day. Especially at the initial stage of the fracture or dislocation, the main purpose of local exercises is practicing active relaxation and contraction of muscles. Such exercises as clenching fists, extending fingers, shrugging shoulders, stretching and flexing toes and ankles, contracting quadriceps muscle of thighs, etc. should be done so as to promote subsidence of swelling and prevent articular adhesion.

Exercises harmful to the stability of the fractured ends must be avoided. Exercises causing shear force, torsion between the fracture ends or angulation should be prohibited. At the middle stage of injury (3—6 weeks after injury), because of the restoration of soft tissues, gradual regeneration of callus, relative stability of fracture ends, the cooperative exercises involving a few joints should be done gradually. At the late stage, due to the clinical healing and removal of external fixation, more and more exercises should be performed until complete functional restoration of the injured limb.

● **Methods of Exercising Different Parts**

1. Exercises of the neck

(1) Bowing and raising the head

During inspiration bow the head down so hard as to make the

chin come very close to the upper border of the manubrium of the sternum and during expiration raise the head and extend the neck to the utmost. Repeat the process 8—10 times (Fig. 2—13).

(2) Left and right movement of the head

Move the head leftward on inspiration, restore it to the normal position on expiration; and then, move the head rightward on inspiration and restore it to the normal position on expiration. The above process should be repeated 8—10 times.

(3) Left-right turning of the head

Turn the head to the left while making a deep inspiration, then turn the head from the left to the right while expiration. Repeat the process alternately 8—10 times.

(4) Rotating the head clockwise and counterclockwise

Rotate the head clockwise and counterclockwise alternately. Rotate it slightly 4—5 times and finally in large amplitude, clockwise and counterclockwise once each.

2. Exercises of the lumbar and back regions

(1) Anteflexion and dorsiextension exercises

Stand upright with the feet apart in shoulder-to-shoulder width and hands akimbo, bend the lumbar region forward and then straighten the back. Be sure to relax the muscles as much as possible during the exercise. Repeat the process 4—5 times.

(2) Lateroflexion of the body to the left and right

Stand with the feet apart in shoulder-to-shoulder width and both arms drooping straight; bend the waist to the left with the left hand drooping as much as possible along the lateral of the left leg; restore to the neutral position, and then curve the body to the right in the same way. The process should be repeated 8—10 times.

(3) Clockwise and counterclockwise movement of the small of the back

Stand with the feet apart in shoulder-to-shoulder width and hands akimbo; rotate the waist clockwise and counterclockwise once each. Repeat the exercise in a rhythmic way from slow to fast and from slight amplitude to big for 4—5 times alternately (Fig. 2

−14).

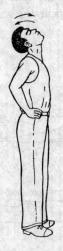

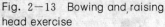

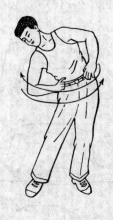

Fig. 2—13 Bowing and raising
head exercise

Fig. 2—14 Clockwise and
counterclockwise movement
of the small of the back

(4) Arched-bridge exercise

Lie on the back with the elbows, hips and knees flexing. With
the head, both elbows and feet as five supporting points, extend
the lumbar region as hard as possible to raise the body into an
arched-bridge (at the beginning with the help of someone's palms
to lift it). Repeat the process many times. The height of the arch
may be increased little by little. After a period of exercise, only
the head and both feet are to be used as three supporting points instead of five with the arms flexed on the chest. During the exercise, the body should be raised into an arch repeatedly. Finally, do
the above exercise with two palms and two feet as four supporting
points (Fig. 2—15).

(5) Flying swallow exercise

Lie in prone position with hands extending by the sides of the
body. Raise the head and shoulders upwards together with two

arms; or stretch both legs straight and lift them upwards. Gradually the above two movements are done at the same time so that the body looks like a flying swallow. Repeat the exercise many times (Fig. 2—16).

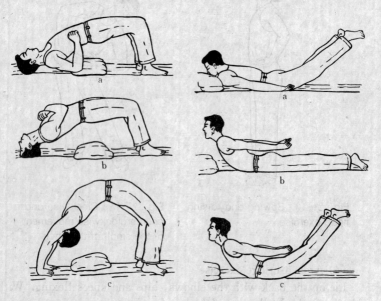

Fig. 2—15 Arch-bridge
dorsiextension exercise

Fig. 2—16 Flying swallow
exercise

3. Exercises of the shoulder and the elbow

(1) Forward extension and backward flexion exercises of the arms

Stand in semi-squatting position with both hands clenched into fists and placed on either side of the loin. Stretch out one arm straight forwards and upwards and then retrieve it with force to restore the original position. Then stretch the other in the same way. The two arms are stretched out repeatedly and alternately for many times (Fig. 2—17).

34

(2) Bending down and drawing circle exercise

Stand with the feet slightly apart, and then bend the body forward with the affected arm hanging down straight. Then begin clockwise and counterclockwise "drawing circle" movements with the affected arm. The movement of circle drawing should be from small to big, from slow to fast and repeated many times (Fig. 2—18).

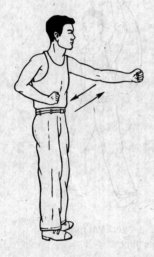 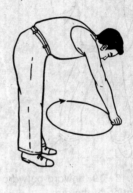

Fig. 2—17 Forward extension and backward flexion of the arms   Fig. 2—18 Bending down and drawing circle exercise

(3) Inward-outward rotation of the arm

Stand in semi-squatting position with both hands clenched into fists, elbow joints flexed and the forearms rotated backwards. Then begin the alternate to and fro "semi-circle drawing" movements with two forearms so that the shoulder joints are driven to make inward and outward rotation. Repeat the movements many times (Fig. 2—19).

(4) Whirling of the upper limb

Stand with the feet apart in shoulder-to-shoulder width and with one hand akimbo and the other hand clenched into a fist. Begin the

clockwise and counterclockwise "circle drawing" movement with
fully straightened arm. The whirling movement should be made
small and slow at first and larger and faster gradually, and the left
and right arms should be exercised alternately. Repeat the process
many times (Fig. 2—20).

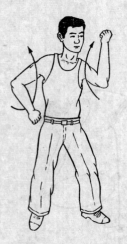 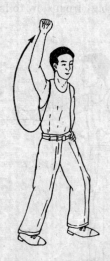

Fig. 2—19 Inward-outward
rotation of the arm

Fig. 2—20 Whirling the
upper limbs

(5) Arm-circling exercise

Stand with one foot in front and the other at the back, and the
affected forearm supported by the unaffected hand. First place the
body's center of gravity on the foot at the back with both elbows
flexing and forearms being close to the chest; then move the
body's center of gravity forward and the forearm of the affected
limb stretches out in a circular clockwise or counterclockwise way
and the center of the body gravity changes alternately from the
foot in front to the foot at the back. Repeat the movements many
times (Fig. 2—21).

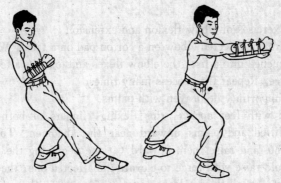

Fig. 2—21   Arm circling exercise

(6) Scorpion climbing-wall exercise of fingers

Stand facing a wall and lay the fingers of the affected hand a-gainst the wall and let them "climb" slowly upward until the arm is lifted to the maximum. Repeat the exercise many times (Fig. 2 —22).

(7) Pulley-aided arm raising exercise

Stand or sit directly under a device with a pulley and hold the ends of a rope passing the pulley, one end in each hand. Pull the rope with the hand of the normal side to raise the affected arm and then let it down. Repeat the exercise many times (Fig. 2—23).

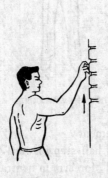

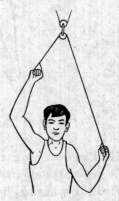

Fig. 2—22   Scorpion climbing-wall exercise of fingers

Fig. 2—23   Pulley-aided raising

(8) Exercises of elbow flexion and extension

Sit with the affected elbow on a cotton pad on a table. With the hand clenched into a fist, the elbow flexes and extends alternately with force. Repeat the process many times.

(9) Supporting the heaven with palms

Stand with feet apart, arms flexing, fingers of both hands cross-knitted and palms upward near the abdomen. Turn the palms 360° and raise them upward (at the beginning the normal arm should raise with force to elevate the affected one; the height the palms can reach should be increased progressively). Look at the palms as they are being raised upwards and finally return the hands to the abdomen. Repeat the exercise many times (Fig. 2—24).

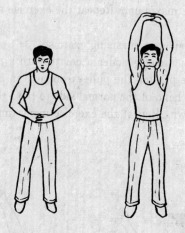

Fig. 2—24 Supporting the heaven with palms

(10) Large-scale arm circling movement

The leg on the affected side makes half step forward, with the affected elbow flexing, hand clenched, forearm in neutral position and the wrist held in the hand of the normal side. Extend the injured arm supported by the unaffected hand toward anterolateral

38

part of the normal side, and at the same time move the center of the body gravity forward, with the knee joint of the affected side flexing and the knee of the normal side straightened. Then take the upper limb back slowly and shift the center of body gravity backwards, the affected knee changes from flexion to extension and the other knee from extension to flexion. The exercise should be repeated many times and the range of movement should be enlarged gradually (Fig. 2—25).

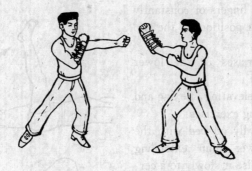

Fig. 2—25 Large-scale arm circling movement

4. Exercises of the forearm and wrist
(1) Forearm rotation exercise
Press the upperarm against the trunk, with the elbow flexing at a 90° angle and a short stick in either hand, and then the forearms rotate inward and outward repeatedly (Fig. 2—26).

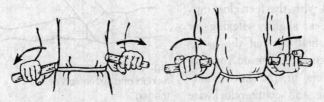

Fig. 2—26 Inward-outward rotation of the forearm

39

(2) Wrist flexion-extension exercise

Clench the hand into a fist and do dorsal extension and palmar flexion of the wrist joint.

(3) Exercise of grasping air to increase strength

Stretch out the fingers energetically and wide apart, then clench the hand into a tight fist and the two steps should be done alternately.

(4) Exercise of ball-rolling by fingers

Hold two small round balls in the hand and roll them unceasingly with the fingers or constantly change their positions of the two balls.

5. Exercises of the lower limbs

(1) Leg elevating, flexing and straightening exercises

Lie dorsally on bed with the injured lower limb extending straight, raise it slowly to a certain height, flex the knee and the hip joint energetically, make dorsal extension of the ankle as much as possible and then straighten the leg energetically. Repeat the process many times (Fig. 2—27).

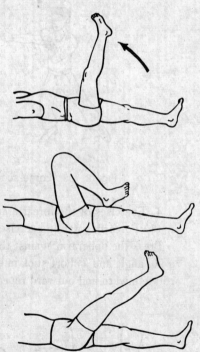

Fig. 2—27 Elevation, flexion and extension of the leg

(2) Moving the knees in circle

Stand with the feet close up, the knees slightly flexing or bending halfway and the hands on the knees. Then do rotatory movements of the knee joints clockwise and counterclockwise to straighten them and flex them alternately. Repeat this process again and again.

(3) Ankle rotation

Lie semirecumbent and rotate the ankle clockwise and then counter-clockwise alternately.

(4) Ankle extension-flexion exercise

Lie on the back or sit and let the foot make dorsal extension and plantar flexion alternately to the maximum.

(5) Rolling a rod to relax muscles and tendons

Sit on a stool with the foot of the injured side treading on a wooden roller and roll it back and forth to perform the flexion-extension exercises of the ankle and knee (Fig. 2—28).

(6) Cycling exercise

Ride on a rehabilitation bike with the feet on the pedals and do cycling movements to exercise all the joints of the lower limbs (Fig. 2—29).

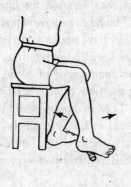
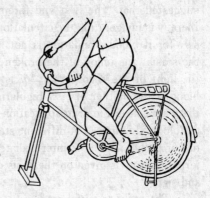

Fig. 2—28 Rolling a rod to relax muscles and tendons

Fig. 2—29 Cycling exercise

Section V Herbal Therapy

Herbal therapy is one of the important therapies in orthopedics and traumatology of TCM with a long history.

In TCM, the human body is deemed to be an integrated organism. If a fracture or dislocation occurs at any part of the body, other parts are usually also involved, and as a result, there will be not only local symptoms but also dysfunction in the solid and hollow viscera, in the meridian channels and collaterals as well as in *qi* and blood. The herbal therapy commonly used in orthopedics and traumalotogy is divided into internal therapy and external therapy.

● **Internal Herbal Therapy**

The guiding ideology of medication in TCM orthopedics and traumatology is proceeding from the body as a whole, taking overall analysis and differentiation of symptoms and signs as the basis for correct diagnosis and proper treatment, setting the regulation of *qi* and blood as the guideline and laying special emphasis on the treatment of blood. It was advocated that "for traumatic injuries, the only thing important is to deal with the blood". It was also suggested that "the first and foremost consideration for internal therapy is invigorating the circulation of blood to remove blood stasis, for if blood circulation is not invigorative enough to remove the stasis, the union of the broken bones will be impossible." In the light of the theory that "*qi* is the commander of blood and blood is the mother of *qi*", regulating the flow of *qi* and blood is the main concern in drug application in TCM orthopedics and traumatology. In clinics, at different stages after injury, namely, initial or early, middle or intermediate and late or natural cure, internal therapy is given on the basis of differentiation of symptoms and signs.

1. The early or initial stage

The stage generally refers to the period of 1 or 2 weeks after an injury. The stagnation of *qi* and blood stasis caused by injury of blood vessels, muscles and joints almost always lead to swelling and pain, for which the following methods are commonly used:

(1) Promoting blood circulation to remove blood stasis and subduing swelling to ease pain

This method is applicable to all cases with local blood stasis,

42

swelling and pain. Most prescriptions are mainly composed of drugs that stimulate blood circulation to remove blood stasis supplemented with drugs which promote flow of *qi* to remove obstruction in the collaterals and they may be modified a little according to whether there is cold, heat, deficiency or excess syndrome. The common recipes are *Taohong Siwu Tang*, *Fuyuan Huoxue Tang*, *Qili San*, *Dieda Wan*, *Huoxue Huayu Pian*, etc.

(2) Promoting the flow of *qi* to remove stagnation and eliminating extravasated blood by catharsis

The method is applicable to cases with local swelling, pain, distending abdominal pain which is aggravated when the abdomen is pressed, and constipation, at the initial stage of the injury. It is effective in removing blood stasis to relax the bowels and promote regeneration. Recipes often prescribed are modified *Taohong Chengqi Tang*, modified *Shunqi Huoxue Tang*, etc.

(3) Clearing away heat and toxic materials

This method is used at the initial stage after injury, suitable for patients with red swelling and burning pain at the injured area or generalized fever. The commonly used recipe is *Wuwei Xiaodu Yin* supplemented with Chinese drugs for promoting the flow of *qi* and blood circulation, or for clearing away heart fire.

(4) Activating blood circulation and tranquilizing the mind to ease mental anxiety

The method is applicable to injury of the head. When there is syncope and unconsciousness, such prescriptions as *Suhexiang Wan*, *Angong Niuhuang Wan*, *Zixue Dan*, *Zhibao Dan*, etc. can be selected for use. After the patient comes to, if headache, dizziness, dysphoria, nausea, vomiting and anorexia are present, it is advisable to use such medicaments as *Tongqiao Huoxue Tang* or *Xiaoyao San* with peach kernel (*Semen Persicae*), safflower (*Flos Carthami*) and abalone shell (*Concha Haliotidis*) for invigorating *yang*, clearing away heat and removing the turbid *qi*, stagnation and obstruction in the channels.

2. The middle or intermediate stage

It refers to the period between 3—6 weeks from the injury. After initial treatment, the swelling and pain are relieved, the bone is knitted but there is still residual stagnation of blood and obstruction of *qi*, the bone union is not firm, and both *qi* and blood are still not in good order and harmony. The therapeutic methods often employed are:

(1) Relieving pain by regulating the nutrient system

Because at the initial stage, *qi* stagnation, blood stasis, swelling and pain are not entirely eliminated and the residual blood stasis hinders the regeneration of new tissues, reunion of bone is difficult, for which reason medicaments should be given to regulate *qi* and blood, remove blood stasis and promote regeneration of new tissues. *Heying Zhitong Tang*, *Dingtong Huoxue Tang*, etc. are of choice.

(2) Promoting reunion of bones, muscles and ligaments

In order to remove blood stasis and promote reunion of osseous and muscular tissues, *Xugu Huoxue Tang*, *Jiegu Zijin Dan*, *Jiegu Dan* and *Daizhang Dan* may be used.

3. The late or natural cure stage

Usually 7 to 8 weeks from injury, clinical healing of fracture takes place. However, due to the injury and long-term external fixation, there are still obstruction of *qi* and blood, disorder or discomfort of bones and soft tissues, various degrees of stiffness of joints or deficiency of both *qi* and blood, and deficiency of liver-*yin*.

The commonly used prescriptions include:

(1) Relaxing muscles and tendons and activating the flow of *qi* and blood to clear obstruction in the channels and collaterals

At the late stage of the injury, deficiency of blood and *qi* and spasm and contracture of muscles are often present, and pathogenic wind-cold-dampness may take the advantage to attack the body leading to aching, numbness, pain, stagnation-syndrome of *qi* and blood, disturbances in movements, etc. This method is used for warming the channels to promote the flow of *qi* and expelling wind and cold. Medicaments such as *Shujin Huoxue Tang*, *Shufeng Yangxue Tang*, *Juanbi Tang*, *Magui Wenjing Tang*, *Da*

Huoluo Dan, *Xiao Huoluo Dan*, *Shujin Pian*, etc. may be prescribed.

(2) Invigorating and tonifying *qi* and blood

At the late stage of injury or in case of long-term confinement in bed, body weakness, deficiency of *qi* and blood and flaccidity of extremities or delayed healing are bound to be present. This method can be used to invigorate *qi* and nourish blood and the common recipes are *Bazhen Tang*, *Shiquan Dabu Tang*, etc.

(3) Strengthening the spleen and the stomach

The spleen is in charge of limbs and muscles. The long-term injury and inactivity may bring about deficiency of the spleen and the stomach, marked by lassitude of limbs, muscular atrophy, indigestion, etc. So it is essential to strengthen the spleen and the stomach so as to promote the conversion of blood and *qi* and accelerate the recovery of bone and muscles. Recipes that can serve the purpose are *Jianpi Yangwei Tang*, *Shenling Baizhu San*, *Guipi Tang*, etc.

(4) Tonifying the liver and kidney

Since the liver is in charge of tendons and the kidney in charge of bones, muscles and bones, therefore, can be strengthened by tonifying the liver and kidney. This method is chiefly used at the late stage of injury and in cases of poor health or old age for delayed union of fracture, osteoporosis, flaccidity in the loin and knees, dizziness and tinnitus. The common prescriptions are *Liuwei Dihuang Wan*, *Zuogui Wan*, *Jingui Shenqi Wan*, *Yougui Wan* and *Zhuangjin Yangxue Tang*.

● External Therapy

It refers to applying medical preparations locally to the injured site. Clinically, the common forms of medical preparations for external use are application, empasma, lotion, fumigant, powder and fomentation, etc.

1. Application

Application refers to ointment paste, plaster, etc. Ointment is prepared in the following processes: Drugs are ground into a fine powder, mixed with such substances as vaseline, maltose, sesame

45

oil, wax, honey, etc. to form a pasty mixture which can be applied directly to the injured site. A plaster is prepared by mixing the fine powder of needed medicinal substances with sesame oil, red lead or bee's wax, etc. and boiling the mixture to the required viscosity. *Dingtong Gao*, *Wulong Gao* and *Quyu Xiaozhong Gao* are used to subdue swelling and alleviate pain. To clear away heat and remove toxic substances, *Jinhuang Gao* and *Shihuang Gao* are applied. During the middle stage of an injury, for relaxing muscles and ligaments, removing obstruction of *qi* in the channels and collaterals and promoting bone reunion, *Jiegu Dan* (for external use), *Shenjin Gao* or *Jiegu Xujin Gao* may be used. At the late stage, the ointments for removing wind-cold, expelling wind-dampness are *Wenjing Tongluo Gao*, *Zhenjiang Gao*, *Goupi Gao*, *Wanling Gao and Wanying Gao*. *Huajian Gao* is used to promote blood circulation, remove blood stasis and soften hard masses and adhesion. For delayed healing of wound, the common prescriptions used to remove necrotic tissues and promote tissue regeneration are *Xiangpi Gao*, *Shengji Yuhong Gao*, *Taiyi Gao* and *Tuoseng Gao*.

2. Empasma

Empasma refers to powder for external use, namely very fine powders of medicinal substances that can be directly spread over the wound or on to a plaster to be applied.

The powders commonly used to arrest bleeding and promoting wound healing are *Taohua San*, *Hualuishi San*, *Rusheng Jindao San*, *Jinqiang Tieshan San*. The powders used to promote tissue regeneration are *Shengji Babao Dan* and *Zhenzhuceng Fen*. The powders used to promote the discharge of necrotic tissues and remove toxic substances are *Baijiang Dan* and *Hongsheng Dan*. The powders used to warm channels and expel cold are *Dinggui San* and *Guishe San*.

3. Wetting agents and liniment

Traditional Chinese drugs may be prepared into liquid forms for local painting, or rubbing the injured part before manipulative maneuvers of injuries. They have the effects of stimulating flow of *qi* and blood, removing obstruction from the collaterals to relieve pain and expel pathogenic wind and cold. *Huoxue Jiu*, *Huixiang Jiu*, *Honghua Jiu*, *Dieda Wanhua You*, *Shangyou Gao*, etc. are commonly used preparations.

4. Lotion and fumigant

Drugs are boiled in water for a hot decoction used to fumigate and bathe the affected part to activate the circulation of *qi* and blood, remove obstruction of *qi* and blood in channels and collaterals, warm channels and expel pathogenic cold. The frequently used preparations are *Haitongpi Tang*, *Sanyu Heshang Tang*, *Huoxue Zhitong San*, *Waixi Yihao Fang* and *Waixi Erhao Fang*. In addition, if there is infection in the wound surface, *Kushen Tang* mixed with *Fanshi Tang* and *Jiedu Xiyao* may be used for local bath.

5. Fomentation

Drugs which activate the circulation of *qi* and blood, warm channels and expel pathogenic cold are heated and packed in a cloth bag to be applied to the injured part to achieve both medical and physical therapeutic effects. For example, prepared iron sand is mixed with vinegar to produce heat as a hot compress treatment. Evodia fruit, rice bran, etc. can be roasted to be applied hot to the affected part.

Chapter 3

Fractures in the Upper Limbs

Section I   Fracture of the Clavicle

The clavicle, also called "the collar bone", is a curved long bone which bridges the sternum and acromion. The lateral 1/3 of the clavicle appears to protrude backward, while the medial 1/3 of it appears to protrude forward. Being very thin in cross section and a junction of both curves, the middle 1/3 segment is mechanically a weak part, where fractures are most likely to occur as well as at the most curved part.

● **Causes and Pathogenesis**

The injury may happen at any age. It is frequently produced by an indirect force when a person falls on the shoulder, elbow or palm but rarely caused by a direct force. The fracture occurs mostly at the middle segment, the lateral 1/3 segment or at the junction of the mid-lateral segment. Oblique and comminuted fractures are frequently seen in adults, in which the lateral proximal end is displaced posterosuperiorly as a result of the traction by the sternocleidomastoid muscle; whereas the distal fractured end is displaced forwards, inwards or downwards due to the traction by the weight of the injured limb and the greater pectoral muscle, leading to overlap of both fractured ends. In cases of comminuted fracture, the fragment which is very much displaced downwards or backwards may compress or stab the subclavian nerve and blood vessels. In cases of greenstick fracture commonly seen in children, the fractured part may look arched and have angulation deformity (Fig. 3—1).

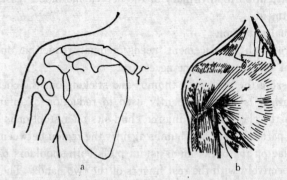

Fig. 3—1 Common types of displacement in fracture of the clavicle

● **Clinical Manifestations and Diagnosis**

1. The patient has a definite history of traumatic injury.

2. Local pain becomes worse while the patient moves his upper limbs. The superior and inferior foveae of clavicle may become full with obvious tenderness because of swelling. The displaced fractured ends can be touched. Bony crepitus is perceptible. Highly protruding angulation deformity can be felt in greenstick fracture.

3. The injured shoulder hangs down and the patient often cups the elbow of the injured member with the hand of the normal side with the head leaning to the injured side to ease pain. The upper limb of the injured side can't be lifted voluntarily (Fig. 3 — 2).

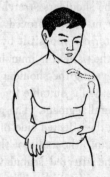

Fig. 3—2 The posture of a patient suffering fromfrac-ture of the clavicle

4. Diagnosis can be established by study of x-ray films in which information about fracture type and displacement may be obtained.

49

5. Pay attention to any injury of the nerves and blood vessels.

● **Treatment**

1. Manual reduction

Fracture with displacement needs manual reduction during which local anesthesia may be necessary.

(1) Pressing the back with thumbs and sticking out the chest

The method is most frequently used in reduction of infantile fracture of the clavicle. The injured child sits on a stool or is carried by its parent. With his thumbs against the region between the two scapulae on the back, an assistant pulls both shoulders backwards respectively with the rest fingers of the two hands. The operator elevates the distal end upwards and presses the proximal end downwards with the thumb, index finger and middle finger of each hand to achieve reduction (Fig. 3—3).

(2) Pushing the back with a knee and sticking out the chest

The patient sits on a stool, sticking out his chest, raising his head and placing his arms akimbo. An assistant puts one foot on the stool and pushes the middle part of the patient's upper back with his knee. Holding the lateral parts of both shoulders with his hands he pulls slowly backward to make the patient's chest stick out and the shoulders stretch. At the same time, the fracture displacement may be improved. If there is still lateral displacement, the operator can reposit it by lifting-pressing maneuver. After reduction, the patient is immobilized for fixation (Fig. 3—4).

(3) Elevating the shoulder from beneath the armpit

The method is suitable for a patient with fracture of the clavicle at the lateral segment. The patient sits up straight. The operator stands by the affected side of the patient, puts his forearm of the same side into the axilla of the affected side and presses the outer part of the affected scapulawith the inner ridge of the hand to make the patient's shoulder stretch posteriorly. Then he lifts his forearm with force and adducts the affected elbow to pull apart the overlapped fractured ends of the clavicle. Finally the operator presses the proximal end of the upward warped fracture down with the thumb of the other hand to achieve the reduction (Fig. 3—5).

50

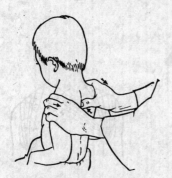

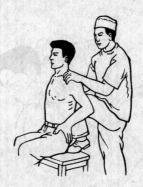

Fig. 3—3 Reduction of
infantile fracture of clavicle

Fig. 3—4 Pushing the back
with a knee and sticking-out
of the chest

2. Fixation

(1) "∞-shape" bandaging

In a case of fracture with obvious displacement, a note-shaped compress should be applied to the affected part. The thicker end is put into the superior hollow part over the clavicle and pressed on the proximal end of the fractured region to make it downward and forward. The thinner end is placed over the clavicle. A plane compress should be placed on top and then fixed with adhesive tapes.

A thick cotton-pad is put under each axilla. Then a bandage is used for fixation starting from the posterior part of the injured shoulder, passing under the axilla of the affected side up to the front shoulder, crossing the back, passing under the axilla of the normal side, then whirling around the front part and the top of the normal shoulder, winding around the back to the axilla of the injured part again. Repeat the above steps to wrap 10—12 layers and the end of the bandage is fixed with adhesive tapes (Fig. 3—6).

51

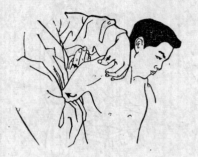 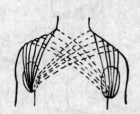

Fig. 3—5 Reduction by elevating   Fig. 3—6 ∞-shape bandaging
the shoulder from beneath the armpit

(2) Two-ring fixation

The compresses are placed in the same way as above. A prepared cotton bandage ring of proper size is harnessed on either of the shoulders. The cotton bandage ring on the injured side must be kept on top of the compress. Pull the two rings from the back tightly, tie two cloth laces respectively to the upper and lower parts of the two rings at the back and knot them. Also fasten the two rings in front of the chest with a cloth lace. Do not pull two rings too tight. If the patient's hands feel numb or the radial artery cannot be felt, loosen the laces properly (Fig. 3—7).

(3) "T-shaped" board fixation

After reduction, a thick cotton pad is placed between the two scapulae. A "T-Shaped" board of proper size (lined with cotton) is put on the back with the top being level with the shoulders. It is fixed to both shoulders, the waist and the back to keep the patient sticking out his chest (Fig. 3—8).

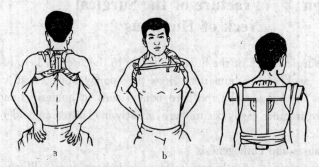

Fig. 3—7 Two-ring fixation   Fig. 3—8 T-shaped board
                                            fixation

3. Herbal therapy

Herbal therapy should be based on the principles of application of Chinese drugs at three stages summarized for fractures in Chapter 2. In a case of mild displacement, plaster can be applied on the injured part before fixation.

4. Dirigation

At the early stage, the patient is advised to practice clenching of his hand and flexion and extension of the elbow joints. After healing and removal of fixation, the patient is encouraged to do exercises of all-direction movements of the shoulder joints.

● **Prognosis**

Generally fracture of the clavicle in children may gain clinical healing in 2—3 weeks, while in adults in 4—6 weeks. So long as the cortices of both ends of the injured bone are not separated, it is rare that patients experience a delayed union or non-union. Mild angulation deformity or overlapping displacement will not leave adverse effects in function in the future. But after clinical healing, unless suitable exercises are taken, restoration of functions of the shoulder is often affected.

Section II Fracture of the Surgical Neck of Humerus

The surgical neck of the humerus refers to the site 2—3 cm below the neck of the humerus. Here the spongy bone (head of humerus) is bounded by the hard bone (shaft of humerus) and therefore fracture easily occurs here, mostly in children and elderly people.

● Causes and Pathogenesis

The fracture frequently results from an indirect force. When a person falls on the elbow or palm, the resultant force may be transmitted up to the superior segment of the humerus, forming shear or torsion force which acts on the surgical neck of the humerus to result in the fracture. The fracture may also result from a direct force, e. g. a fall on the shoulder or hitting on the shoulder, but it is rather rare.

Different postures of the upper limbs during a fall may lead to different types of fracture: abducent or adducent.

1. Abducent type

On falling, the patient's body leans toward the injured side with the upper arm in an abducent position and the palm and elbow touching the ground first. The surgical neck of the humerus is broken by the load of shear. The broken ends often present themselves as anterior or medial angulation deformity, with the proximal end adducted and distal end abducted. Some cortices of the distal end are often impacted into the spongy bones of the proximal end, resulting in slight overlapping (Fig. 3—9—a).

2. Adducent type

This type of fracture occurs because the patient falls on the elbow or hands with upper extremities abducted. The injured ends protrude laterally to form angulation deformity with the distal end adducted, the proximal end abducted, impaction on the fracture

54

ends medially and the injured ends separated laterally. In a fracture with severe displacement, the surface of the two fractured ends are even vertical with the broken ends separated (Fig. 3—9 —b).

3. Fracture without displacement

The fracture caused by a direct force of the shoulder is usually below the periost, presenting simple fissure fracture. Also, fracture of surgical neck without displacement but with impaction of the fractured ends may occur when one falls on a palm with slight abduction of the upper limb (Fig. 3—9—c).

4. Fracture associated with dislocation of the shoulder joint

This type of fracture is rare clinically. When the upper limb is in abduction and extortion position and subjected to a violent force, impacted fracture with abduction may result. If the force continues to act on the head of the humerus, anteroinferior dislocation of the head of the humerus may occur (Fig. 3—9—d).

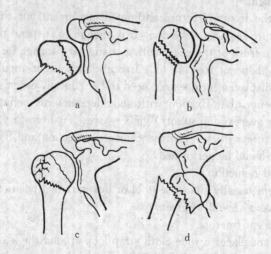

Fig. 3—9 Types of fracture of the surgical neck of humerus

● **Clinical Manifestations and Diagnosis**

The patient has a definite history of traumatic injury. There is local swelling, pain, ecchymosis and tenderness. When the longitudinal axis of the upper limb is tapped, sharp pain can be felt in the fractured part. Except in the fracture without displacement, bony crepitus, abnormal movement and deformity may be present. Sometimes, the manifestations of an abduction fracture are quite similar to those of dislocation of shoulder joint except that the shoulder remains plump, which differs from the "square shoulder" type of shoulder dislocation. In fracture of the surgical neck of the humerus complicated by shoulder dislocation, even if the part below the acromion is hollow, signs of elastic fixation cannot be found.

Radiographic examination can determine the type and the degree of displacement of the fracture and make a judgment about whether the fracture is accompanied with dislocation, so x-ray film in anteroposterior view should be taken. Attention should be paid to whether the nerves and blood vessels are damaged.

● **Treatment**

Neither the fissure fracture without displacement nor the impacted fracture requires reduction. It is enough to suspend the injured limb in front of the chest with a triangular bandage for 2—3 weeks. An abducent fracture or a fracture with slight angulation and lateral displacement does not need to be reduced, especially in elderly patients, but fixation with shoulder-humerus connecting splint (joint-overpassing splints) for 3—4 weeks is necessary. In a case of fracture with severe displacement, reduction and fixation afterwards should be performed.

1. Manual reduction

The patient usually sits on a stool or lies in dorsal position and local anesthesia should be given.

(1) Abducent fracture

An assistant places a wide cloth strap loop around the shoulder of the patient's affected side and pulls the shoulder upwards with the patient's elbow flexed at 90 degrees and the forearm in the neutral position. Another assistant holds the patient's forearm and elbow. The two assistants perform counter-pulling. The second assistant should perform traction first along the direction of the longitudinal axis of the distal end. The operator stands by the fractured side with both thumbs pushing against the greater tubercle of the humerus and the rest fingers surrounding the medial side of the fractured lower end. When the two assistants pull the impaction and overlapping of the fractured ends apart, the operator presses and pushes hard with his thumbs the proximal end inwards and with the rest of the fingers he pulls forcefully the distal end outwards. At the same time, the assistant holding the patient's forearm moves the injured elbow towards the body trunk so that any angulation and malposition can be corrected. The operator's pushing-pulling maneuvers must be well coordinated with the traction and adduction of the two assistants (Fig. 3—10).

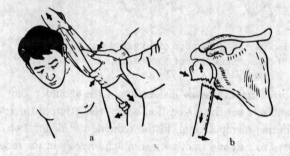

Fig. 3—10 Reduction of abducent type
of fracture of surgical neck of humerus

(2) Adducent fracture

The assistant pulls the upper arm and the operator takes the same position as described in (1) above, but the direction of the force used is different. The assistant holding the forearm applies traction first in the direction of the longitudinal axis of the distal end of the fracture. The operator presses the distal end with both thumbs and holds the proximal end from the medial aspect with other fingers. He presses and pushes the distal end inwards with thumbs and pulls the proximal end outwards with other fingers.

After adducent traction, the assistant holding the forearm slowly moves the upper arm to perform abducent traction. In this way reduction can be achieved. If the displacement is severe, the assistant holding the forearm should raise the injured limb over his head under continual traction so that the operator can correct the malposition by the pushing-pulling maneuver (Fig. 3—11).

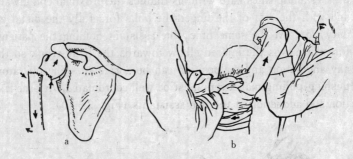

Fig. 3—11 Reduction of adducent type of fracture of the surgical neck of humerus

(3) Fracture complicated by dislocation of the shoulder joint

It is advisable to set the dislocation before reduction of the fracture with routine manipulation. In the reduction of dislocation, it is unnecessary to pull and tract with so much force as in the reduction of ordinary dislocation of the shoulder joint. A cloth strap is wound half around the upper end of the humerus and is pulled outward by an assistant. Another assistant holds the patient's wrist and tracts the upper arm in its own direction. The operator holds the humeral head with the fingers of both hands to pull it into the glenoid cavity. In cases difficult to reposit with manual reduction, it is advisable to perform surgical reduction early and use internal fixation.

2. Fixation

(1) Abducent fracture

After reduction, a cotton-pad is applied over the shoulder, and the fracture is fixed with a shoulder-coaptation splint. An L-

58

shaped board is placed to the superolateral side of the shoulder, with two long boards put to the anterolateral and posterolateral sides, two short boards placed to the posteromedial and anteromedial sides and tied up with bandages. The forearm is suspended before the chest with a splint under it and a bandage round the neck (Fig. 3—12).

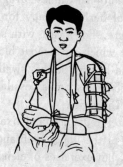

Fig. 3—12 Fixation of abducent type of fracture of the surgical neck of humerus

(2) Adducent fracture

If the fractured ends are stable, a shoulder-coaptation splint can also be used for fixation, before which the elbow should be clapped several times with a fist along the longitudinal axis of the humeral shaft to impact the injured ends close together.

If the fractured ends are unstable or still tend to develop angulation or displacement, abduction-splint may be used for fixation because it is beneficial to the stability of the fracture. After 2—3 weeks or so, shoulder coaptation splint can be used instead depending on the conditions (Fig. 3—13).

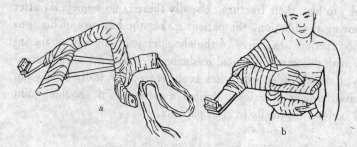

Fig. 3—13 Fixation of adducent type of fracture of the surgical neck of humerus

3. Herbal therapy

59

Traditional Chinese drugs can be prescribed based on the principles of herbal therapy for the initial, middle and late stages of fracture. For a case with severe local swelling, greater dosage of drugs which can remove blood stasis and promote blood circulation should be used so that swelling and ecchymosis can be subdued and absorbed as soon as possible.

4. Dirigation

After reduction and fixation of the dislocated fracture, movement of the upper limb and elbow should be restricted within 10 days, but exercises of clenching fist can be done, for it is good for subduing local swelling. Later on, exercises of the shoulder and elbow can be taken progressively but exercises of the shoulder which may affect the stability of fracture should be avoided. For example, the patient with abducent fracture should avoid abducent exercises of the shoulder while the patient with adducent fracture must avoid adducent movements of the shoulder. The patient shouldn't do all-direction movements of the shoulder until the fracture has healed to prevent adhesion of the shoulder joint.

● **Prognosis**

Because there is good blood circulation at the surgical neck of the humerus and the fractured ends usually have impaction, so the fracture is easy to heal. It takes adults 4 weeks and children 3 weeks to heal their fracture. Usually there is no sequela if, after removing the fixation, the patient makes the best use of his time to do functional exercises of the shoulder joint and bathes the injury with decoction of herbal medicine. For patients with dislocation of the shoulder which has been treated surgically or has not received proper exercises, limited movements of shoulder joint may be left, especially in aged patients.

Section Ⅲ　Fracture of the Greater Tuberosity of Humerus

The greater tuberosity is a protrusion of the lateral sponge bone of the upper end of the humerus and the end of supraspinous, infraspinous and teres minor muscle. The anteromedial end of greater tuberosity of the humerus is the intertubercular sculus through which passes the long-head tendon of the biceps muscle of the arm. In most cases the fracture of greater tuberosity of the humerus is a complication of dislocation of the shoulder joint and fracture of the surgical neck of the humerus, and is usually of avulsion type.

● **Causes and Pathogenesis**

The fracture is usually produced by an indirect force. When a person falls on his arm which is in an outward position, the resultant load may be transmitted upwards along the arm, the greater tuberosity of the humerus will strike against the acromion, the rotator cuff muscle will contract suddenly and avulsion of greater tuberosity will take place. Since the broken fragment is small, it may be displaced upwards by the traction of the supraspinous muscle.

Under a strong force, the fracture may happen accompanied by dislocation of shoulder joint or fracture of the surgical neck of the humerus. The torn fragment caused by the injury is greater and displaced upwards (Fig. 3—14).

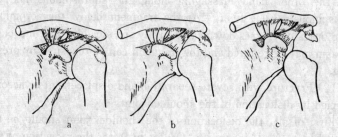

Fig. 3—14   Types of fracture of the great tuberosity of humerus

● **Clinical Manifestations and Diagnosis**

The patient has a definite history of traumatic injury, local swelling and pain, swelling of the lower part of acromion, restricted movements of shoulder joint, especially severe dysfunction in abduction and external rotation. There is distinct tenderness below the acromion and bony crepitus can sometimes be perceptible to the touch.

When the fracture is associated with fracture of the surgical neck and displacement of the shoulder joint, besides the symptoms and signs of the fracture and displacement mentioned above, both swelling and pain below the acromion are severe.

X-ray examination can help establish the diagnosis and make judgment about whether there is complication and the type of injury.

● **Treatment**

Fissure fracture without displacement does not call for reduction, but only a triangular sling or bandage is needed to hang the injured arm in front of the chest.

1. Manual reduction

(1) Fracture with minor displacement

The patient sits on a stool or takes the dorsal position. The reduction is carried out under local anesthesia or without anesthesia at all. The operator stands by the injured side, one hand holding the affected elbow and abducting the patient's limb and the thumb of the other hand massaging along the supraspinous and infraspinous muscle fibers. At the fragment below the acromion, the operator presses downwards firmly and steadily. The muscular spasm may be relieved and the fragment can be reposited by pressing.

(2) Fracture with severe separation and displacement or accompanied by dislocation of the shoulder joint

First of all, the dislocation of the shoulder joint should be reduced by manual maneuvers. Generally, after the reduction of the shoulder joint, the fragment of greater tuberosity is also reposited immediately. In case of severe separation of fragment, the method described in (1) above can also be used, but the injured arm must be abducted to a larger angle and the fragment can usually be pressed back to its original position. In case of severe displacement that is difficult to reduce, surgery can be considered (Fig. 3—15).

(3) Fracture of the surgical neck of the humerus associated with fracture of the greater tuberosity

In this kind of fracture, the fractured fragment has become a part of the humerus. It may be dealt with in the same way that the fracture of surgical neck of the humerus is treated.

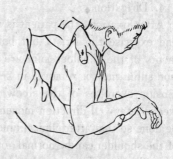

Fig. 3—15 Reduction of fracture of the great tuberosity of humerus

2. Fixation

(1) After the reduction of the fracture with displacement of smaller fragment, shoulder-coaptation splint should be applied for fixation, with the elbow flexed at 90 degrees and the forearm suspended with a triangluar sling before the chest.

(2) After reduction of the fracture with displacement of bigger fragment, a cotton-pad is placed on the fragment and then the fracture is fixed with abduction splints which should be changed to shoulder-coaptation splint two weeks later.

(3) For the fracture associated with displacement of the shoulder joint and fracture of the surgical neck of the humerus, after reduction, the fixation is performed in much the same way that the fixation for the dislocation with fracture of the surgical neck of the humerus is done.

3. Herbal therapy

Herbal medication should be given according to the therapeutic principles for the early, middle and late stages of fractures. Modified recipe of *Fuyuan Huoxue Tang* or *Dieda Wan*, *Sanqi Pian*, etc. can be prescribed for patients at the early stage. *Shenjin Gao* can also be used externally. While the patients do exercises at the late stage, hot lotion of *Erhao Xiyao* can be used to bathe the injury.

4. Dirigation

After fixation, the patient is advised to practice hand clenching and exercise the wrist, but both abducent and extorsion movements of the shoulder joint are prohibited. The shoulder-coaptation splint may be removed in 2—3 weeks and then flexion and extension exercises of the elbow and shoulder can be done. Four weeks later, all-direction movements of the shoulder joint should be done so that after clinical union of the fracture, the movements of the shoulder can be normal; otherwise, it may be difficult to restore the normal movements of the shoulder.

● Prognosis

There is a rich blood circulation at the greater tuberosity of the humerus. Good reduction generally leads to quicker union. Clinical union may occur within 3—4 weeks but such troubles as functional disturbances in abduction and extorsion of the shoulder joint may remain. They are due to:

1. Local stasis of blood and organization of hematoma result in adhesion of tissue, which is likely to occur in fracture associated with dislocation of the shoulder joint. So at the early stage, it is indispensable for the patient to take Chinese drugs which can stimulate blood circulation and remove blood stasis. It is desirable to subdue the swelling within a week.

2. When the fracture fragment is big and the reduction is undesirable, the fracture line may involve the intertubercular sulcus of the humerus to affect the sliding of muscular tendon in the sulcus.

3. If a big fragment displaces superomedially and is healed there, it will come against the acromion during abduction of the shoulder and prevent the abduction of shoulder joint.

4. Delayed removal of fixation and dirigation may cause rigidity and adhesion of the joint, resulting in functional disturbances of the joint. Therefore, the external fixation should not be kept over 4 weeks and after removing the fixation, dirigation must be performed in time.

Section IV Fracture of the Humeral Shaft

Humeral shaft refers to the tubular bone below the surgical neck of the humerus and above the medial and lateral epicondyles of the humerus. It is cylindrical with the upper segment thick but the middle segment thin. The lower segment gradually becomes oblate and slightly inclined forwards, so fractures are most likely to occur at the middle segment, and then at the lower segment, commonly seen in adults.

After the radial nerve leaves the axilla, it goes round to the posterior side of the middle segment, along the radial groove closely against the humeral shaft and come obliquely from the medioposterior part down to the anterolateral part. So when a fracture occurs in the middle or lower third, it is often associated with radial nerve injury.

● **Causes and Pathogenesis**

The middle and upper parts of the humeral shaft are of a hard texture. Fracture there is often caused by a direct force such as hitting, machine impact or crush and so on. The common forms are transverse or comminuted. Spiral or oblique fracture resulting from a transmitting force commonly occur in the thin lower segment of the humeral shaft. The fracture in the mid-lower third is often caused by the twisting violent force, called throwing fracture. For example, on throwing a hand grenade, etc., the upper arm is kept at abduction and extorsion of 90° with the elbow flexed at 90° and the apex of the elbow pointing superolaterally. On throwing something, the abrupt strong contraction of greater pectoral muscle, teres major muscle and the broadest muscle of the back makes the arm rotate inwardly but the lower end of the humerus is still in an extorsion position because of the action of gravity of the object being thrown and the forearm. At that time, the rotating violent force caused by the forces in opposite directions in the upper and lower parts may lead to the spiral fracture.

There are rich adherent muscles around the humeral shaft and displacement in a fracture is closely related to the muscular traction. Here are some common patterns: When a fracture occurs above the insertion of the deltoid muscle, the proximal end of the fracture is likely to displace forward or inward due to the contraction of greater pectoral muscle, broadest muscle of the back and teres major muscle, while the distal end is likely to displace upward and outward because of the traction by deltoid muscle. The fractured ends form inward angulation accompanied with overlapping. When a fracture occurs below the insertion of deltoid muscle, the proximal end of the fracture is likely to displace forward and outward because of the traction by deltoid muscle and coracobrachial muscle while the distal end is likely to displace superiorly owing to the contraction of brachial triceps muscle and biceps muscle of the arm. There is forward and outward angulation of the fracture accompanied with overlapping (Fig. 3 — 16).

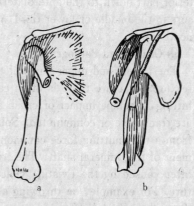

● **Clinical Manifestations and Diagnosis**

After an injury, the upper arm swells and feels a severe pain. There is apparent tenderness and longitudinal percussion pain. If the fracture is accompanied with displacement, the injured arm looks apparently shorter with angulation and rotational deformity, bony crepitus and abnormal movements. The patient often carries the fractured arm close to the chest with the normal one and does not dare to move it, and the injured arm loses its functions.

Fig. 3—16 Displacement in fracture in the upper 3rd and middle 3rd of the humeral shaft

X-ray films can help ascertain the site and type of the fracture, and the degree and direction of displacement.

66

Attention should be paid to whether the nerve and blood vessels are injured. In case of fracture in the mid-lower part of the humerus accompanied with injury of the radial nerve, wrist drop may occur, the thumb is unable to stretch, and the metacarpophalangeal articulations fail to extend straight and skin hypoesthesia or anesthesia on the radial side of the back of the hand occurs (Fig. 3—17).

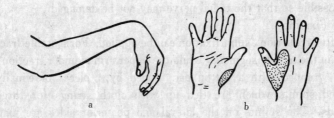

Fig. 3—17   Clinical signs of injury to the radial nerve
a. fracture in the middle   b. fracture in the lower segment

● **Treatment**

1. Manual reduction

Under brachial plexus block or local anesthesia, the patient sit on a stool or takes the dorsal position. One assistant pulls the upper arm upward by passing a long wide cloth strap from under the axilla of the injured side (or alternately, for fracture in the lower part of the humerus, the assistant may hold the upper segment of the injured arm with both hands) while another assistant holds the patient's elbow and forearm with both hands (keeping the elbow flexed at 90° and the forearm in neutral position). The two assistants apply counter-traction slowly but forceful traction should be avoided. Standing beside the injured part of the patient, the operator manipulates by pressing-pushing or pulling-lifting the fractured ends according to the different conditions. In case of a fracture above the insertion of the deltoid muscle, the operator presses the distal end of the fracture inwards with both thumbs and pulls the proximal end of the fracture outwards with other fingers encircling the arm. The two opposite forces push and pull to squeeze the fractured ends together. In case of a fracture below the insertion of the deltoid muscle, the operator presses the proximal end inwards with two thumbs, but pulls the distal end outwards with the other fingers. The reduction can be achieved through the cooperation of the operator and the assistants. During the reduction, if radiating symptoms of the hand occur, they suggest that the radial nerve is squeezed. The maneuvers should be as gentle and steady as possible so that the radial nerve may not be damaged.

2. Fixation

After reduction, splintfixation can be applied. For a stable fracture in the middle segment, while the upper arm is under traction, it is wrapped with a cotton pad topped by 4 pieces of equally spaced splints which are tied up with cloth strings for three rounds. The splints on the lateral and posterior sides are long ones, the anterior splint should be a little shorter while the medial one should be short. For the fracture in the upper third, the upper end of the lateral splint should be curved and go beyond the shoulder joint. For the fracture in the lower third, the lower end of the splint should be curved to pass the joint of the elbow (Fig. 3—18).

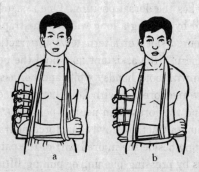

Fig. 3—18 Splinting of fracture of the humeral shaft

For unstable fracture, in the light of different displacement tendency, compresses are placed by double-spot or triple-spot compression method and then fixed with splints in the same way as mentioned above. Care should be taken that the brachial artery and radial nerve are not compressed.

After fixation, the elbow should be fixed at 90° and the forearm in neutral position. The forearm is kept suspended in front of the chest with a supporting splint or triangular sling.

The arm and chest can also be wound together horizontally for several rounds with bandages to strengthen the fixation and prevent the abduction of the injured arm. After fixation, supporting the injured arm from beneath the elbow with one hand, the operator pats the upper part of the affected shoulder with the other hand for a few times along the direction of the longitudinal axis of the injured arm to make the fractured ends in close contact.

In addition, for a fracture with unstable broken ends that cannot be fixed satisfactorily with the above methods or a fracture with severe swelling that is unsuitable for manual reduction, skeletal traction through olecranon of ulna together with splint fixation may be adopted as treatment. Attention should be paid to the traction weight (not over 4—5 kg) to prevent separation of the injured ends. The method is generally unfit for transverse fracture (Fig. 3—19).

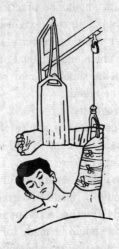

Fig. 3—19 Skeletal tractionr for fracture of the humeral shaft

3. Herbal therapy

Medication should be prescribed in accordance with the therapeutic principles for each of the three stages of fracture treatment. At the early stage, it is preferable for the patient with severe swelling to take decoction which can hasten the subsidence of swelling. In cases of unstable fracture or delayed healing, *Jiegu Dan* should be applied externally and then fixed with splints to promote fracture union.

4. Dirigation

Proper exercise may speed up the union of the fracture, prevent joint stiffening and promote restoration of functions. At the early stage, flexion-extension and rotation exercises of the wrist joint, and clenching the hand are recommended. Depending on the patient's condition, active muscular relaxation and contraction exercises of the affected upper arm may be practiced but the movements of the joints of the shoulder and elbow should be avoided because the exercise may increase the squeezing force of the fractured ends on the longitudinal axis. Rotatory exercises of the upper arm is prohibited so as to prevent redisplacement.

Two to three weeks later flexion-extension exercises of the elbow joint should be practiced to prevent stiffening of the elbow joint. Slight flexion-extension exercises of the shoulder joint and shoulder rotation exercise should also be done gradually. After clinical union and removal of the fixation, more all-direction exercises of the shoulder joint such as "Arm Circling Exercise", etc. should be taken.

● **Prognosis**

In most cases, fracture of the humeral shaft gets a good result after manual reduction and splint fixation. Clinical healing generally occurs in 5—6 weeks. The weight of the forearm and elbow is likely to induce separation of the fractured ends, so x-ray examination should be made to correct any misalignment.

For the fracture accompanied with injury of the radial nerve, observation should be made for 2—3 months; if it is not healed, surgical exploration may be considered.

For a fracture with delayed healing because of improper treatment, severely destroyed blood supply, or impaction of soft tissues between the broken ends, *Jiegu Gao* should be applied externally. For a fracture which fails to heal, the fractured part should be cut open, reduced and fixed internally, or bone grafting be performed.

70

Section V Supracondylar Fracture of the Humerus

The lower end of humerus is flat, broad, and like a fish tail. There is the coronary fossa at its anterior side and the olecranal fossa at its posterior side. Between the two fossae is only a very thin layer of bone. The lower end of the humerus appears slightly anteverted and is the border between the cancellous bone and consistent bone, therefore fractures easily occur there. The supracondyle of the humerus lies 2cm above the internal and the external condyli. The brachial artery and vein and the median nerve run from the medial side of the lower segment of the upper arm into the anterior fossa of the elbow and then pass through the bicipital aponeurosis into the forearm. When supracondylar fracture happens here, the brachial artery and vein and median nerve may be stabbed and compressed.

● Causes and Pathogenesis

Different kinds of wound mechanism result in different types of fracture which may be divided into extension type and flexion type. Extension type is most common, approximately amounting to 90% or so but the flexion type is rare. Most supracondylar fractures occur in children at the age of 5—12 years old.

1. Extension type

When one falls on a palm with the elbow joint in semi-extension or full extension position, the violent force is transmitted upwards along the forearm, acting on the lower segment of the humerus and pushing the condyle backwards; meanwhile the body weight presses and pushes the upper segment of the humerus forwards to lead to fracture at the lower end of the humerus where the bone is thin and weak. The fracture line is oblique, going from the upper part in the front to the upper part of the back. Transverse or comminuted fractures may also occur. In severe cases, blood vessels and nerves may be injured (Fig. 3—20—a).

71

2. Flexion type

The fracture is mostly caused by a direct force, or results from a fall with the elbow joint flexed and the back of the elbow against the ground. The violent force is transmitted from the elbow to the lower end of the humerus. The fracture line is oblique, going from the upper part of the back to the upper part of the front. The distal end of the fracture is displaced forward and upward (Fig. 3—20—b).

Both types of the fracture may be complicated by radial or ulnar displacement. In a case of fracture with radial displacement, there is inward angulation accompanied with lateral displacement of the distal end, because when the injury occurs, there is also a torsive force which makes the humerus rotate from the medial side to the lateral side and causes compression or produces small comminuted fragments at the lateral part of the fractured ends. In a case of fracture with ulnar displacement, there may also be outward angulation accompanied with medial displacement because when the injury takes place, there is also a violent torsive force which makes the humerus rotate from the lateral side to the medial side to result in compression or produces comminuted fragments at the medial side of the fractured ends (Fig. 3—20—c).

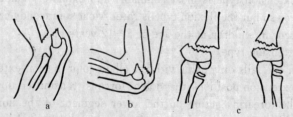

Fig. 3—20 Types of supracondylar fracture of the humerus

The forward displacement of the proximal end occurring in supracondylar fracture of the humerus, especially in the extension type, may directly compress or irritate blood vessels or cause large hematoma. It also brings an excessively high pressure below the antecubital deep fascia, which compresses the blood vessels to

72

bring about the severe result of ischemia in the forearm. Sometimes injury to the median nerve and ulnar or radial nerve may occur too.

If the force is not too violent, greenstick fracture or extension or flexion type of fracture with only slight displacement may form.

● **Clinical Manifestations and Diagnosis**

After injury, there is pain, swelling and sometimes ecchymosis and tension blisters at the injured elbow. Obvious local tenderness and functional disturbances of the elbow joint are present. Abnormal movements and bony crepitus can be noticed in complete fracture.

Extension type of fracture is marked by deformity of backward protrusion called boot-shaped deformity. The elbow is frequently seen in semi-flexion position and the protrusive proximal end of the fracture may be felt in the antecubital region. The flexion type of fracture is characterized by a hemisphere shape at the back of the elbow. The highly protrusive proximal end of fracture may be felt at the posterior region of the elbow. In a case of fracture with radial displacement a pit on the lateral side of the fracture and a slight process on the medial side may appear. On the contrary, a fracture with ulnar displacement shows the signs just opposite to those mentioned above. Though there is deformity in the supracondylar fracture of the humerus, the triangle (i. e. with the elbow flexed at 90°, the three points of the medial epicondyle, the lateral epicondyle and olecranon may be linked into an isosceles triangle) remains unchanged. It can be used to distinguish this injury from dislocation of the elbow joint (Fig. 3 —21).

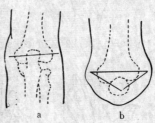

a   b

Fig. 3—21 The normal postcubital triangle

X-ray films of the elbow joint in anteroposterior and lateral views can confirm the diagnosis and show the type of fracture and the condition of displacement.

Radial and ulnar arteriopalmus, peripheral circulation in the forearm and the sense and movements of hand should be examined to make sure whether there are injuries of blood vessels and nerves. Injuries to the median nerve and the ulnar nerve are clinically common. In a case of the median nerve injury, the feeling of three and half fingers on the radial side and the skin feeling of the palm on the radial side become weak or absent. With the passing of time, atrophy of the major thenal muscle occurs.

If the ulnar nerve is injured, the skin sensation of the little finger and the ulnar side of the ring finger becomes weak or absent. With the passing of time, atrophy of interosseous muscle and minor thenal muscle happens. The joints of the little and ring fingers become flexed and the metacarpophalangeal joints become hyperextended. The wrist is unable to make ulnar flexion, the fingers are unable to separate or come together, and the thumb has difficulty in abduction (Fig. 3−22,23). As for the signs and symptoms of the injury of radial nerve, see Section Ⅳ.

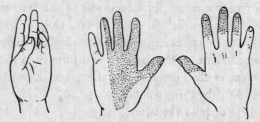

Fig. 3−22 Clinical signs of injury to the median nerve

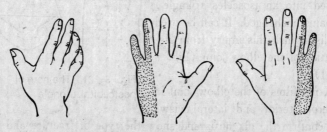

Fig. 3−23 Clinical signs of injury to the ulnar nerve

74

● **Treatment**

1. Manual reduction

Local anesthesia or brachial plexus block may be given according to the actual condition.

There is no need of reduction for greenstick fracture without apparent angulation and fracture without displacement. For fracture with displacement, perfect reduction is required to correct the deformity completely.

The patient is seated on a stool or takes dorsal position. An assistant holds the upper arm in both hands, another assistant holds the wrist and forearm with two hands and with the patient's elbow half-flexed, they perform slow steady countertraction which may correct the overlapping displacement and angulation deformity. The operator should cross-knit the fingers of both hands together and pinch the fractured part with both palms to correct the lateral displacement (Fracture without lateral displacement does not need correction). For fracture with ulnar displacement, the operator presses the lateral part of the proximal end of the fracture with the 2nd to 5th fingers and presses hard with the thumbs the medial part of the distal end towards the lateral part to correct the displacement. For a fracture with radial displacement, the method is the same as above, but the sites pressed by the fingers and thumbs and the direction of the pressing are just the opposite to those used in the correction of fracture with ulnar displacement. After correction of lateral displacement, the anteroposterior displacement should be corrected. In the reduction of extension type, the operator presses the distal end forwards with two thumbs and pulls the proximal end backwards with the rest of the fingers. At the same time, the assistant holding the wrist and the elbow is asked to make continual traction and flex the elbow to 60°—70°. Generally the fracture can be reduced (Fig. 3—24).

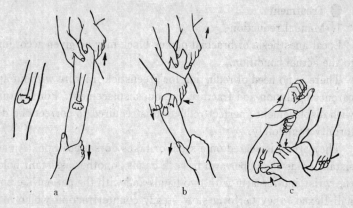

Fig. 3-24   Reduction of extension type of supracondylar fracture

For the flexion type, the corrective direction in the reduction is opposite to the above, that is, the operator presses the distal end backwards with two thumbs and pulls the proximal end forwards with the rest of his fingers.

Meanwhile the assistant holding the forearm is asked to gently extend the injured elbow straight, when reduction can be achieved (Fig. 3-25).

2. Fixation

(1) Upper arm fixation with splints overpassing elbow

Four splints for the anterior, posterior, medial and lateral sides are made of thin willow boards or bark of China fir. The upper ends of all the

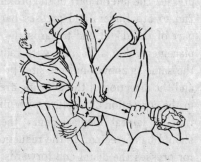

Fig. 3-25   Reduction of flexion type of supracondylar fracture

four splints extend to the site 2-3cm below the axiallary fossia. The lower end of the anterior splint extents to the elbow joint. The lower end of the posterior one should be made arched and go beyond the olecranon. The lower ends of the splints on both the

76

medial and lateral sides extend 1—2cm below the medial and lateral epicondyles of the humerus. Both the anterior and posterior splints are cured to have a 90° bend at the elbow part so that the elbow can be fixed in flexion of 90°. In the fixation of the extension type, the fracture is first wound several rounds with bandages. A compress is placed at the anterior side of the proximal end and another placed at the posterior side of the distal end. In a case with ulnar displacement a compress should be placed at the lateral side of the proximal end and the medial side of the distal end (As for fracture with radial displacement, the vice versa). Then after being covered with cotton pads or with a few layers of bandages, four pieces of splints are put in order and fastened with four pieces of cloth laces. For the extension type of fracture, the elbow is fixed in flexion position of 90° while for the flexion type, it is fixed at semi-flexion (A week later, changed to flexion of 90°). The forearm is suspended before the chest with a supporting splint or a triangular sling (Fig. 3—26).

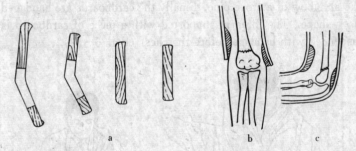

Fig. 3—26 Fixation of extension type of supracondylar fracture

(2) Fixation with cardboard overpassing the elbow
Four pieces of hard cardboard are used in the following way: The cardboard on the anterior and posterior sides is curved with an angle of 70°—90°, extending far beyond the elbow. Both the medial and lateral cardboard is cut into an " L " shape with a curvature of 70°—90°. The cardboard should be lined with cotton pads or

several layers of bandages. Compresses may be used according to the actual needs and in the same way as described in (1) above. After the four pieces of cardboard are in place, two pieces of string are used to fasten the cardboard above and below the elbow. On top of the cardboard a bandage is wound in ∞-shape. The angles of fixation for extension and flexion types of fracture are the same as described in (1) above and the forearm is also hung in front of the chest.

(3) Fixation with arched cardboard

Four pieces of long trapezoidal cardboard with a proper arch are prepared. First, compresses are placed in the same way as described in (1) above at the fractured location and then covered with cotton padding. Two pieces of cardboard are placed on opposite side of the upper part of the forearm and the other two on the lower end of the upper arm. The cardboards should be overlapped and then fastened with four pieces of cloth strings. On both sides of the elbow, the two cloth strings close to the elbow are tied tightly and obliquely with a piece of string so that the arm looks like an elbow of a stove pipe. Finally the cardboards are bandaged in ∞-shape. The forearm supported with a piece of cardboard is suspended with bandage before the chest (Fig. 3—27).

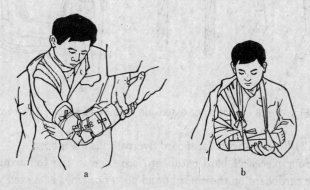

a   b

Fig. 3—27 Fixation of flexion type of supracondylar fracture with arched cardboard

In the fixation of flexion type of unstable fracture, a cotton pad is wrapped at the lower segment of the arm and upper segment of the forearm, a long wooden board (or a plaster or hard cardboard support) is placed at the back of the injured limb and a long arched cardboard is put at the antecubital region. They are tied up with the elbow in extension position. One or two weeks later, the fixation will be changed with the elbow in flexion position.

The external fixation with cardboard has many advantages: it is more reliable, the materials are cheap and convenient to obtain and compression injuries are less likely to occur (Fig. 3—28).

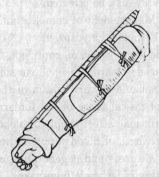

3. Herbal therapy

Fig. 3—28 Fixation of exten -sion type of supracondylar fracture with cardboard

The fracture mostly occurs in children. Patients with less severe swelling may take *Sanqi Pian* and *Huoxue Quyu Pian*. If they are difficult for a child to take, *Yunnan Baiyao*, *Xuejie Fen* or *Sanqi Fen* may be mixed with honey for oral use. In case of severe swelling, Chinese medicinal herbs which can promote blood circulation, remove blood stasis, relieve pain and subdue swelling such as modified *Taohong Siwu Tang* may be decocted for oral use. Also, large dosage of medicinal herbs for promoting blood circulation to remove blood stasis along with herbs for inducing diuresis to reduce edema should be prescribed, such as cogongrass rhizome (*Rhizoma Imperatae*), stem of manshurian aristolochia (*Caulis Aristolochiae Manshuriensis*), etc. At the middle stage, *Jiegu Pian* can be taken. At the late stage, Chinese medicinal herbs for promoting blood circulation and relaxing muscles and tendons should be used both internally and externally such as *Shujin Pian* for oral use and *Erhao Xiyao* for external local bathing.

4. Dirigation

Shoulder shrugging, fist clenching and wrist extension-flexion exercises should be taken at the initial stage. Immediately after union of the fracture, exercises of the shoulder joints should begin. After clinical union and removal of fixation, timely extension-flexion exercises of the injured elbow should start to strive for functional restoration of the elbow within 2—3 weeks. Otherwise, the functions may be affected.

5. Management of complications

(1) Ischemic myospasm

The stimulation or contusion by the proximal end of fracture displaced towards the palmar side or too tight external fixation may cause injury and spasm of the brachial artery, and hypertension of fasical space of the forearm resulting from swelling of the forearm may affect supply of blood. These troubles may all lead to disturbances of blood supply in the forearm. If ischemia lasts a bit long, necrosis and degeneration of muscular tissues will happen, resulting in ischemic myospasm. At the early stage of the complication, a sharp pain may occur as a result of ischemia and anoxia of muscular tissues. If the ischemia continues, nerve fibers will lose their conducting function, which causes numbness, attenuation or disappearance of superficial sensibility. If ischemia lasts 6 to 8 hours, contracture caused by muscular degeneration occurs because the connective tissues take the place of muscular tissues. First the flexor group in the forearm is involved so that the fingers are able to flex but unable to extend. Only on flexion of the wrist, the fingers can be extended. In a severe case, stiffness of interphalangeal joints of the hand also appears (Fig. 3—29).

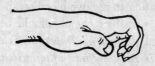

Fig. 3—29 Typical deformity from ischemic myospasm

It is very important to prevent or deal with the complication at the early stage. Within 6 to 8 hours of ischemia, effective measures such as operation or removal of the external fixation should be taken to eliminate the causes. If ischemic muscular contracture has already appeared, the mild cases may be treated internally and externally with Chinese medicinal herbs for promoting blood circulation to remove blood stasis, relaxing muscles and tendons and activating the flow of *qi* and blood in the channels and collaterals, such as *Shentong Zhuyu Tang*, *Haitongpi Tang* or *Huoxue Zhitong San* for local bathing. Massage and physiotherapy can also be given. A device for elastic dirigation of the wrist and fingers fixed at the forearm also has some effect. In severe cases, a proper operation may be performed.

(2) Nerve injury

The injuries of the median or radial nerves are caused by hypertraction of displacement of fracture or manual reduction. Injury of the ulnar nerve is rare. Most injuries are due to contusion and recovery will begin in 2—3 months or so. Chinese medicinal herbs for promoting blood circulation and activating the flow of *qi* and blood in channels and collaterals, such as *Tongqiao Huoxue Tang*, *Bushun Zhuangjin Wan* or *Da Huoluo Dan* may be taken. External bathing with *Shujin Tang and Erhao Xiyao* or external rubbing with *Zijin Jiu* can promote the recovery of nerves. If the symptoms are not improved in 3 months, surgical exploration should be considered.

(3) Cubitus varus

Cubitus varus is a common complication of the fracture. When the fracture occurs, the epiphysis is also injured, which results in imbalanced development of the medial and lateral sides of the lower end of the humerus. In a case of fracture with ulnar displacement, if the medial part of the broken end is squeezed to result in collapse or defect and the distal end is intorsed, cubitus varus may occur several months or years after the union of the fracture. When it occurs, the outward portable angle will be changed into varus angle, and if the deformity is severe, the function may be affected. Clinically prevention should be put first. Efforts should be made to reduce the fracture properly and avoid overlapping and rotation of the fractured ends. Especially for the fracture with ulnar displacement, a thorough correction or even "overcorrection" should be done in order that there might be a radial displacement of less than 1/4 of the broken end or a separation of less than 2mm in width between the fractured ends on the medial side to produce an extroversion of the distal end of limb. For cubitus varus which hinders the normal function, an operation may be indicated.

● **Prognosis**

There is a good blood supply at the supracondyle of the humerus. Generally within 3 — 4 weeks, the ends of fracture are linked firmly. For deformed union or inversion of the elbow which results from improper treatment or other causes and affects the normal functions, an operation should be performed to correct it.

Section VI Intercondylar Fracture of the Humerus

Intercondylar fracture of the humerus is also known as "T" or "Y" shape fracture of the supracondyle of the humerus, belonging to intraarticular fracture.

There is a coronary fossa before the intercondyle of the humerus and an olecranon fossa behind it. Between the capitulum of the humerus and the trochlea of the humerus at its lower end is a longitudinal groove which is a weak part and is susceptible to longitudinal split when subjected to a violent force. When this site and the weak part of the supracondyle both suffer from injury, intercondylar fracture is likely to develop.

● **Causes and Pathogenesis**

In most cases the fracture occurs as a result of an indirect force, for example, when one falls on the palm with the joint of the elbow extended or half-flexed. The violent force is transmitted from the forearm to the lower end of the humerus to produce supracondylar fracture of the humerus. When the violent force is too great and intensified by the gravity of the body, it may cause the proximal end of fracture to strike the distal end where the bone is spongy. In addition, the upward force from the forearm makes the radius and semilunar incisure of the ulna collide respectively with the capitulum of the humerus and the trochlea of the humerus. These upward and downward forces in opposite directions result in the split of the medial and lateral condyles. The fracture line resembles a "T" or "Y" shape (Fig. 3—30).

When the elbow is struck by a direct force or during a fall on the elbow which is in flexion, the violent force passes through the olecranon and capitulum radii to cause fractures of both the condyles and the supracondyle.

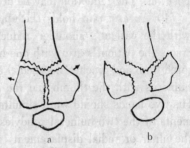

When an injury happens, the elbow may be flexed or extended, so the line of intercondylar fracture is similar to

Fig. 3—30 Displacement in intercondylar fracture of humerus

that of the extension type or flexion type of supracondylar fracture. Therefore, the intercondylar fracture is also called "special type" or "comminuted type" of supracondylar fracture of the humerus.

● **Clinical Manifestations and Diagnosis**

There is local swelling, severe pain, blue skin, ecchymosis or blisters at the elbow. Apparent local tenderness is present and the elbow is out of shape. Clear bony crepitus and abnormal movements can also be noticed. Abnormality of the postcubital triangle and loss of mobility of the elbow joint occur. Rotary movements of the forearm are restricted.

Because of the severe local stasis of blood, it is common for generalized symptoms such as fever, anorexia, thirst, constipation, pavor, insomnia, etc. to appear. Sometimes the ulnar nerve may be injured, so corresponding symptoms may be seen. X-ray films should be taken to observe the displacement of fragment and if

83

there is any small bone fragments in the articular cavity.

● **Treatment**

Because the intercondylar fracture of the humerus with displacement is of a comminuted nature, it is very difficult to treat.

1. Manual reduction

The reduction should be performed under local anesthesia or brachial plexus block. The patient sits on a stool or takes dorsal position. The reduction may be done in two ways:

(1) An assistant holds the upper segment of the injured arm with the patient's shoulder abducted at 60°—80°. The operator tracts the patient's arm with one hand holding the wrist of the injured limb and pinches the medial and lateral supracondyles of the humerus with the thumb and the rest fingers of the other hand. His two hands should work simultaneously to make the bone fragments of the two humeral condyles come together. On this basis, the ulnar or radial displacement, if any, should be corrected by pinching. In case of ulnar displacement, the distal end should be pressed hard towards the lateral side, and on the contrary in radial displacement, the distal end should be pressed towards the medial side. Then with the elbow flexed at 90° (in extension type) or slightly flexed at about 40° (in flexion type), the operator pulls the proximal end forwards while pinches (for extension type) or pushes the distal end backwards (for flexion type) to reduce the forward and backward displacement in supracondylar fracture. The maneuver mentioned above may be helped by flexing and extending the elbow (Fig. 3—31).

(2) With the shoulder of the patient abducted at 60° or 80°, an assistant holds the upper segment of the affected arm with both hands to perform countertraction with another assistant holding the lower segment of the forearm. With the fingers of the two hands cross-locked, the operator squeezes the medial and lateral supracondyles of the humerus with two palms from two opposite sides. The direction of squeezing force and the method are the same as described in (1) above. The vertical intercondylar fracture of the humerus, the ulnar or radial displacement and supracondy-

84

lar fracture should be reduced in turn. The assistant holding the forearm should cooperate with the operator by flexing or extending the elbow joint while performing continual traction (Fig. 3—32).

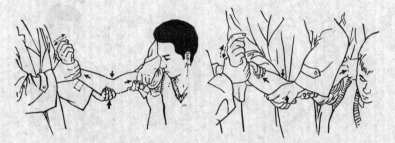

Fig. 3—31 Reduction of intercondylar fracture with pinching maneuver by one hand

Fig. 3—32 Reduction of intercondylar fracture with pinching maneuver by both hands

2. Fixation

Upper arm tripod-shaped splint fixation, upper arm superarticular splint fixation or arch-shaped cardboard fixation may be chosen according to the individual conditions (see Section V: Supracondylar fracture of the Humerus). Tripod-shaped splint fixation: Four splints made of willow board are used with the medial, lateral and posterior splints starting from the plane of the axillary fossa at the upper ends and extending 3cm beyond the elbow, and with the anterior splint extending from the plane of the axillary at the upper to the cubital fossa at the lower. Two holes are drilled at the lower end of each of the four splints, each hole being 1cm away from the edges. During fixation, traction should be maintained to keep a good apposition after reduction. A compress should be placed at both the medial and lateral epicondyles of the humerus. The four spilnts should first be covered with a cotton pad or several layers of bandages, then placed in order and finally tied up at the two ends and in the middle with cloth strings. The cloth string at the lower end should go through each hole in the four splints and after being tightened and knotted, it is fastened at the subcubital part. With the elbow flexed at 90° or 60°, the forearm is hung in front of the chest with a triangular scarf or supporting board and bandage (Fig. 3—33).

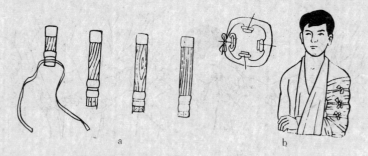

Fig. 3—33 Four-splint fixation

Unstable fracture of flexion type (with the fragment displaced forwards and an oblique fracture line of supracondyle going upwards from the posterosuperior part to the anterosuperior part) may be fixed at the extension position. For muscular patients or those with severe swelling or unsatisfactory reduction, skeletal traction through olecranon of the ulna as well as splint fixation mentioned above may be applied. A small hole is drilled at the lower end of both the medial and lateral splints in order that the needle to be used in skeletal traction can pass through.

3. Herbal therapy

The principles of herbal therapy is the same as those for supracondylar fracture of the humerus. At the early stage, large blisters may be punctured and drawn up with a sterilized needle and syringe. Thereafter gentian violet is painted externally. After the removal of fixation, Chinese medicinal herbs are to be decocted in water to bathe the affected region to relax muscles and tendons, activate collaterals, ease joint movement and prevent rigidity of the joint.

4. Dirigation

At the early stage, the patient may practise flexion-extension exercises of the wrist and finger joints but clenching fist with force should be restricted to prevent fracture displacement that may be caused by contraction of extension-flexion muscular groups in the forearm. At the middle stage, the patient should practice exercises of shoulder joints. Three weeks later when fixation is removed, flexion-extension exercises of cubital joints should start and be increased progressively, for at that time, the fracture is only roughly united but still not very firm. To exercise the elbow joint as early as possible plays an important role in the molding of the articular surface of the capitulum of the humerus and trochlea because the exercise is not only beneficial to the restoration of anatomic form of the medial and lateral condyles of the humerus, but also to the prevention of traumatic arthritis. Moreover, since there is severe blood stasis in the elbow, early exercises are good for the prevention of organization and adhesion of soft tissues and the rigidity of joints. However, exercises of cubital joints should be done in an orderly way and step by step and at the beginning they should not be done with much force. Also, the patient is not to do the same type of exercises as the fracture type, i. e. , the patient with extension type of fracture should avoid full extension exercises while the patient with flexion type of fracture should avoid flexing his elbow fully.

● **Prognosis**

Because of a good blood supply at the condyles of the humerus, a quick union can be expected. However, since the fracture is within the joint, traumatic arthritis tends to happen, for which the best prevention is a good apposition of the fracture. Three to five days after the first reduction and fixation, x-ray films should be ordered for a check. If displacement occurs, early correction should be made to guarantee a good anatomic apposition. Moreover, lack of functional movements at the early stage and exercises at the late stage frequently results in the disturbances of articular functions.

Section VII　Lateral Condylar Fracture of the Humerus

Fracture of the capitellum, also known as separation of epiphysis of capitellum, is common in children of 5 — 10 years old, because the epiphysis of the lower end of the humerus in children is not very strong before synostosis. The extensor muscles of the forearm adhere to the lateral condyle of the humerus, so the muscular pulling is also likely to cause fracture and displacement there.

● **Causes and Pathogenesis**

The fracture is generally produced by an indirect force. When one falls with an elbow slightly flexed and extorted, the palm touching the ground and the forearm pronated, the violent force is transmitted to the upper end of the ulna and the radius. The impact force of capitulum radii and the wedging force of the border of the ulnar semilunal incisure lead to the lateral condylar fracture of the humerus. The fragments include the epiphysis of capitulum of the humerus, the lateral part of the trochlear epiphysis and part of the metaphyses. The degree of the displacement of fragments is dependent upon how great the force is and how the fragments are pulled by the muscles in the forearm. The displacement can be divided into three degrees: fissure fracture without apparent displacement, fracture with outward displacement but without resupination of the fragment and fracture with both displacement and resupination of fragment in which the fragment may turn over more than 90° around the sagittal axis, the fracture faces the lateral side and the articular surface of capitulum humeri faces inwards (Fig. 3—34).

Sometimes the fragment may displace by rotating along the longitudinal axis and the condition of displacement is rather complicated varying with the elbow in extension or in flexion position when the injury takes place. The lateral condylar fracture of the humerus accompanied with injury of nerve and blood vessels are uncommon.

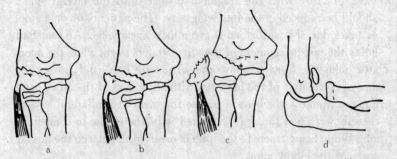

Fig. 3—34　Types of displacement in lateral condylar fracture

● **Clinical Manifestations and Diagnosis**

After injury, there is swelling on the lateral part or even the whole elbow, local skin cyonosis and ecchymosis, loss of functions and pain which is aggravated by movement. The elbow joint stays at the semi-flexion position and there is obvious tenderness on the lateral side. When separation displacement takes place, moving fragment and bony crepitus at the lateral part of the elbow may be felt. The postcubital triangle becomes abnormal.

X-ray films in anteroposterior and lateral views can help determine the condition of fracture and the direction of displacement. In children only the ossification center of the epiphysis can be shown on x-ray films, so the fragment may appear much smaller on x-ray films than it really is. Since the fracture belongs to intraarticular type, improper treatment may give rise to severe deformity and dysfunction of the limb.

● **Treatment**

Lateral condylar fracture of the humerus asks for a good anatomic apposition in only one reduction and proper fixation afterwards, otherwise it is easy to cause damage to the blood supply of fracture fragment and cartilagines of epiphyses, resulting in cubitus extroversion, etc.

89

1. Manual reduction

(1)Fissure fracture without displacement needs no reduction.

(2)Fracture with the fragment displaced to the lateral side should be reduced in the following way. The patient sits on a stool or takes dorsal position and is given local anesthesia. An assistant holds the middle segment of the affected upper arm while the operator holds the forearm above the wrist with one hand, raises the medial epicondyle of the humerus with all fingers of the other hand but the thumb, which rests on the fragment at the lateral side of the elbow. Then the arm is tracted with the elbow in semi-flexion. While being tracted, the limb is inverted to enlarge the lateral space of the elbow joint.

Meanwhile the operator presses the fragment hard with the thumb to reposit it, and then flexes and extends the affected elbow several times to make the reposited fragment stable (Fig. 3 — 35).

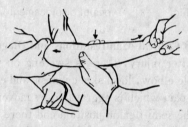

Fig. 3—35 Reduction of lateral condylar fracture with outward displacement of fragment

(3) The reduction of lateral condylar fracture of the humerus with displacement and resupination of the fragment should be carried out as follows: First, two assistants perform countertraction in the same way as mentioned above and the operator should find out, by feeling with the thumb resting on the lateral part of the humerus, the outward fracture surface and the condition of the resupination and rotation of the broken fragment. Then with the affected elbow in a 45° flexion, the forearm is rotated backwards to render great inversion and enlarge the lateral joint space. The wrist should be kept at dorsiextension to relax the extensor muscles. Immediately after that the operator presses the upper edge of the fragment from the anterolateral upper part to the posteromedial lower part with his thumb tip to correct its re-

supination and displacement. Finally he should press the fracture fragment inwards, and flex and extend the affected elbow several times so as to correct the residual displacement. In the reduction of this type of fracture, the operator needs great patience and care but forceful and abrupt maneuvers must be avoided lest the injury of the fracture may be worsened (Fig. 3—36).

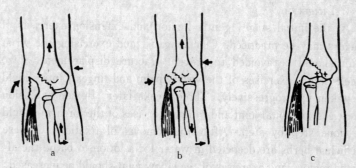

Fig. 3—36 Direction of the force used for repositing the resupinated fragment of lateral condylar fracture

Another method is to insert a sterilized steel needle under fluoroscopy of x-ray. The upper edge of fracture fragment is poked with the needle to turn it over to its original position and then the outward displacement is corrected (Fig. 3—37).

2. Fixation

After reduction, a square plane compress is placed on the lateral condyle of the humerus, fixed with adhesive tape and cov-

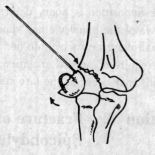

Fig. 3—37 Needle-poking reposition of lateral condylar fracture

ered with a cotton pad. The forearm is rotated backwards and slightly abducted with the cubital joint at semi-flexion. Then the fracture is fixed with splint or cardboard passing beyond the elbow

91

and the forearm is hung before the chest. Two weeks later, refix the fracture with the elbow flexing at 90° till clinical union.

3. Herbal therapy

Herbal therapy is given with reference to the principles of medication for the three stages of fractures and according to the actual condition.

4. Dirigation

At the initial stage, gentle flexion and extension exercises of fingers may be practiced. Clenching fist and exercising the wrist joint should be avoided to prevent fracture displacement. Two weeks later, exercises of the wrist, palm and finger joints should be taken up progressively. Three weeks later, flexion-extension exercises of cubital joint and rotary exercises of the forearm should be done step by step. After the removal of fixation, Chinese medicinal herbs are decocted in water for a lotion to bathe the affected region, and exercises of the elbow joint should be increased.

● **Prognosis**

In general, the prognosis is good. If the apposition of the fracture is properly done, the fixation can be removed in 3—4 weeks. If the apposition is poor, deformity of prominence of the lateral condyle of the humerus may appear. Early fusion of epiphysis and fish-tail deformity which do not affect the functions of the cubital joint require no special attention. Slight eversion or delayed ulnar neuritis may occur at the late stage in some cases.

Section Ⅷ   Fracture of the Medial Epicondyle of Humerus

Fracture of the medial epicondyle of humerus is also called epiphysis separation of the medial epicondyle of humerus. The medial epicondyle of humerus is the point of attachment of flexor muscles of forearm and round pronator muscles and the ulnar nerve passes from behind it.

● **Causes and Pathogenesis**

The disease is usually caused by an indirect force, often occurring in youngsters when they fall on a palm with the affected elbow at an overextension and abduction position, and the medial part of the elbow is subjected to an eversive stress. Also, when one throws an object or lifts a heavy thing with a sudden strong movement, the medial epicondyle of the humerus may be lacerated as a result of traction by the sudden contraction of the flexor muscles of the forearm. The fragment is pulled towards the anteromedial side or even has rotated. The fracture may be divided into four types according to the displacement of fragment.

First-degree fracture: Fissure fracture or fracture with minor displacement and part of the periost unbroken.

Second-degree fracture: fracture with separation or slight rotatory displacement but with the fragment still above the horizontal plane of the elbow joint.

Third-degree fracture: fracture with rotary displacement and with the fragment impacted into the joints. Because of a strong eversive force to the affected limb, the fragment is sucked by the negative pressure into the articular cavity from the rupture of the joint capsule and jammed tightly between the ulnar semilunal incisure and trochlea of the humerus.

Fourth-degree fracture: fracture with separation and rotation displacement of fragment and associated with dislocation of the elbow joint towards the radial and posterior sides. The fracture plane of the fragment faces the trochlea. This type of fracture is likely to be mistaken for simple dislocation of the elbow joint and reduced as such so that the fragment is impacted between the trochlea of the humerus and semilunal incisure, becoming a third-degree fracture (Fig. 3—38).

93

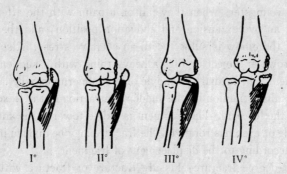

I° II° III° IV°

Fig. 3—38 Types of displacement in medial condylar fracture

● Clinical Manifestations and Diagnosis

There is swelling, ecchymosis and apparent tenderness on the medial aspect of the elbow, and dysfunction of the elbow joint. The elbow is in semi-flexion position. Pain is present which becomes worse when the elbow is moved. In the case of fracture with separation displacement, loose fragments and bony crepitus may be felt or heard on the medial aspect of the elbow. If the fragment is impacted into the humeroulnar articulation, it can not be felt but the flexion and extension of the elbow are obviously restricted.

In cases of the first-degree and second-degree fractures, there is only occasional dragging pain in the medial side with slight disturbance in flexion and extension of the elbow joint. In a case of a third-degree fracture, there is apparent disturbance of flexion and extension of the elbow. In a fourth-degree fracture, there is severe swelling and obvious deformity at the elbow with changes of the triangle at the back of the elbow and elastic fixation. Both the third-degree and fourth-degree fractures may be complicated by injury of the ulnar nerve. At the late stage, the compression of callus and roughness of the groove of the ulnar nerve may also injure the ulnar nerve.

X-ray films in anteroposterior and lateral views may help to de-

94

termine the fracture type and the condition of fragment displacement. However, in children under six, diagnosis can't depend solely upon x-ray films because their epiphyses have not appeared yet. Diagnosis should be made on the basis of clinical examinations.

● **Treatment**

1. Manual reduction

For reduction of a second-degree fracture, brachial plexus block is given or no anesthesia is used. The patient sits on a stool or takes the dorsal position. An assistant fixes the upper arm. Holding the forearm in one hand and making the affected elbow flexed at 90 degrees, the operator presses and pushes with his thumb and forefinger of the other hand the displaced fragment towards the posterosuperior part. When there is a rough frictional sense, it suggests that the fragment has been reposited.

For a third-degree fracture with the fragment impacted into the humeroulnar joint, the operator fully extends the affected elbow with one hand, rotates the forearm backwards and abducts it to cause eversion of the elbow so as to enlarge the space in the medial aspect of the elbow joint and benefit the fragment reduction. He should also force the finger and the wrist joints of the affected limb to make extreme dorsiextension so that the flexor muscles of the forearm will be tight enough to pull the fragment out from the humeroulnar articulation. Then the reduction can be performed in the same way that the second-degree fracture is done.

In a case of a fourth-degree fracture with articular dislocation of the elbow, the dislocation should be reduced first. A second assistant is commissioned to hold the lower segment of the patient's forearm and adduct it as much as possible so as to narrow the joint space in the medial aspect of the elbow and prevent the fragment from entering the articular cavity. The operator corrects the lateral dislocation of the elbow joint by pushing and squeezing to convert the fracture into a first-degree or second-degree one and then performs reduction in the same way as described above.

After reduction, x-ray check should be done in time. If manual

95

reduction fails, a steel needle can be inserted to poke the fragment out and then reduction may be carried out in the same way that a first-degree or second-degree fracture is done. An operation may also be considered to cut the joint open for reduction.

2. Fixation

After successful reduction, a square flat fixation pad is placed on the anteromedial part below the fracture fragment and fixed with adhesive tape. Cover the injured area with a cotton pad or bandage and fix splints or cardboard which should extend beyond the elbow with the elbow flexed at 90°. The arm is hung before the chest.

3. Herbal therapy

Chinese medicinal herbs can be prescribed for internal or external application following the principles of medication described in Section V, Chapter 2.

4. Dirigation

Within a week after reduction and fixation, only slight flexion and extension exercises of fingers may be practiced. Clenching fist and rotary movements of the forearm must be avoided. Three weeks later, flexion and extension of the elbow joint can begin. After removal of fixation, medicinal herbs are decocted in water for a hot lotion to bathe the injured area and more flexion and extension exercises of the elbow joint should be taken.

● **Prognosis**

After proper treatment and fixation for 3−4 weeks, the fracture will be fused and the fixation can be removed. Generally no functional disturbances will be left. A fracture with severe injury of soft tissues may have temporary limitation in flexion and extension of the elbow joint, which will disappear after fumigation and bathing with the decoction of Chinese medicinal herbs combined with more exercises. Injury of the ulnar nerve accompanying the fracture will recover in approximately 3 months.

Section IX Fracture of the Olecranon

The olecranon assumes a curved form and lies at the proximal end of the ulna. The olecranon process connects with the coronary process to form the semilunal incisure. This articular surface and the trochlea of the humerus constitute the humeroulnar articulation. The tendon of brachial triceps attaches to the olecranon. Because the olecranon is very shallow, strong contraction of brachial triceps of the humerus or hitting is likely to cause olecranal fracture. As the olecranon in children is short and thick and the substances of the bone are hard, olecranal fracture occurs less frequently in children than in adults.

● **Causes and Pathogenesis**

The olecranon may be lacerated by the strong traction of brachial triceps of the humerus when one falls on his palm with his elbow in flexion position. The fractured fragment most frequently displaces upwards. A direct force striking against the olecranon process may result in comminuted fracture, which usually does not displace and is uncommon clinically (Fig. 3 — 39).

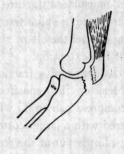

Fig. 3—39 Displacement in fracture of olecranon

● **Clinical Manifestations and Diagnosis**

After injury, there is obvious swelling, pain and local tenderness at the back of the elbow. Functional disturbance of the elbow joint develops. In a case of fracture with displacement, a separation gap is palpable. X-ray films can help make a definite diagnosis.

● **Treatment**

As the olecranal fracture belongs to intraarticular type, a good reduction is very important. Otherwise, the articular flexion and extension of the elbow will be affected.

1. Manual reduction

A fracture without displacement or with separation of less than

2mm needs no reduction. A fracture with displacement over 2mm is to be reduced under local anesthesia. The patient takes sitting position. An assistant fixes the affected arm with the elbow in extension position. The operator holds the olecranon process tightly between a thumb and an index finger and pushes and squeezes it towards the distal end along the ulnar longitudinal axis. In the course, he may shake the elbow gently until the bony crepitus produced by the two fracture ends disappears and the fragment becomes stable. If the separation of the fracture is too wide to be dealt with by manual reduction, open reduction and internal fixation should be adopted.

2. Fixation

For an undisplaced fracture or a fracture without clear displacement, cardboard or splint fixation starting from the upper arm and extending beyond the elbow should be used with the elbow in mild flexion or full extension.

After reduction of a fracture with displacement, the operator should press on the reposited fragment and place a horseshoe-shaped compress pad on it, which will be fixed with adhesive tape and covered with a larger cotton pad or several layers of bandage. A wood splint is put at the dorsal side of the effected limb (up to subaxilla and down to metacarpophalangeal articulation) and arched cardboard at the palmar side. The splint and cardboard are tied with cloth strings and bandaged. The elbow should be in extension position (Fig. 3—40).

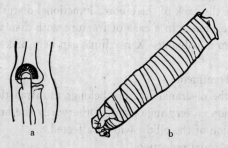

Fig. 3—40 Fixation of fracture of olecranon

3. Herbal therapy

At the initial stage, Chinese medicine for promoting blood circulation, removing blood stasis, subduing swelling and alleviating pain such as *Heying Zhitong Tang* or *Sanqi Pian* may be prescribed for oral use. *Xiaozhong Zhitong Gao* may be prescribed for external application. At the middle stage, Chinese medicine for promoting reunion of bones, muscles and tendons and regulating the nutrient system to benefit regeneration of tissues should be prescribed, such as *Zhuangjin Yangxue Tang* and *Jiegu Dan* for internal use and *Jiegu Gao* for external application. At the late stage, medication for relaxing muscles and tendons, activating the flow of *qi* in the channels and collaterals and strengthening bones, tendons and muscles, such as *Liuwei Dihuang Wan* and *Shujin Pian* may be taken. *Haitongpi Tang* is recommended for external local fumigation and bathing.

4. Dirigation

After fixation, exercises of the finger, wrist and shoulder joints can start immediately. Four weeks later when fixation is removed, flexion and extension of the elbow joint can be done progressively but forceful flexion of the elbow must be avoided.

● **Prognosis**

Clinical healing may occur within 3 — 5 weeks in cases of good apposition and reduction. Nonunion of fragment or traumatic arthritis may happen in patients with fragment separation and displacement which are poorly appositioned. Severe comminuted fracture is likely to leave adhesion, so it is important to do exercises early to produce a good articular moulding and prevent articular dysfunction and traumatic arthritis.

Section X　Fracture of the Radial Head

Fracture of the radial head refers to fracture of the head, neck and epiphysiolysis fracture of the head of the radius. The head of the radius and the capitulum of the humerus form the humeroradial articulation and the head of the radius and radial notch of the ulna form the upper ulnoradial articulation. Annular ligament surrounds the head of the radius and adheres to the posterior margin of the radial notch of the ulna. The head and part of the neck of the radius lies in the articular capsule. The radial nerve is divided into superficial and deep branches at the antecubital region. The fracture is mostly seen in youngsters and if it occurs to victims between the age of 5 to 15, it is most probably epiphysial type.

● **Causes and Pathogenesis**

Fracture of the radial head is mostly produced by a direct violent force. When one falls on the palm with the elbow in full extension and the forearm in pronation, the force is transmitted up to compel the head of the radius to ram the head of the humerus; meanwhile over-eversion of the elbow occurs, which forces the head of the radius to clash upwards and towards the ulnar side. In the process the radial head is compressed to produce the fracture. According to the mechanism of injury and different fracture forms, the fracture is often divided into:

1. Fissure fracture

A less violent force only produces a fissure in the head and neck of the radius.

2. Impacted fracture

A greater vertical violent force produces longitudinal impaction in the neck of the radius, but no significant displacement.

3. Fracture with oblique displacement

A strong force from extroversion results in lateral collapse of the head of the radius. The fragment split off is displaced towards the lateroinferior part and the condition is vividly described as "a hat worn askew".

4. Resupinated fracture

A great violent force causes the fragment to turn and displace with the articular surface looking outward, or even with complete separation of the two fractured ends.

5. Epiphysial fracture

It is common that the entire epiphysis on the head of the radius displaces laterally, often along with a small triangular piece of

100

metaphysis (Fig. 3—41).

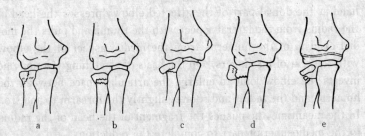

Fig. 3—41 Types of fracture of radial head

● **Clinical Manifestations and Diagnosis**

After injury, there are pain and clear lateral swelling in the elbow. If the hematoma is wrapped by articular capsule, there may be no apparent swelling. When the forearm is supinated, obvious pain may be felt and there is tenderness at the head of the radius. Sometimes, bony crepitus and moving fragment may be felt. X-ray films are to be ordered to make clear the diagnosis and condition of displacement.

● **Treatment**

The fissure fracture of the head of the radius needs no reduction. In the reduction of fracture with a fragment less than one third of the articular surface and only mild displacement, or oblique displacement within 30° and collapse fracture being less than one third of the circumference of the head of the radius, anatomic apposition is not absolutely required, for in the future, the functions of the elbow joint remain intact.

1. Manual reduction

In case of fracture with significant displacement, efforts should be made to achieve a good reduction so as to restore the flexion, extension and rotation functions of the elbow joint.

The patient sits on a stool or lies on his back. Local intrahematoma anesthesia should be given and the upper arm is fixed by

101

an assistant. The operator stands by the patient on the injured side, holds the forearm with one hand, extends the elbow joint straight and performs stretching traction; he then places the other hand at the dorsal part of the affected elbow, presses the head of the radius from the lateral aspect with the thumb and pulls the medial condyle of the humerus from the medial aspect of the elbow with the rest of his fingers. On the basis of stretching traction, he inverts the elbow joint to enlarge the articular space between the humerus and the radius and rotates slightly the forearm to and fro. In the meantime, he pushes the fragment of the head of the radius to the mediosuperior part to complete the reduction.

It is more difficult to reposit a fracture in which the fragment has turned so much (over 90°) that the articular surface of the head of the radius faces the lateroinferior aspect, the head of the radius is dislocated from the ring ligament or the ring ligament is lacerated. The above method may be tried, but the operator should press the medial edge of the articular surface of the head of the radius with the thumb and push it to the mediosuperior aspect. Meanwhile, he pushes the lateral edge of the articular surface (i. e. the lower part of the fragment) upwards with the other thumb to turn the fragment back. Afterwards, the reduction is performed in the way described above.

For fracture with severe displacement or difficult to reduce manually, on the basis of the above method, needle-poking reposition can be used and usually a satisfactory result can be obtained. On reduction by poking with a needle, the operator must be familiar with the local anatomy so that the radial nerve and the articular surface of the head of the radius will not be damaged. Attention should be paid to strict aseptic manipulation in the process (Fig. 3 —42).

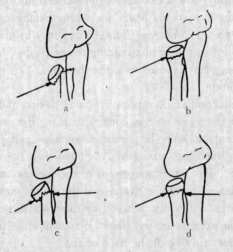

Fig. 3—42 Needle-poking reposition of fracture of the radial head

2. Fixation

Shenjin Gao may be applied externally for fissure fracture. Then with the elbow flexed at 90°, the arm is hung before the chest with a triangular bandage for 2 — 3 weeks. After reduction of a displaced fracture, an arch-shaped rectangular compress pad is laid on the lateral aspect of the head of the radius. With the elbow flexed at 90° and the forearm rotated, four splints which should extend beyond the elbow should be fixed on the forearm and beyond the elbow with the upper end of the lateral splint covering the compress pad. The forearm is suspended and fixed for 3 — 4 weeks.

3. Herbal therapy

At the early stage, it is advisable to use drugs which promote blood circulation, remove blood stasis, subdue swelling and relieve pain such as *Huoxue Zhitong Tang* and *Huoxue Quyu Pian*. *Shenjin Gao* or *Dingtong Gao* may be applied externally. At the middle stage, medication for promoting reunion of fractured bones and injured muscles such as *Zhuangjin Yangxue Tang* or *Jiegu Pian* may be taken orally. *Jiegu Gao* may be prescribed for external application. At the late stage, drugs for strengthening muscles, joints and bones such as *Shengxue Bushui Tang* may be prescribed for oral use. A lotion prepared according to the recipe *Shangzhi Shunshang Xifang* may be used to bathe the arm.

4. Dirigation

After reduction and fixation, articular flexion and extension of the fingers and wrist may be done. Clenching fist and exercises of shoulder joints may also be practiced, such as exercises of "Grasping Air to Increase Strength", "Supporting the Heaven with Palms", etc. But rotary movement of the forearm must be avoided. Mild flexion-extension exercise of the elbow joint may be done 2 weeks later. After the removal of fixation, flexion, extension and rotation exercise of the elbow joint should be increased, for example, over-turning of the hand or fist.

● **Prognosis**

A good prognosis for fracture of the head of the radius without displacement or with only mild displacement may generally be expected. But since the fracture is of an intraarticular nature, if there is severe displacement and the reposition is poor, disturbance of flexion and extension of the elbow and rotation of the forearm may be left over. In some cases of fracture with severe epiphysiolysis, deformity of secondary cubitus valgus may result. For very few cases of severe functional disturbances, resection of the head of the radius should be done.

Section XI Fracture in the Proximal 3rd of the Ulna Associated with Dislocation of Radial Head

Fracture in the proximal 3rd of the ulna associated with dislocation of the radial head is common among injuries. The injury refers to fractures of the upper segment below the semilunal incisure of the ulna, associated with dislocation of the humeroradial articulation and the proximal radioulnar articulation while there is no dislocation of the humeroulnar articulation.

● **Causes and Pathogenesis**

Fracture in the proximal 3rd of the ulna associated with dislocation of the radial head may be caused by either a direct force or an indirect force, with the latter being more common. It may occur at any age but clinically is more frequently seen in children. According to the direction of the causative force and the condition of displacement, the fracture can be classified as extension type, flexion type, adduction type and peculiar type (Fig. 3—43).

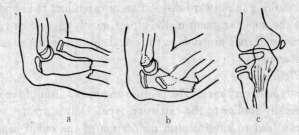

a　　　　　　　b　　　　　　　c

Fig. 3—43　Types of fracture in the upper 3rd of the ulna associated with displacement of the radial head

1. Extension type

This type mostly occurs in children. The patient falls with his elbow joint in an extension or over-extension position, his forearm rotating backwards and his palm against the ground. The violent force is transmitted through the ulna and the radius from the palm to the anterosuperior part of the ulna and radius producing dislocation of the radial head towards anterolateral part and fracture of the proximal 3rd of the ulna. The fractured ends protrude towards the palmar and radial sides respectively to give rise to angulation or displacement.

2. Flexion type

This type mostly happens in adults. The patient falls with his elbow joint in a half-flexion position, forearm suspending forward and the palm against the ground. The violent force is transmitted from the palm, through the ulna and the radius, to the elbow, causing dislocation of capitulum radii to the posterolateral part and fracture of the proximal 3rd of the ulna. The broken ends protrudes toward the back and radial sides forming angulation or displacement.

3. Adduction type

This type mostly occurs in children. When the patient falls with the elbow joint extended and adducted, the forearm rotated backwards and the palm against the ground, the violent force is transmitted from the palm, through the ulna and the radius, to the elbow, resulting in outward dislocation of capitulum radii and fracture of the upper segment of the ulna (mostly greenstick type) . The fractured ends protrude to the radial side producing angulation or displacement.

4. Peculiar type

This type is very rare. The posture and mechanism of the injury are basically similar to the extension type. Only a greater violent force can lead to anterolateral dislocation of the radial head and fracture of both the ulna and the radius.

Each type mentioned above forms angulation towards the radial side, which not only has something to do with the direction of the inducing force but also has a close relationship with the traction of the supinator and ancoeus muscles. Moreover, each type of dislocation of capitulum radii is usually associated with laceration or rupture of annular ligament. Sometimes the condition is complicated by damage of the deep branch of the radial nerve.

● **Clinical Manifestations and Diagnosis**

After injury, there is swelling and pain in the elbow and the forearm plus obvious tenderness at the fractured part and bony crepitus. In the cases with apparent displacement, ulnar angulation deformity may be seen. At the posterior and lateral sides, dislocated radial head is palpable. Sometimes, signs which indicate injury to the radial nerve may develop, such as inability of the thumb to perform dorsal extension and abduction, wrist drop, etc. Whenever x-ray films of the displaced fracture involving only the radius or the ulna are ordered, the elbow and wrist joints should be included so that the dislocation of the upper and lower joints of the radius and ulna may not be overlooked in making the diagnosis. Sometimes the dislocation of the radial head may be reposited automatically and when the patient goes to see a doctor, x-ray films show only the fracture but no dislocation. In such cases, if the fixation of the radial head is neglected, redislocation may happen.

● **Treatment**

1. Manual reduction

On doing manual reduction, the dislocation of the radial head should be set first, followed by the reduction of fracture of the ulna. The patient sits on a stool or lies in dorsal position. Local anesthesia or brachial plexus block should be given. While one assistant holds the patient's upper arm, the operator should first reduce the dislocation of the radial head before repositing the fracture, for which the ways of reduction and fixation vary with different types.

(1) Extension type

Holding the upper part of the wrist of the injured limb with one hand, encircling the elbow with the other hand and pressing the radial head with the thumb, the operator does countertraction with the patient's elbow extending straight, then supinates the forearm and at the same time presses hard the radial head inwards and backwards; he then quickly flexes the affected elbow to the utmost with the other hand and the radial head will be reposited. At this time the radial head may be used as a support, the fractured end of the ulna may often be reduced owing to the traction of interosseous membrane. If there is still mild lateral displacement, lifting-pressing maneuvers may be used to correct it (Fig. 3—44).

(2) Flexion type

With the affected elbow in semi-flexion, the operator performs traction, pronates the forearm, presses the radial head inwards and forwards with the thumb of one hand, quickly extends the patient's affected elbow straight with the other hand and turns the forearm into extreme supination. After all these maneuvers, the radial head can be reposited. The angulation and transposition of the broken ends of the ulna can be corrected at the same time (Fig. 3—45).

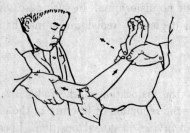 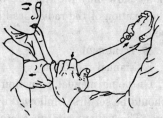

Fig. 3—44 Reduction of the extension type

Fig. 3—45 Reduction of the flexion type

(3) Adduction type

Stretching traction should be performed first with the affected elbow in full extension. The operator presses the radial head inwards with a thumb, and makes the forearm supinate and abduct slightly, then the radial head and the upper segment of the ulna will be reposited.

2. Fixation

(1) Extension type

After reduction, a rectangular compress is applied to the anterolateral aspect of the radial head (Fig. 3—46) to exercise pressure on the radial head in a semiarch shape and is wrapped with a cotton pad. A long splint is placed at the anterior, posterior, medial and lateral aspects of the upper-middle segment of forearm; the proximal end of the lateral one must cover the compress on the radial head so as to prevent outward dislocation. Fasten the splints with three laces at the upper, middle and lower parts respectively. The elbow is in flexion with an angle smaller than 90° and the forearm

108

is supported with a board and hung with a sling before the chest (Fig. 3—47).

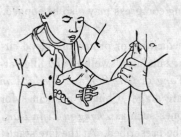

Fig. 3—46 The site of compress placed in extension type

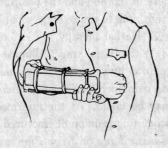

Fig. 3—47 Fixation with small splints in extension type

(2) Flexion type

After reduction, apply a small compress to the posterolateral aspect of the radial head and cover it with a cotton pad. Fix the forearm and elbow in extension with 4 superarticular splints and the lateral splint must cover the compress to fix the radial head (Fig. 3—48).

Two to three weeks later when the fracture is stable, the fixation should be redone with the elbow in semi-flexion and can be removed in another 2 — 3 weeks.

(3) Adduction type

After reduction, the fixation is all the same as that for the flexion type except that the compress is applied

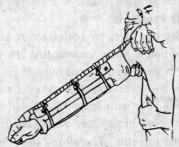

Fig. 3—48 Fixation with small splints in flexion type

to the lateral aspect of the radial head. After 2 — 3 days of fixation, x-ray films must be taken for a check with due attention to the position of the radial head. Due to the traction of muscles or interosseous membrane, there is likely to be angulation formed by fractured ends of the ulna in the dorsal or radial aspect. The tightness of fixation and the position of the compress should be checked from time to time. Bone-separating compress may also be applied.

3. Herbal therapy

At the initial stage, Chinese medicines for promoting blood circulation by removing blood stasis, subduing swelling and alleviating pain such as *Taohong Siwu Tang* or *Qili San* and *Dieda Wan* may be taken. At the intermediate stage, Chinese medicines for promoting reunion of fractured bones such as *Zhenggu Zijin Dan*, *Huoxue Tang* or *Jiegu Pian* may be prescribed. At the late stage, medicines for strengthening muscles and bones, e. g. *Zhuangyao Jianshen Wan*, *Liuwei Dihuang Wan*, etc. are of choice.

4. Dirigation

During fixation, flexion and extension exercises of the metacarpophalangeal joints and interphalangeal joints may be done. The forces for clenching fist should be increased progressively and all-direction movements of the shoulder joint can be performed. After the removal of fixation, movements of elbow and rotation exercise of the forearm should be enhanced gradually.

● **Prognosis**

Because there are both fracture and dislocation in the injury, the condition is rather complicated. However, after manual reduction, the reposition is satisfactory in most cases. Generally, children take 3—4 weeks to heal and adults need 4—6 weeks. If the reduction is poor with apparent angulation in the radial side, radial and ulnar bone bridge may occur, resulting in loss of rotatory function of the forearm. Therefore, the restoration of ulnar strength line should be paid attention to in the treatment.

Section XII   Fracture of the Shaft of Radius and Ulna

Fracture of the shaft of the radius and ulna is a common injury.

The bones in the forearm consist of radius and ulna arranged side by side. The ulna is bulged at the upper end but thin at the lower end and is an important bone composing the elbow joint. The radius is just the opposite, small at the upper and bulged at the lower end, and is the major bone constituting the wrist joint. Both the radius and ulna are long, slightly arched bones. From the front view, the ulna is relatively straight while the radius has an approximately 9.3° curvature to the radial aspect along its shaft. From the side view, there is a 6.4° curvature to the dorsal aspect in both. The ulna is the axis of the forearm. It is connected with the radius by interosseous membranes and proximal and distal radioulnar articulations, the joint movements of which endow the forearm with the rotatory function.

There are fibrous interossous membranes between the two bones. The fibers originate from the crista of the radius, extend oblique to the inferomedial side and are attached to the crista of ulna. These fibers play an important role in the stabilization of proximal and distal radioulnar articulations and maintenance of the rotatory movement of the forearm. When the forearm is in the neutral position, the space between the two bones is the widest and all the interosseous membrane is tight like an unfolded stretcher; when the forearm is in the supinated position, the space is slightly narrower; if the forearm is in pronation and the two bones cross each other at the mid-upper 3rd, the interosseous space is most narrow and the membrane relaxes.

● **Causes and Pathogenesis**

The fracture may be produced by a direct force, an indirect force or a torsional force. The fracture caused by direct forces such as hitting or a crush show fracture lines at the same level, mostly in comminuted or transverse forms. An indirect force, for example, during a fall on the palm, is transmitted upwards along the radius to cause fracture of the middle or upper segment of the radius. Meanwhile the residual force is transmitted to the ulna through interosseous membrane, leading to fracture of the ulna at the lower level, mostly transverse or oblique fracture. Fracture of the radius and ulna caused by torsional forces often present oblique fracture lines towards one side, usually from the medio-superior part to the lateroin-ferior part. The fracture line of the ulna usually appears at the upper part, being spiral in most cases (Fig. 3—49).

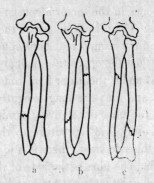

Fig. 3—49 Types of fracture of the shafts of both the radius and ulna caused by different foreign violent force

⬤ **Clinical Manifestations and Diagnosis**

After injury, there are local swelling, pain and functional loss of the forearm. In a case of complete fracture, angula-tion deformity, abnormal movement and bony crepitus are present. In cases of greenstick fracture in children, only angulation deformity occurs. X-ray films can help establish the diagnosis, but the elbow and wrist should be included in x-ray examination so that rotatory displacement or dislocation of proximal and distal joints may not be neglected in making the diagnosis.

⬤ **Treatment**

1. Manual reduction

The patient with displaced fracture sits on a stool or lies in the dorsal position. Under local anesthesia or brachial plexus block, the patient's shoulder is abducted at 90 degrees and elbow flexed at 90 degrees. For fracture of the lower-middle 3rd, the forearm should be kept in neutral position. For fracture of the upper 3rd, the forearm should be supinated. Two assistants holding the upper arm and the wrist respectively perform countertraction to correct angulation and overlapping displacement. The operator restores normal width of the space between bones by separating and pinch-ing bones (Fig. 3—50), then holds the proximal end of the frac-ture with one hand and the distal end with the other hand to cor-rect rotatory displacement. The assistant holding the wrist must perform rotation simultaneously. The operator may correct the lateral displacement by elevating-pressing maneuver. If the fractured ends are transverse or serrated and the overlapping is difficult to tract apart, contra-angular flexion maneuver may be applied (Fig. 3—51). During the reduction, the interosseous membrane must be pulled as tightly as possible, and by the traction of the interosseous membrane, the ulna and radius may be reduced at the same time like one bone; or the reduction of one bone is performed first and the other bone will be reduced automatically. If the stability of the radius and ulna is different, the more stable bone may be reduced first and fixed, followed by the reduction of the other bone.

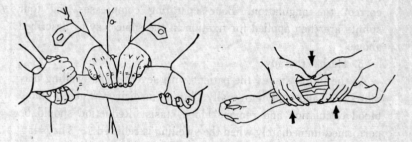

Fig. 3—50 Reduction of the fracture in the shaft of both the radius and ulna by separating and pinching bones

Fig. 3—51 Reduction of fracture in the radius and ulna with contra-angular flexing maneuver

2. Fixation

After reduction, under steady traction, a bone-separating compress is applied to the dorsal aspect and a plane compress is applied to the palmar aspect, fixed with adhesive tape. When there is lateral displacement, in line with double-spot compression method, square compresses are applied to the proper location. Four splints covered with cotton pads are placed respectively at the anterior,

113

posterior, medial and lateral aspects of the forearm and fastened with laces near both ends and in the middle. Support the forearm with a board in a neutral position and suspend it with a sling before the chest (Fig. 3—52).

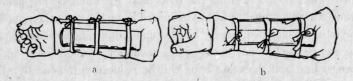

a   b

Fig. 3—52 Fixation of fracture of the radius and
ulna with small splints

As for greenstick fracture with angulation in children, under proper traction, contra-angular flexion maneuver should be used to correct the angulation. Bone-separating compresses and four splints are then applied for fixation in the same way as described above.

3. Herbal therapy

At the initial stage, the patient with severe local swelling may take orally and apply externally Chinese medicines which promote blood circulation and remove blood stasis. Reduction should be performed immediately when the swelling is relieved 2—3 days later. At the middle stage, bone-knitting tablets may be taken. For fractures slow in healing, bone-knitting medicines for tonifying the kidney such as *Liuwei Dihuang Wan* supplemented with calcined pyrite (*Pyritum*), ground beetle (*Eupolyphaga seu Steleophaga*), dragon's blood (*Resina Draconis*), etc. should be prescribed. At the late stage *Erhao Xiyao* for local bathing may be used to promote functional restoration of the elbow joints.

4. Dirigation

At the initial stage, appropriate exercises of shoulder joints and fist-making may be done. Three to four weeks later, proper flexion-extension exercise of elbow joints in small range may be practiced. At the late stage, after the removal of fixation, flexion-ex-

114

tension exercise of elbow joints and rotatory movements of the forearm may be strengthened, and weight-carrying training may be performed gradually.

● **Prognosis**

Generally, it takes adults 4 or 6 weeks and children 3—4 weeks to obtain clinical healing. A few patients with partial lateral displacement may also have good functions so long as there is good alignment and bone space between the radius and the ulna. Poor reposition and improper fixation may lead to deformity and affect functions. In case of delayed healing or nonhealing, sometimes it is necessary to cut the injury open to perform reduction and internal fixation.

Section XⅢ Fracture of the Shaft of Radius

The upper 3rd of the shaft of the radius is made up of hard bone and covered by rich muscles so fractures are less likely to occur here but easy to happen at the middle or the lower 3rd of the shaft of the radius because there are less muscles there. The physiological curvature is greatest at the lower-middle 3rd of the radius and therefore more fractures occur there. Simple fracture of the radius is seldom seen in clinical practice and mainly occurs in the youngsters.

● **Causes and Pathogenesis**

In most cases, the injury is produced by an indirect force. For example, when a person falls on a palm, the violent force is transmitted to the shaft of the radius. The most common forms are transverse or oblique fractures. A direct force may also produce fractures of the radial shaft usually resulting from hitting or crushing the radial side of the forearm by heavy objects. The common forms of this type are transverse or oblique fractures. The greenstick fracture is relatively common in children.

The affected shaft of the radius presents angulation to the ulnar aspect as a result of the traction by the interosseous membrane and

115

rotatory displacement happens due to muscular traction. If a fracture happens at the upper 3rd of the radius and the fracture line is above the end of round pronator muscle, the proximal end is often supinated as a result of the traction by the biceps muscle of arm attached to the tubercle of the radius and the supinators adhering to the upper 3rd of the radius whereas the distal end is pronated as a result of the traction by the round pronator muscles and quadrate pronator muscles adhering to the middle and lower parts of the radius. When the fracture occurs at the middle or lower-middle 3rd of the shaft of the radius and the fracture line is below the end of the round pronator muscle, the proximal end is in the neutral position because the supinated tendency of biceps of the arm and supinator is counteracted by the pronating traction of the round pronator muscle while the distal end is in forward rotary displacement as a result of the traction by quadrate pronator muscle (Fig. 3 — 53).

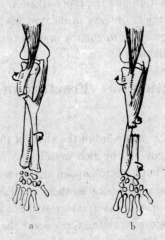

Fig. 3—53　Sites of fracture of the radius and displacement

● Clinical Manifestations and Diagnosis

After injury, there are local swelling, pain, tenderness and apparent functional restriction of the forearm. When passive rotation of the forearm is performed, the pain worsens, the radial head doesn't rotate and bony crepitus may appear. X-ray films may help establish the diagnosis and determine the fracture type and displacement direction.

● Treatment

1. Manual reduction

Undisplaced fracture and greenstick fracture with mild angula-

116

tion need no reduction. Displaced fracture and greenstick fracture with greater angulation require manual reduction.

The patient takes dorsal position with the shoulder of the affected side abducting at 90° and the elbow flexing at 90°. One assistant holds the upper part of the elbow while another holds the wrist and they perform countertraction. When the fracture occurs at the upper 3rd of the radial shaft, the traction is performed with the forearm first in neutral position and gradually changed to supination so that the distal end of the fracture which has displaced to the ulnar aspect and in a pronated position can be turned to the radial aspect and in a supinated position and be close to the proximal end. Then the operator applies pushing-squeezing maneuvers to rectify the lateral displacement.

If the fracture of the radial shaft happens at the middle 3rd or the lower 3rd, the traction should be performed with the forearm in neutral position to correct overlapping displacement. If there is angulation to the ulnar aspect or displacement, first apply bone-separating maneuvers and then rectify the lateral displacement. If the fractured ends displace to the dorsal and palmar sides, the elevating-pressing manipulation may be used in reduction. The operator lifts the end displaced to the palmar side towards the dorsal side with one hand and presses the end displaced to the dorsal side towards the palmar side with the thumb of the other hand to reposit them.

2. Fixation

After reduction, a bone-separating pad is applied to both the palmar and dorsal aspects of the forearm. According to the actual conditions of the lateral displacement, other compresses may be placed and covered with cotton pads. Four splints are placed and fastened for fixation (Fig. 3—53). If fracture of the radius occurs at the upper 3rd, the forearm should be suspended in slight supination or full supination. If fracture of the radius occurs at the middle 3rd or the lower 3rd, the forearm is fixed in the neutral position. Generally the fixation lasts 4—6 weeks.

3. Herbal therapy

Traditional Chinese drugs can be prescribed in each of the three stages of the fracture injury on the basis of overall analysis and differentiation of symptoms and signs. See "Herbal therapy" in Section XII of this chapter.

4. Dirigation

At the initial stage, fist-making exercise may be practiced. When the swelling has basically disappeared, exercises of the shoulder and elbow joints may be done gradually. After the removal of fixation rotatory exercises of the forearm should be increased.

● **Prognosis**

Fracture of the shaft of the radius is easy to heal but poor reduction of rotatory or angular displacement may work on the rotatory functions of the forearm after union.

Section XIV Fracture of the Shaft of Ulna

The ulnar shaft is thick at the upper part and thin at the lower part, especially below the middle segment. And moreover there are no muscles at the medial and dorsal aspects to protect it, so it is easy to be subjected to the action of violent force and sustain fracture, which is seldom seen in clinical practice, though.

● **Causes and Pathogenesis**

The fracture is mostly produced by such direct forces as hitting, crushing and contusion, and is usually of transverse or comminuted types. After injury, because of the support by the radius and the link of the interosseous membrane, there is usually not much displacement of the injured ends. However, the proximal end may be displaced forward as a result of the traction by the biceps muscle of the arm while mild displacement of the distal end to the radial or palmar aspect may occur as a result of the traction by the quadrate pronator muscle. The ulna has a physiological projection to the dorsal side, so when fracture occurs, there is angulation to the dorsal side.

● **Clinical Manifestations and Diagnosis**

118

After injury, there is local swelling, pain and ecchymosis, sometimes angulation to the dorsal aspect, obvious tenderness and longitudinal impact pain. Abnormal movement and bony crepitus may be present. The fractured ends may be felt at the dorsal subcutaneous part of the ulna. X-ray films should be ordered to help make a definite diagnosis and determine the condition of displacement. The upper and lower radioulnar articulations should be included in x-ray examination so as to ascertain whether there is dislocation.

● **Treatment**

1. Manual reduction

The fracture without displacement needs no reduction. When there is angulation or rotatory deformity, manual reduction should be performed to correct it. The patient takes dorsal position or sits on a stool. One assistant holds the lower segment of the upper arm and another holds the carpometacarpal part. With the patient's shoulder abducted at 90° and the elbow flexed at 90°, the two assistants perform countertraction. In case of fracture of the ulna at the upper or middle 3rd, the traction is done with the forearm in the neutral position, whereas for fracture of the ulna at the lower 3rd, the traction is done with the forearm in pronated position so as to correct its rotatory and shortening displacement. If the fracture forms angulation to the dorsal aspect, the operator presses the angular protrusion to the palmar aspect with both thumbs and with the other fingers of both hands encircling from the concave side pulls the arm to the dorsal aspect. If lateral displacement is also present, after applying bone-separating maneuver, the operator holds the proximal end of the fracture with one hand and holds the distal end with the other to correct the anterior-posterior displacement with elevating-pressing maneuvers or the medial-lateral displacement with pushing-squeezing maneuver.

2. Fixation

After reduction, traction should be maintained. If the fracture is accompanied with angular displacement, compresses may be placed with triple-spot compression method. If there is anterior-posterior displacement, a plane compress is applied to both the palmar and dorsal aspects; for medial-lateral displacement, a bone-separating compress is applied to both palmar and dorsal aspects at the injured part. Then four splints are used for external fixation (same as the fixation of the fracture of the radial shaft). In cases of fracture of the ulna at the lower 3rd, the forearm is fixed in pronated position; for the fracture at the upper or middle 3rd, the forearm is fixed in the neutral position and suspended before the chest. Generally the fixation lasts 4—6 weeks, but should be prolonged properly in case of delayed healing.

3. Herbal therapy

Traditional Chinese drugs may be prescribed in each of the three stages of fracture on the basis of overall analysis and differentiation of symptoms and signs. See "Herbal therapy" in Section XII of this chapter.

4. Dirigation

At the initial stage, flexion-extension exercise of fingers and fist-making may be practiced. At the middle stage, movement of the shoulder and elbow joints may be done step by step. After removal of fixation, rotatory exercises of the forearm may be performed.

● **Prognosis**

Generally, the healing of fracture of the ulna takes place rather slowly, especially at the middle 3rd and lower 3rd, because there are not many muscles there and the blood supply there is poor. Every effort should be made to procure a good reposition and reliable fixation.

Section XV   Fracture of the Radius at the Lower 3rd Associated with Dislocation of the Lower Radioulnar Joint

This is a common injury in the upper limbs and may occur in

both adults and children, especially in men at the age of 20—40. The shaft of the radius changes gradually from very thin at the middle segment to thick at the lower 3rd and presents a great curvature toward the lateroposterior side. This curved part is a weak point to a stress. The connection and stability between the lower radioulnar joints are chiefly maintained by the strong triangular fibrocartilage and the weak ligaments of the lower inferior radioulnar joints at the palmar and dorsal sides.

● **Causes and Pathogenesis**

This disease is mostly produced by an indirect force, e. g. when the patient falls forwards with palms against the ground, the force is transmitted to the lower 3rd of the radius, producing a fracture. The fracture line is usually transverse or short and oblique. Direct forces can also bring about this injury, e. g. the fracture resulting from the hitting or crushing of the forearm by heavy objects, in which case the fracture is mostly transverse or comminuted. In the fractures mentioned above, upward displacement, or displacement to the palmar or dorsal aspect, of the distal end, may often occur. The laceration of triangular fibrocartilage together with the ulnar ligaments of the wrist or avulsion of styloid process of the ulna results in the dislocation of the inferior radioulnar joints.

● **Clinical Manifestations and Diagnosis**

After injury, there is pain and swelling in the forearm and wrist, apparent tenderness and longitudinal tapping pain in the lower middle part of the forearm. Angulation to the palmar or dorsal aspect at the injured part may form, protrusion of the small head of the ulna may protrude to the ulnar or dorsal side, the wrist may assume deviating deformity to the radial side, the forearm shows functional disturbances and the inferior radioulnar joint is loose.

When x-ray films are taken, the inferior radioulnar joint should be included so as to determine the fracture type and dislocation condition.

● **Treatment**

1. Manual reduction

For unstable fracture of the radius at the lower 3rd associated with dislocation of the inferior radioulnar joint, the overlapping, angulation and lateral displacement of the fracture should be dealt with first, followed by reduction of the separation dislocation of the inferior radioulnar joints.

The patient sits on a stool or takes dorsal position and local anesthesia is applied. With the patient's shoulder in an abducent position and the forearm in neutral position, one assistant holds the affected elbow while another holds his hand to make the forearm in a slightly supinated position, and the two assistants perform countertraction. The operator first corrects the inward displacement of the distal fractured end with bone separating maneuver, then presses the distal end to the dorsal side with thumbs, pulls and elevates the proximal end to the palmar side with the remaining four fingers so as to correct the anterior displacement of the distal end. If the distal end displaces to the dorsal side, the direction of the reduction should be done in the opposite way. The operator clamps the reposited fracture end with one hand and presses down the high protrusion of the distal end displaced to the parlmar or dorsal side with the other hand, then squeezes the radial and ulnar sides of the wrist with the thumb and the forefinger to reposit the separated inferior radioulnar joints.

2. Fixation

After reduction, a bone-separating compress is put between the radius and the ulna at the lower 3rd of the forearm and an arched compress is placed on both sides of the distal ends of the radius and the ulna, covered with cotton pads and fixed with four splints. The lower ends of the medial and lateral splints should go about 2cm beyond the wrist joint so as to fix the inferior radioulnar joint. Then with the elbow flexed at 90°, the forearm is suspended before the chest.

3. Herbal therapy

Traditional Chinese medicines should be prescribed for internal and external use in each of the three stages of a fracture on the basis of overall analysis and differentiation of symptoms and signs.

122

4. Dirigation

After reduction and fixation, flexion-extension exercises of the finger joints can start immediately but rotatory exercise of the forearm should be avoided. At the middle stage, exercise of elbow joints may be done. Only after the removal of fixation can rotatory exercises of the forearm be performed.

● **Prognosis**

As a rule, clinical healing of the injury takes place in 4 weeks, but the healing of the triangular fibrocartilage is difficult, so pain in the wrist and restriction to wrist movement are often left over.

Section XVI　Fracture of the Distal End of Radius

This disease refers to the fracture occurring within 3cm of the inferior end of the radius, which is the enlarged part of the inferior end of the radius, the junction of spongy bone and hard bone, and a weak spot to stress. Fractures are easy to happen here, mostly in adults, especially old people.

● **Causes and Pathogenesis**

Fracture of the distal end of the radius is usually produced by an indirect force and sometimes by a direct force. By the posture of the wrist in the course of injury and condition of displacement, the fracture is clinically divided into the following two types:

1. Extension type

When one falls with the wrist in dorsal extension, the forearm in pronation and the palm against the ground first, a fracture occurs as a result of convergence of the reactive force from the ground and the body gravity at the distal end of the radius. If the indirect force is not very strong, the fracture may be accompanied by only slight impaction but when the force is great, the distal fractured end may displace to the dorsal side and the radial side or even overlapping displacement may be produced, the hand and wrist may assume a "fork-shaped" deformity (Fig. 3—54) accompanied by dislocation of the inferior radioulnar joints and laceration of the triangular fibrodisc. In old patients, owing to osteoporosis, the fracture is often comminuted and the fracture line involves the articular surfaces.

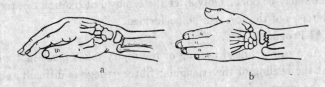

a
b

Fig. 3—54 Displacement in extension type of fracture of the distal end of radius

2. Flexion type

When one falls, the wrist joint is in palmar flexion, the dorsum of the hand strikes the ground first, the transmission force will produce a fracture at the distal end of the radius. The distal fractured end displaces to the palmar and the radial sides and the wrist and hand assume "slice-shaped" deformity. If the dorsal side of the wrist is hit by a direct force, this fracture may also be produced, but it is seldom seen in clinical practice.

● **Clinical Manifestations and Diagnosis**

In the fracture without displacement, there is only mild local swelling and pain. The displaced fracture is marked by apparent swelling, pain, tenderness and longitudinal percussion pain at the upper part of the wrist. Wrist movement may be restricted. From the lateral view of the extension type of fracture, " fork-shaped" deformity can be seen whereas from the front view, "bayonet-shaped" deformity may appear. From the lateral view, the flexion type of fracture may assume "slice-shaped" deformity (Fig. 3—55).

X-ray films may reveal the type of fracture and condition of displacement.

● **Treatment**

Fractures without displacement and greenstick type need no reduction and only require fixation with splints for 2—3 weeks. The displaced fractures should be reduced in line with the fracture type.

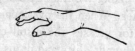

1. Manual reduction

(1) Exterior type

Here are the common reduction maneuvers:

① Two-person reduction method

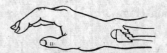

Fig. 3—55 Displacement in flexion type of fracture of the proximal end of radius

After local anaesthesia, the patient sits on a stool or takes the dorsal position with the affected limb abducting. An assistant holds the inferior extremity of the upper arm and the operator holds the hands of the affected side with one hand to perform countertraction with the assistant. His thumb of the other hand presses the distal end of the fracture from the dorsal aspect and the other four fingers raise the proximal end from the palmar aspect. At the same time of this pressing and raising maneuvers, the wrist is made to flex to the palmar aspect to correct the displacement of the distal end to the dorsal aspect. Then the operator pushes the distal end of the fracture from the radial side with the thumb and pulls the lower segment of the ulna simultaneously with the other four fingers to correct the displacement of the distal end of fracture towards the radial side. At the same time of pushing-pulling, the affected hand is made to flex to the ulnar aspect to facilitate the reposition (Fig. 3—56). The displacement to the radius may also be reduced before the reduction of the anterior-posterior displacement.

② Contra-angular flexing reduction method

The patient sits on a stool or lies in dorsal position with the affected limb abducted. An assistant holds the lower end of the upper arm with both hands and the operator holds the palm with both hands, presses with his two thumbs from the dorsal aspect on the distal end of the fracture and performs stretching traction for 3—4 minutes. When the overlapping displacement is pulled apart, the operator presses the distal end of the fracture downwards with both thumbs, lifts and props the proximal end of the fracture upwards with two index fingers. Meanwhile, he quickly makes the wrist joints flex to the palmar by the ulnar aspect to achieve the reposition (Fig. 3—57).

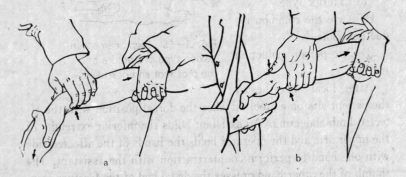

Fig. 3—56 Two-person reduction of fracture in the distal end
   a. Correction of the displacement of the distal end to the dorsal aspect
   b. Correction of the displacement of the distal end to the radial aspect

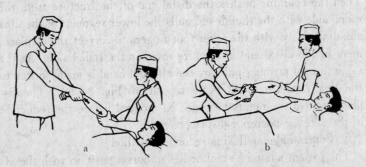

Fig. 3—57 Reduction of extension type of fracture in the distal end of the radius with contra-angular flexing maneuver

126

③ Three-person reduction method

The patient sits on a stool or lies in dorsal position. One assistant holds the patient's upper arm while another holds the patient's hand and they perform countertraction to correct the overlapping displacement. The operator holds the patient's carpometacarpal part to push the distal end of the fracture to the ulnar aspect with one hand and holds the proximal end of the lower segment of the forearm and push it toward the radial aspect with the other hand and squeezes from the two sides to correct radial displacement of the distal end of the fracture. Then the operator presses the distal end of the fracture with two thumbs, holds the proximal end with the other fingers, applies the lifting-pressing maneuver to correct the displacement to the palm-dorsal side and at the same time the assistant holding the hand makes the affected wrist flex to the palmar aspect (Fig. 3—58).

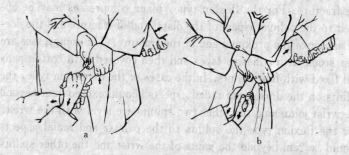

Fig. 3—58 Three-person reduction of extension type of fracture in the distal end of the radius

(2) Flexion type

The patient sits on a stool. One assistant holds the elbow with the forearm of the affected side in supination, another assistant takes the patient's hand and they perform countertraction for 3—5 minutes. The operator presses the distal end of the fracture from the palmar to the dorsal aspect with two thumbs, lifts the proximal end of the fracture from the dorsal aspect to the palmar aspect with the other fingers.

Meanwhile under steady countertraction, the assistant holding the hand makes the affected wrist extend to the dorsal aspect and incline to the ulnar aspect so that it can be reduced (Fig. 3 — 59).

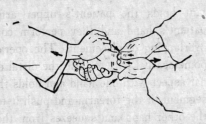

Fig. 3—59 Reduction of flexion type of fracture in the distal end of radius

2. Fixation

All fractures of the distal end of the radius may be fixed with splints. According to the displacement condition of the injured end, compresses may be applied. For the extension type, plane compresses may be applied to both the dorsal and radial aspects of the distal end and the palmar aspect of the proximal end of the fracture. For the flexion type, plane compresses may be applied to the palmar aspect of the distal end of fracture and the dorsal aspect of the proximal end of the fracture. The compresses are first stuck with adhesive tapes and then covered with cotton pads and fixed with four splints. In the cases of the extension type, the splints on the dorsal and radial aspects should exceed 1cm beyond the wrist joints and the other two splints are level with the wrist. For the flexion type the splints to the palmar and radial aspects should be 2cm beyond the joints of the wrist and the other splints be level with the wrist. The splints should be fastened for 3—4 rounds with cloth laces. The forearm is hung in front of the chest. Usually the fixation should be kept for 4 weeks (Fig. 3—60, 61).

3. Herbal therapy

At the initial stage, a patient with severe swelling may take modified *Taohong Siwu Tang*, *Fuyuan Huoxue Tang*, etc. to subdue swelling, alleviate pain, promote blood circulation and remove blood stasis. At the middle stage, the patient may take *Xinshang Xuduan Tang*, *Jiegu Pian*, etc. to promote the regeneration of tissue by regulating the nutrient system and rejoin the fractured bone and restore the soft tissues. At the late stage, after the removal of fixation, patients with deficiency of blood and *qi* or impaired liver-kidney essence may take *Bushen Zhuangjin Tang*, *Shiquan Dabu Wan*, etc. orally and use *Erhao Xiyao* to bathe the affected part externally so as to relax muscles and tendons and activate the flow of *qi* and blood in the channels and collaterals.

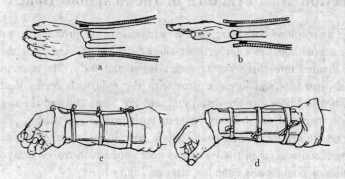

Fig. 3—60 Compress placement and splinting
in the extension type of fracture

4. Dirigation

Right after reduction and fixation, flexion exercises of interphalangeal and carpometacarpal joints, and functional exercises of the shoulder and elbow may begin. After the removal of fixation, exercises of flexion and extension of the wrist joints and rotatory exercises of the forearm should be strengthened.

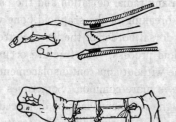

Fig. 3—61 Compress placement and splinting in the flexion type of fracture

● Prognosis

Generally, the disease has a

good prognosis and the functional restoration is usually satisfactory. However, comminuted fracture, especially when the fracture line infringes the articular surface, restriction of functions or pain in the wrist joints may remain. A poor reduction of the fracture may cause slight deformity of the wrist joints or separation of inferior radioulnar joints so that functions may be limited.

Section XVII Fracture of the Scaphoid Bone

The scaphoid bone lying on the radial side of the proximal row of the carpal bones is a larger boat-shaped oval bone. The bone may be divided into three parts: node, waist and body. Its proximal end protrudes and forms a joint with the radius. It forms joints with other bones at the distal end and the ulnar and radial sides. Most parts of the bone is covered with articular cartilage. The blood supply to the scaphoid bone is poor because there are only tiny blood vessels in the waist and node, for which reason delayed union or nonunion is common after an injury here.

● **Causes and Pathogenesis**

The injury is mostly produced by an indirect force. For example, when one falls, if his wrist joints are in extreme dorsal extension and radial deviation and the palm strikes against the ground, the breaking of the scaphoid bone will occur due to the impact by the dorsal border of the lower extremity of the radius or border of styloid process. The fracture occurs at the waist of the scaphoid bone without apparent displacement but a space. This type of fracture is more common. Sometimes the injury happens in the node and the fragments may be displaced to the radial side but this type is rarely seen clinically. The fracture may also occur at the proximal end of the scaphoid bone (Fig. 3—62).

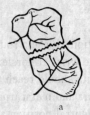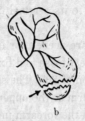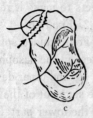

a b c

Fig. 3—62 Types of fracture of scaphoid bone
a. fracture at the waist   b. fracture at the proximal end
c. fracture at the node

● **Clinical Manifestations and Diagnosis**

After injury, there are swelling and pain at the dorsal aspect of the wrist. Dorsiextension of the wrist joints and movements to the radial aspect are restricted. There is obvious tenderness at the nasopharyngeal fossa and pain of carpus on percussion or pressing along the longitudinal axis of the second metacarpal bone. X-ray films in anteroposterior and lateral views, plus a film in oblique view of ulnar deviation of the hand must be taken to make a definite diagnosis. If clinical signs suggest a fracture but the x-ray films show a negative result, it is necessary to make another radiographic examination 1—2 weeks later, because by then the bone substance will have been absorbed and the fracture line will be distinctly visible in the films. Occasionally it should be distinguished from congenital double scaphoid bones.

● **Treatment**

1. Manual reduction

The fracture without displacement needs no reduction but splintage only. In the reduction of the displaced fracture, the patient is told to sit on a stool. The operator holds the upper part of the wrist with one hand, presses the snuffpot with the thumb of the other hand and encircles the patient's thumb of the affected hand in his other four fingers. Then both hands perform countertraction in ulnar deviation. On this basis, the operator presses the dis-

131

placed distal end with the thumb towards the ulnar and palmar aspects to make it return to its original place.

2. Fixation

Four molded splints are needed for fixation. Place a round compress in the nasopharygeal fossa and fix the wrist at dorsiextension of 30° and ulnar deviation of 30°. The splints should reach the middle segment of the forearm at the upper part and metacarpal cervix at the lower part. Keep the forearm in a neutral position and hang it with a sling for 7—10 weeks. If a check shows that healing of the fracture has not been achieved, the fixation should be kept till clinical union (Fig. 3—63).

Cardboard fixation may also be performed in the same way as far as the range and posture is concerned. Some doctors prefer that the wrist should be fixed at palmar flexion of 30° and ulnar deviation of 10° so as to reduce the shear force to the fractured ends, increase the longitudinal pressure and benefit the union of the fracture.

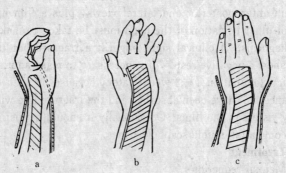

Fig. 3—63 Fixation with small splints for fracture
of scaphoid bone
a. the wrist at dorsiextension of 30°   b. anteroposterior view
c. the wrist at deviation of 10°

3. Herbal therapy

At the initial stage, the principle of medication is promoting blood circulation to remove blood stasis and regulating the flow of *qi* to subdue swelling. It is advisable for the patient to take *Huoxue Zhitong Tang* and *Dieda Wan*. Because the union of the fracture occurs slowly the patient should also take Chinese medicines which can promote reunion of bone, muscle and ligament such as *Zhenggu Zijin Dan*, etc. At the late stage, after the removal of fixation, *Wujiapi Tang* or *Erhao Xiyao* may be used for external local bathing.

4. Dirigation

At the initial stage, exercises of finger, shoulder and elbow joints may be practiced but movements of the wrist joints to either the radial or ulnar side must be avoided. At the middle stage, fist-making exercises may be done. After the removal of fixation, enough functional exercises of the wrist joints must be performed.

● **Prognosis**

The prospects of the union of fracture of the scaphoid bone are related to the location and type of fracture. As a rule, union will occur in 3 months. The fractures at the waist and node heal easily while the union of the fracture at the proximal end is poor. Especially when the fracture is not properly fixed, cysticosteoporosis may appear, which is the manifestation of delayed union, but still the fracture may be knitted given that subsequent proper fixation is performed and internal and external Chinese drugs are used. In very few cases the fracture line widens and a sclerotic belt appears which are indications of non-union and in such cases an operation is sometimes necessary.

Section XVIII   Fracture of Metacarpal Bones

There are five metacarpal bones in the palm. The first metacarpal bone is thick and short and has a relatively large range of movement, so its base is susceptible to fracture, which is sometimes accompanied by articular dislocation of the carpometacarpal joint. The second and third metacarpal bones are both thin and long. Fractures in them usually result from hitting something with the fist. The fourth and fifth metacarpal bones are thin and short. Fracture in the fifth metacarpal bone happens when it suffers from hitting. These fractures are mostly seen in adults.

● **Causes and Pathogenesis**

Fracture of metacarpal bones may be produced by either a direct force or an indirect force.

1. Fracture at the base of the first metacarpal bone

The fracture is mostly incurred in a fall with the patient's thumb against the ground or by the impaction of the metacarpal bone a-gainst the trapezium resulting from the longitudinal hitting by an external force on the first metacarpal bone, often occurring at the site 0.5—1cm from the proximal end of the first metacarpal bone. It is usually in transverse form with the distal end displaced to-wards the ulnar and palmar aspects and angulated at the radial and dorsal aspects. This fracture is of articular type.

If the fracture line is oblique, it may go obliquely from the mediosuperior part of the metacarpal base to the lateroinferior part and extends further into the intracarpometacarpal joint and a trian-gular bony fragment is formed at the medial aspect of the base and so the fracture belongs to intraarticular type. Owing to its de-creased stability and traction by the long abductor and the short flexor of the thumb, the distal end of the fracture is dislocated to-wards the radial and dorsal aspects and flexed towards the palmar aspect (Fig. 3—64).

2. Fracture of the metacarpal shaft

The fracture may be seen in one or more metacarpal bones, mostly caused by a direct force. The common forms are transverse or comminuted fracture. The broken ends are angulated towards the dorsal aspect and displaced towards the lateral aspect as a re-sult of the traction of digital flexor and interosseous muscle.

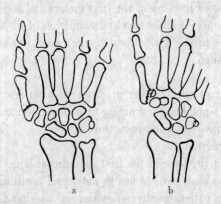

Fig. 3—64 Types of fracture at the base of the 1st metacarpal bone
a. fracture line does not pass articular surface   b. fracture line passes
the carpometacarpal joint surface

3. Fracture at the metacarpal cervix

Such a fracture is often produced by a force acting directly on
the head of the metacarpal bone when one hits something with the
fist and is mostly seen in the fourth or fifth metacarpal bone. Since
this sort of fracture often occurs in boxers, it is often referred to
as boxing fracture. The distal broken end is angulated towards the
dorsal aspect because the
traction by the interosseous
muscles and lumbrical muscle render the head of
metacarpal bone rotate towards the palmar aspect
(Fig. 3—65).

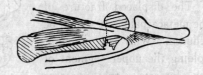

Fig. 3—65 Displacement in
fracture of the metacarpal cervix

● **Clinical Manifesta-
tions and Diagnosis**

After injury, there is local swelling, pain, restriction of movement, obvious tenderness and longitudinal tapping pain. A fracture with displacement may show bony crepitus. In a case with

135

shortening deformity, collapse of the head of metacarpal bone may be seen. In a case of fracture of the first metacarpal bone, there is apparent disturbance of abduction and adduction of its thumb and movements of the palm. X-ray films in anteroposterior and oblique views must be taken.

● **Treatment**

The treatment of the fracture at different locations should be carried out with a good understanding of its condition and the particular needs to ensure a good reduction.

1. Manual reduction

(1) Fracture at the base of the first metacarpal bone

The patient sits on a stool or lies in the dorsal position. The operator holds the patient's affected wrist in one hand with the thumb pressing on the protruding part at the base of the first metacarpal bone towards the ulnar and palmar aspects, stretches the patient's injured thumb with the other hand and turns the head of the first metacarpal bone towards the dorsal and radial aspects making the first metacarpal bone abduct and extend slightly towards the dorsal aspect. The displacement of the fracture and dislocation can be corrected by the manipulation of the two hands (Fig. 3—66).

(2) Fracture of the metacarpal shaft

The displaced fracture of the metacarpal shaft should be reduced. With an assistant holding the upper segment of the forearm, the operator holds the affected finger with one hand to perform countertraction. With the other hand he corrects the fracture angulation by lifting and pressing the broken ends and corrects lateral displacement by pinching from

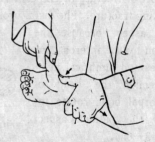

Fig. 3—66 Reduction of fracture at the base of the 1st metacarpal bone

the two sides of the injured bone (Fig. 3—67).

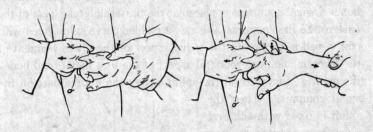

Fig. 3—67   Reduction of the fracture at shaft of metacarpal bone
a. Correction of the backward-forward displacement of the fractured ends
b. Correction of the inward-outward displacement of the fractured ends

(3) Fracture at the metacarpal cervix

The operator fixes the patient's affected palm with one hand, holds the proximal end of the fracture between the fingers, holds the affected finger with the other hand and makes the metacarpophalangeal joint flex to 90° so that the lateral paraligament becomes tonic and the proximal end of the proximal phalanx lies against the metacarpal head. Then he pushes the proximal phalanx along the direction of its longitudinal axis toward the dorsal aspect and presses the proximal broken end of the metacarpal bone towards the palmar aspect with the thumb and the fracture is set right (Fig. 3—68).

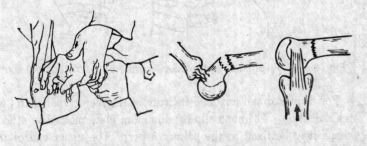

Fig. 3—68   Reduction of fracture at the metacarpal cervix
a. reduction maneuver   b. sketch map

137

2. Fixation

After reduction of the fracture at the base of the first metacarpal bone, a small compress is placed at the posterolateral aspect of the base of the first metacarpal bone, a molded curve splint lined with cotton pad is applied to the radial aspect of the lower segment of the forearm and posterolateral aspect of the first metacarpal bone, the greatest curvature of the splint covers the injured part on the small compress. Then the splint is fixed with adhesive tapes or a bandage to keep the first metacarpal bone in extension position (Fig. 3—69). For undisplaced or stable fracture of the metacarpal shaft, a bone-separating compress is ap-

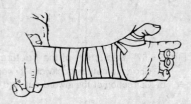

Fig. 3—69 Fixation of fracture at the base of metacarpal bone

plied to either side of the dorsal aspect of the fracture and a hard square cardboard is applied on both the dorsal and palmar aspects of the metacarpal bone and fixed with bandage (Fig. 3—70).

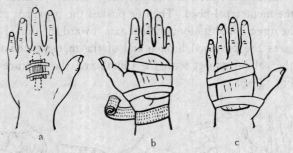

Fig. 3—70 Fixation of undisplaced fracture of the metacarpal shaft

For displaced and unstable fracture of the metacarpal shaft, after reduction, a bamboo slip or aluminum plate molded in a hook shape may be fixed to the palmar aspect. The upper end of the splint reaches the lowder-middle part of the palmar aspect of the forearm and the lower end extends to the finger with a piece of

138

cardboard placed on the upper part of the splint. The curvature of the splint should be such as allows the injured finger in the functioning position. It is then bound up with cotton padding and bandages (Fig. 3—71).

After reduction of the fracture at the metacarpal cervix, a right-angled bamboo or aluminum slip may be applied to the dorsal aspect of the carpometacarpal part as well as the injured finger to keep the metacarpophalangeal and proximal interphalangeal joints flexed at 90°. The slip

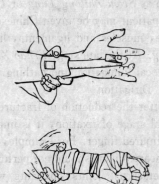

Fig. 3—71 Fixation of fracture in the metacarpal shaft with a hook-shaped splint

and finger are then bound up with cotton pad and bandages (Fig. 3 —72,73).

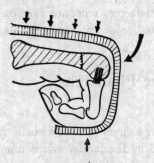

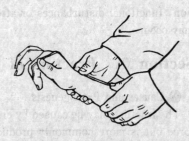

Fig. 3—72 Sketch map of the fixation of fracture at the metacarpal cervix

Fig. 3—73 Fixation of fracture at the metacarpal cervix

3. Herbal therapy

At the initial stage, the patient may take Chinese drugs which

139

promote blood circulation, remove blood stasis and alleviate pain such as *Siwu Zhitong Tang* or *Dieda Wan*. At the middle stage, the patient may be given Chinese drugs for promoting reunion of bone, muscles and ligaments, like *Jiegu Pian* or *Xugu Huoxue Tang*. At the late stage *Erhao Xiyao*, etc. should be administered for local fumigation and bathing.

4. Dirigation

After the reduction of fracture of the metacarpal bones, at the initial stage of fixation, it is improper for the patient to exercise the injured finger. For example, patients with fracture of the first metacarpal bone should not perform adducting exercises of the carpometacarpal joints; patients with fracture at the metacarpal cervix are not allowed to do finger extension exercises and patients with fracture of the metacarpal shaft are advised against fist-making exercises, etc. But proper exercises of elbow and shoulder joints should be encouraged. After 4—6 weeks when the fixation is removed, functional exercises of the fingers and wrist joints should be increased gradually.

● **Prognosis**

Clinical union of fracture of the metacarpal bone usually takes place in 4—6 weeks. In cases of unsatisfactory reduction and fixation, functional disturbances or attenuation of grip strength, etc. may occur.

Section XIX   Fracture of the Phalanges

● **Causes and Pathogenesis**

The fracture may be caused by either a direct force or an indirect force but is more commonly produced by the former and is often open comminuted type. The fracture produced by an indirect force is mostly of transverse and oblique types.

In a fracture of the proximal phalanx, the broken ends often protrude to the palmar aspect to form angulation due to the traction by the interosseous muscles and lumbrical muscles. The fractured ends of the phalangeal cervix also form angulation toward the palmar aspect and the distal end rotates 90° dorsally as a result of the traction by the central part of the extensor tendon, making the dorsum of the distal end face the surface of the proximal end. The dorsal base of the distal phalanx is the end point of expansion of finger extensor tendon. When the finger is in extension position, the finger end is impacted by the force, avulsion fracture at the dorsal base of the proximal phalanx may occur, in which case the distal phalanx fails to extend straight actively, presenting a hammer shape and is called as such (Fig. 3—74).

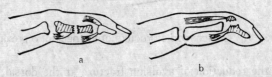

Fig. 3—74 Displacement of fracture at different sites of phalanges

● **Clinical Manifestations and Diagnosis**
After injury, local swelling, pain, ring tenderness and longitudinal percussion pain arise. Bony crepitus and abnormal movement may be present. Angulation or protrusive deformity may appear in the case of noticeable fracture displacement. X-ray films may determine the type and condition of fracture displacement.

● **Treatment**
Every effort should be made to achieve anatomic reduction so as to prevent functional disturbances of any degree of the finger.

1. Manual reduction
During reduction, the patient sits on a stool. An assistant holds the affected palm and the proximal end of the finger. The operator picks up the distal end of the fracture with one hand and tracts it to correct angulation. Meanwhile he pinches the broken ends with the thumb and index finger of the other hand to correct the anterior-posterior or medial-lateral displacement. In setting a fracture at the cervix of the proximal phalanx, the operator first enlarges the angle of the broken ends and then with the contra-angular flexing skill tracts the distal end toward the dorsal aspect at 90°. Then he

141

quickly flexes the patient's affected finger and meanwhile pushes
the proximal end from the palmar aspect toward the dorsal aspect.
Thereupon th reduction is completed (Fig. 3—75).

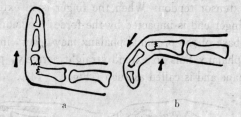

a   b

Fig. 3—75   Sketch map of fracture of the neck of a proximal phalanx

In the reduction of avulsion fracture at the dorsal base of the
distal phalanx, the operator flexes the proximal interphalangeal
articulation, makes extreme extension of the distal interphalangeal
articulation and presses the fragment towards the palmar aspect
with the thumb.

2. Fixation

For undisplaced fracture of the proximal and middle phalanxes,
after the injured finger is wound with several turns of bandage
round it, it is fixed with cardboard (two pieces of hard arched
cardboard), small slip splints or aluminum plate. Generally the
finger is fixed in the functional position (Fig. 3—76—a).

For avulsion fracture at the dorsal base of the distal phalanx,
molded small bamboo splint or an aluminum plate is applied to the
palmar aspect of the affected finger making the distal interphalangeal joint flexed at 90° and the proximal interphalangeal joints
in overextension. A small square compress is applied to the dorsal
aspect of the injured part covered with an arch-shaped cardboard
and bound up with adhesive tapes so as to benefit the relaxation of
extensor tendon and stability of fragments (Fig. 3—76—b).

142

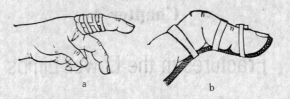

Fig. 3—76 Fixation of fracture of a phalanx

3. Herbal therapy

The principle of medication at the initial stage is promoting blood circulation ιo remove blood stasis and the patient may take *Qili San* and *Huoxue Quyu Pian*. At the middle stage, *Jiegu Dan* may be prescribed for oral use. At the late stage, *Shangzhi Xifang* may be prescribed for external local fumigation and bathing.

4. Dirigation

At the initial stage of the fixation, under the condition that the stability of the injured finger is not affected, exercises of other fingers and wrist joints may be practiced. After the removal of fixation, functional exercises must be strengthened so as to restore the normal functions as early as possible.

● **Prognosis**

If the reduction and fixation of fracture of the phalanxes are well done and exercise is prompt and proper, satisfactory functional restoration can usually be obtained. Disturbances of functions or even stiffness of joints may appear in patients with deformed union due to poor reduction and fixation, in which case the functions of the hand may be severely affected.

143

Chapter 4

Fractures in the Lower Limbs

Section I　Fracture of the Femoral Neck

The femoral neck is just below the femoral head and above the femoral shaft. There is an included angle between the femoral neck and the shaft, called collodiaphysial angle, normally being 125°—130° in adults. When the collodiaphysial angle is greater than the normal range, coxa valga is suggested. On the contrary, coxa vara is suggested if the angle is smaller than the normal range. The forward inclination of the femoral neck is known as anterior slope angle, being 12°—15° or so in adults. As most parts of the femoral neck lie in the joint capsule and it has a poor blood supply, it is difficult for a fracture of the femoral neck to heal or even ischemic necrosis may occur.

● **Causes and Pathogenesis**

This is a common disease, mostly affecting the old people, for they often suffer from osteoporosis and are weak in constitution, and the bearing capacity of their femoral neck has become decreased. Sometimes even a slight external force may result in the fracture in them, such as in a fall, sudden torsion of the lower limb, etc. The injury occurring in the young and robust adults is mostly produced by a powerful force, such as a fall from heights.

Fracture of the femoral neck is often divided into adduction type and abduction type based on the mechanisms of injury. The fracture of adduction type occurs when the coxa is in adduction. The angle formed between the fracture line and the vertical line of the longitudinal axis of the femoral shaft is larger than 50° and the collodiaphysial angle smaller than normal. Since the distal fractured end is frequently adducted and displaced upwards and the blood supply to the joint capsule is greatly damaged, the fracture is difficult to heal and the rate of necrosis of the femoral head is high. When the coxa is in abduction, fracture of the abduction type may occur with the fracture line below the femoral head and with little displacement or impaction of the fractured ends. The angle of inclination formed by the fracture line and the vertical line of the longitudinal axis of the femoral shaft is often smaller than 30°. The broken ends are usually stable due to very little shear force at the fractured part. As a rule, the intracapsular blood supply is seldom damaged so the fracture is easy to heal (Fig. 4—1, 2, 3).

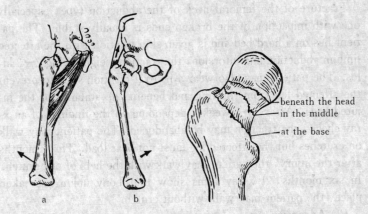

Fig. 4—1 Fracture of femoral neck
a. abducent type b. adducent type

Fig. 4—2 The common sites of fracture of the femoral neck

beneath the head
in the middle
at the base

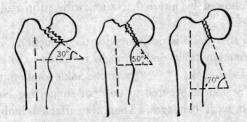

Fig. 4—3 The inclination angle of fracture line of the femoral neck

● **Clinical Manifestations and Diagnosis**

The injury mostly occurs in old people. The patient has a history of trauma with pain in the affected hip, tenderness at the greater tuberosity, and longitudinal tapping pain. The injured leg remains in extorsion position and looks shorter in a case with apparent displacement. Functional disturbances of the affected leg appear in most cases. X-ray films are of help in the determination of the location of the fracture and condition of displacement.

● **Treatment**

1. Manual reduction and fixation

(1) Stable abduction type

Fracture of the femoral neck of the abduction type, especially one with impaction of the broken ends is usually stable. The patient lies on a hard bed and is given skin traction with the affected limb in abduction and intorsion, the traction weight being 2—3 kilos. The patient may also wear a neutral-position shoe to prevent the affected leg from rotating and benefit the stability of the injured ends. After 5—7 weeks, depending on the findings of an x-ray check, the traction may be abandoned. The patient may walk on crutches but the affected leg must not bear load. Three months after the injury, the patient may walk with the help of one crutch. In six months, if x-ray films show that bony union has taken place, the patient may walk without crutch.

(2) Adduction type

Clinically, this type of injury is common. In most cases the fracture is unstable with displacement. It is often treated with manual reduction followed by internal fixation with trifin nails or three steel needles.

Peridural anesthesia is necessary for the reduction. The patient lies on a traction table and is made to extend the normal leg straight and abduct at 20°—30° with the ankle joints in the neutral position. The foot is secured to the foot supporting board of the traction bed with bandages. Then the affected limb is pulled straight and the foot is also secured in the same way. The operator holds the foot of the affected limb and tracts the limb slowly together with the supporting board so as to restore the normal length of the affected limb. Then the traction is maintained by the traction bed. The affected limb is intorsed to make the fractured end surfaces meet with each other. At the above posture, the affected limb is gradually abducted at $20° - 30°$ to ensure that the fracture ends closely contact with each other and will not displace again.

X-ray films of the coxa in anteroposterior and lateral views should be taken to check the reduction result. If the reduction fails, another method of reduction may be used: Holding the ankle of the affected leg with one hand and laying another at the popliteal fossa to make both the knee and coxa joints flex at 90°, the operator performs traction by lifting and pulling the knee and hip upwards. Under steady traction the operator makes the coxa abduct at $20° - 30°$ and extend the limb straight while intorting it. The "palm-heel test" may be done to find out whether the reduction is achieved or not (the heel of the affected side is cupped with the palm and if it does not extort, reduction is successful). Then the foot is fixed to the supporting board. X-ray films should be ordered to confirm the reduction. Finally, internal fixation with a trifin nail or three steel needles should be performed in the light of the actual need (Fig. 4—4).

2. Herbal therapy

As the symptoms of internal injury is severe, the patient is usually confined to bed for a long time, there tend to be complications and as the fracture is difficult to heal, it is very important to prescribe Chinese medicines for oral use. At the initial stage, stress should be laid on promoting blood circulation to remove

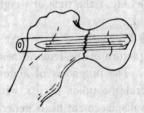

Fig. 4—4 Internal fixation of fracture of the femoral neck with a trifin nail

blood stasis, subduing swelling and alleviating pain and the patient

147

may take such Chinese medicines as *Huoxue Quyu Tang* plus *San-qi Fen*. In cases with stagnation of *qi* in the intestines and the stomach, modified *Shunqi Huoxue Tang* should be prescribed for oral administration. At the middle stage, Chinese medicines for tonifying the kidney and the liver and strengthening bones, tendons and muscles like *Liuwei Dihuang Wan*, etc. as well as *Jiegu Dan* should be taken.

3. Dirigation

After fixation, the patient is encouraged to exercise the upper limbs and the healthy lower leg to prevent various complications. However, body turning-over and leg crossing are forbidden. Flexion and extension exercises of ankle and toe joints of the injured limb may be done at the early stage. Relaxation and contraction exercises of quadriceps muscle of the thigh may be performed step by step. At the late stage, after the removal of fixation, flexion-extension exercises of the hip and knee joints should be gradually increased, starting while the patient is still in bed, but external rotation and adduction of the affected hip must be avoided. After the union of fracture, the patient may get out of bed and move about on crutches and take weight-carrying walks progressively. If x-ray films show some phenomena of ischemic necrosis like increase in density of the substance of bone in the femoral head, collapse, etc., the time of weight- carrying exercise should be postponed.

● **Prognosis**

Fracture of the femoral neck is one of the fractures difficult to heal. The prognosis of abduction-impaction type is good and in general the union occurs within 3 months. The adduction type with displacement heals generally in 3—6 months if the treatment is proper. But in a few cases delayed union, non-union and aseptic necrosis of the femoral head may occur or such sequelae as traumatic arthritis, adhesion and stiffness of the coxa may be left.

Section II Fracture of the Intertuberosity of the Femur

As the bone between the large tuberosity and small tuberosity of the femur in old people is in rarefaction, so even a mild force may produce a fracture. The injury is very common in old people.

● **Causes and Pathogenesis**

When an old person falls with the tuberosity of the femur against the ground or suffers an external force, this fracture may arise from the extorsion, intorsion or inversion of the involved limb. According to the direction and location of the fracture line, it may be divided into three types:

1. Positive fracture of the intertuberosity

The fracture line begins from the top of the large tuberosity, goes obliquely downwards to the upper part or slightly lower part of the small tuberosity. The direction of fracture line parallels with the spine of the intertuberosity. In this type of injury, the inversion of the hip is usually not severe and sometimes a small fragment may be split off from the small tuberosity. This injury is one of the most common stable fractures.

2. Negative fracture of intertuberosity

The fracture line begins at the small tuberosity and the base of the femoral neck, goes obliquely outwards to the lower part of the large tuberosity. The deformity of coxa vara may appear. This type is unstable.

3. Fracture below the tuberosity

The fracture line passes through the lower parts of both the large and small tuberosities. This injury is also unstable.

4. Comminuted fracture

The comminuted fracture produced by a violent force may occur in any type of fractures mentioned above. The cortex of bone on the large or small tuberosity and the medial part is comminuted, coxa vara is severe, upward displacement of the distal broken end

149

may occur and the fracture is unstable (Fig. 4−5).

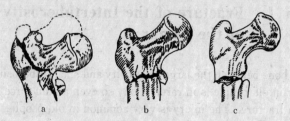

Fig. 4−5　Types of fracture of the intertuberosity of the femur
　　　　a. along the intertuberosity　b. against the intertuberosity
　　　　c. below the intertuberosity

● **Clinical Manifestations and Diagnosis**

After injury, there are local swelling and pain, the victim cannot sit up or walk, movements of the coxa are restricted, and
shortening, adduction or extorsion deformity of the lower limb
may be seen. On tapping the large tuberosity, sharp pain occurs.
Sometimes bony crepitus may be noticed on touch. X-ray films are
of help in making a definite diagnosis. The common complications
are pneumonia and other infections.

● **Treatment**

1. Manual reduction

The undisplaced fracture with impaction needs no reduction.
The patient lies in dorsal position for bed rest with the affected
limb abducting (about 30°−40° and the affected foot in "neutral-
position shoe" or with the affected limb kept in neutral or slightly
inverted position with the help of sand bags. After 4−6 weeks,
the patient can sit up and do exercise in bed and try to walk on
crutches gradually. Only after the knitting of bone can the affected
limb bear weight.

Displaced fracture needs reduction. Under local anesthesia the
patient lies in dorsal position. An assistant performs upward traction by pulling both armpits of the patient with both hands. Another assistant performs downward traction by holding the upper
part of the ankle of the affected limb. After the overlapping dis-

150

placement is corrected, the operator encircles the medial side of the upper part of the thigh with a wide strip of cloth and pulls the thigh towards the lateral aspect with one hand and simultaneously pushes the upper part of the large tuberosity towards the medial aspect with the other hand. At the same time, the assistant holding the ankle abducts and intorts the affected limb and thereupon the reduction is completed.

2. Fixation

After reduction, a thick cotton pad is applied to the large tuberosity and the lateral aspect of the affected limb is covered with cotton. All the protrusive parts should also be lined with cotton pads. A long molded splint is applied to the lateral aspect and then secured with bandages. The long splint should reach the 6th to the 7th ribs at the top and 2cm beyond the foot with the arched part at the tuberosity. This fixation is simple and easy to do but not very stable.

Fixation by skin traction with the affected limb in abduction is better. The traction weight is about 4 — 7 kilos. Sand bags are placed on the lateral aspect of the affected limb so as to keep the leg in the slight intorsion position or neutral position. As a rule, after 5 — 6 weeks of fixation, the patient can start exercises while still in bed. Eight weeks later, he can get up and move about on crutches.

3. Herbal therapy

Chinese medicines can be prescribed for internal use in each of the three stages on the basis of overall analysis and differentiation of symptoms and signs. At the initial stage, bone-knitting plaster may also be applied to the large tuberosity externally. This plaster should be changed every 3 — 4 days. Complications, if any, should be dealt with on the basis of overall analysis and differentiation of symptoms, signs, causes, nature, etc.

4. Dirigation

During fixation, proper exercises of the healthy limb and extension-contraction exercises of the phalangeal joints and quadriceps of the thigh should be taken. The patient must avoid lying on his

151

sides and crossing his legs. After the removal of fixation, articular flexion-extension exercises of the affected limb should be practiced before getting up. The patient cannot take weight-carrying walk until the union of fracture.

● **Prognosis**

Because there is a rich blood supply at the tuberosity of the femur, so the union of the fracture occurs quickly. It is rare to find non-union cases. Coxa vara or shortening of the affected limb may appear in cases with displacement or improper fixation, which usually will not affect the functions much though the patient may limp to some extent.

Section Ⅲ Fracture of the Femoral Shaft

The femoral shaft is a long tube-like bone with smooth surface. Its substance of bone is thick and solid. There is a good blood supply for the femoral shaft.

● **Causes and Pathogenesis**

Fracture of the femoral shaft is mostly seen in young and robust adults or in children, and men are more vulnerable to it than women. It is mainly produced by a strong direct force or an indirect force. A direct force may result in comminuted or transverse fracture while an indirect force may lead to oblique or spiral fracture, all belonging to unstable type. As the fracture is often accompanied by severe injuries of soft tissues, severe internal hemorrhage often ensues, which sometimes results in shock. In children the fracture may also be seen as greenstick or incomplete.

The relatively typical displacement of the broken ends often occurs due to the muscular traction and action of the gravity. In the cases of fracture in the upper third of the femoral shaft, the proximal end of the fracture presents abducent, extorsive and flexing displacement as a result of the traction by the middle gluteal muscle, least gluteal muscle, iliopsoas muscle and extortor muscle. The distal end presents a medial and upward displacement due to the action of adductor. In the cases of fracture in the middle third

152

of the femoral shaft, the injured ends usually form angulation in the anterolateral aspect or form other displacement. If the fracture is in the lower third of the femoral shaft, the distal end usually displaces backward because of the traction by gastrocnemius muscle and articular capsule. Sometimes lesion of the sciatic nerve and vessels in the popliteal fossa may arise (Fig. 4—6)

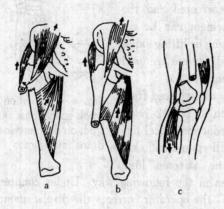

Fig. 4—6 Relationship between displacement of fracture at different sites of the femoral shaft and muscular traction

● **Clinical Manifestations and Diagnosis**

After injury there is severe pain, swelling, tenderness and dysfunction of the affected limb often associated with shortening, angular or rotatory deformity, bony crepitus and abnormal movement. In the cases of fracture in the lower third of the femoral shaft, injuries to the popliteal veins, arteries and nerves may be incurred. Shock may occur in patients suffering from severe pain and hemorrhage. X-ray films can reveal the fracture displacement.

● **Treatment**

1. Manual reduction and fixation

(1) Stable fractures without displacement need no reduction but only local fixation with small splints plus a long splinting board outside or small splints plus skin traction.

(2) For displaced fractures in children under five, manual re-

153

duction, skin traction by suspending the lower limbs, and fixation with small splints are necessary. After $1-2$ days of suspension traction, the overlapping or angulation deformity can generally be corrected and the lateral displacement can be reduced by pressing or lifting skill. Then four small splints are used for fixation (Fig. 4-7).

(3) In cases of displaced fracture in children of $6-12$ years old, manual reduction, local fixation with small splints and skin traction of the affected limb

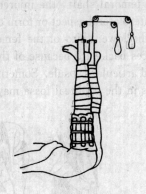

Fig. 4—7 Fixation with small splints plus skin traction and suspension of the lower limbs

should be given in the following way: Under countertraction by two assistants, the operator corrects the displacement by lifting-pressing manipulation with two hands. Then the fracture is fixed with four small splints and skin traction should be performed.

(4) In cases of displaced fractures in adults, manual reduction, fixation with small splints and skeletal traction may be used. For fractures in the upper or middle third of the femur, skeletal traction through supracondyle of the femur should be done. For fractures in the lower third of the femur, skeletal traction through tibial tubercle or through supracondyle of the femur may be selected according to the actual condition (Fig. 4-8). After the pin for skeletal traction penetrates through the bone, manual reduction is done under proper anesthesia. During the reduction of fractures in the upper third of the femur, an assistant keeps the pelvis in place and another assistant carries the leg of the affected side from the posterior aspect of the upper segment of the shank with a forearm, holds the ankle with the hand of the other side to perform upward traction by pulling and lifting the thigh with the patient's knee and coxa in flexion and the thigh in a little extorsion and abduction. In

154

cases of fractures in the lower third, only the patient's knee and coxa are flexed during traction. For fracture in the middle third, the traction may be performed with the leg stretching straight. Then with regards to different locations and displacement directions of fractures, the operator may apply such manipulations as pulling, lifting, pushing, pressing or rotating, etc. to correct different kinds of displacement of the fracture (Fig. 4—9).

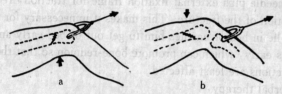

Fig. 4—8 Skin traction of fracture at different sites of the lower segment of the femur
a. through the supracondyle for flexion type
b. through tibial tubercle for extension type

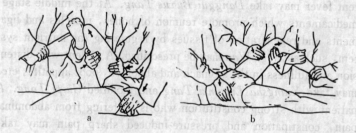

Fig. 4—9 Reduction of fracture of the femoral shaft
a. the upper 3rd b. the lower 3rd

After reduction, necessary small compresses should be placed at proper sites, the fracture is fixed with six small splints and bandages and then skeletal traction is performed with a weight varying from 7 to 10 kilos. During traction, x-ray examination should be made in proper time to check the fracture reposition so as to regulate the tightness of the splinting and traction weight from time to time, ensure the effect of fixation and prevent overtraction.

In cases with extraordinarily rich muscles, severe overlapping displacement or fracture too difficult to correct with manual reduction, skeletal traction for 3—5 days may precede manual reduction and fixation with small splints. The traction usually lasts 6—8 weeks. If closed reduction fails, open reduction and internal fixation may be applied. In recent years, many experts have adopted the technique of closed internal penetration of fractured bone with a steel needle plus external fixation frame for traction, reduction and fixation of the fracture. This makes it unnecessary for the patient to lie in bed or enables him to get out of bed early and start exercises early, which can promote bone-reunion so that the articular functions are least affected.

2. Herbal therapy

Shock resulting from massive bleeding is the manifestation of insufficiency of blood and exhaustion of *qi*. Besides blood transfusion and fluid infusion, the patient may take *Shengmai San*, *Dushen Tang* or *Shenfu Tang*. Patients with massive bleeding and persistent fever may take *Danggui Buxue Tang*. At the middle stage, medicaments which promote reunion of bones, muscles and ligaments and regeneration of tissues by regulating the nutrient system, such as *Jiegu Wan* may be prescribed. A patient with distension and fullness in the stomach and abdomen, poor appetite, etc. may take *Xiangsha Liujunzi Tang* and modified *Guipi Tang*. A patient with strong constitution who is suffering from abdominal pain, constipation and pressure-induced sharp pain may take *Dachengqi Tang*. At the late stage, it is sensible to give the patient *Zhenggu Wan*, *Bazhen Tang*, *Liuwei Dihuang Wan*, etc. to invigorate *qi*, enrich blood, nourish both the liver and the kidney and strengthen bones, tendons and muscles. After the removal of fixation, *Erhao Xiyao* may be used for external local bath to relax muscles and tendons and activate the flow of *qi* and blood in channels and collaterals to speed up the restoration of functions.

3. Dirigation

After reduction and fixation, articular flexion and extension of the ankle and relaxation-contraction of quadriceps muscle of the

156

thigh may be performed. After 3 or 4 weeks when the fracture becomes stable, arm-bracing and hip-raising exercises under the traction may be done to make flexion-extension of the hip and knee joints. The patient bends his knee of the healthy leg, pulls the cross bar over the traction table with both hands and erects the upper part of his body half way but the affected limb is not to exert itself or do levelraising. After the removal of traction, splintage should be maintained and exercises of the hip and knee and other joints may be practiced in bed. After reunion of the fracture, the patient may get out of bed and progressively practice weight-carrying walk on crutches to strive for an early restoration of the functions of the affected limb.

● **Prognosis**

As a rule, fracture of the femoral shaft will be knitted with a good prognosis. It usually takes babies 3—4 weeks to reach clinical healing, children, 4—5 weeks, and adults, 7—8 weeks. After the fracture of the femoral shaft, children's molding ability is very strong, and so, except rotatory deformity, forward angulation within 10° or overriding within 2.5cm may all be corrected automatically. In adults the molding ability is rather poor. After long time of fixation and possibly delayed functional exercise, rigidity and function limitation of the joints of knee and ankle may develop. In case of malunion which affects functions severely, open reduction and internal fixation should be performed.

Section Ⅳ Fracture of the Femoral Condyle

● **Causes and Pathogenesis**

The fracture may be caused by either an indirect force or a direct force. For example, when one falls from a high place on the feet, supracondylar fracture of the femur may occur. If the violent force goes on, the proximal end of the fracture will impact between the two condyles of the femur to split them apart leading to T-shaped or Y-shaped fracture, accompanied in most cases with severe displacement. Sometimes a force may act directly on the condyles of the femur resulting in fracture of a single condyle, mostly found in the external one (Fig. 4—10).

● **Clinical Manifestations and Diagnosis**

After injury, swelling, pain, and functional disturbance at the upper part of the knee appear. Because of the possible intraarticular hematocele, the knee joints may swell remarkably. If the severe local hematoma com-presses or injures the popliteal

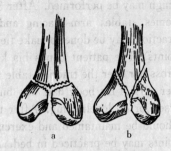

Fig. 4—10 T-shape and Y-shape fractures at the femoral condyles

artery, weakening or disappearance of pulsation of the dorsal artery of the foot or the posterior tibial artery may arise. X-ray films in anteroposterior and lateral views should be taken to find out the type and displacement of fracture.

● **Treatment**

1. Reduction and fixation

Undisplaced fracture needs no reduction. Under aseptic manipu-lation, the operator draws up the intraarticular hematocele up, then applies supra-articular splinting. The lower end of the anteri-or splint reaches to the superior border of the knee-cap and the lower end of the posterior splint extends to the middle part of the popliteal fossa. Movable and with axles, the two lateral splints should go beyond the knee joints. The fixation for the leg is also done in the same way. Four cloth laces may be used to bind up the splints above the knee and three or four cloth laces bind up below the knee. Skeletal traction through tibial tubercle may be per-formed with the leg on the traction stand and the knee flexed by 50 degrees.

Displaced fracture requires reduction. In cases of fracture with separation of the internal and external condyles, intraarticular hematocele is first extracted before the traction of the condyle of the femur with ice tongs. Under the traction, the operator squeezes both condyles with his palms from opposite sides to reposit the fragments, which is followed by fixation with supraarticular splints. The position of the subsequent traction is the same as above.

The fracture of a single condyle may be reposited by manual reduction. Take the fracture of external condyle as an example. After anesthesia, the patient takes dorsal position, an assistant fixes the pelvis and another assistant holds the ankle of the affected side. The operator, with a hand on the displaced fragment in the lateral aspect of the upper part of the affected knee, presses from the laterosuperior part to the inferomedial part to make it return to the original place. Then supraarticular splints will be applied to fix the knee joints in a flexion and mild inversion position.

For a fracture of the condyle of the femur which is difficult to reposit by manual reduction, needle-poking reduction and closed internal fixation with crossing steel needles under aseptic manipulation may be adopted. Since the fracture is of intraarticular type, it requires anatomical reduction. When closed reduction is unsatisfactory, open reduction and internal fixation should be considered.

2. Herbal therapy

At the initial stage of the fracture, as there is much internal bleeding and severe swelling, Chinese medicines for promoting blood circulation to remove blood stasis, e. g. *Fuyuan Huoxue Tang*, should be prescribed in large dosages. Patients with blood stasis, fever and thirst may take Chinese medicines for clearing away heat and toxic materials and removing heat from blood. If there is severe intraarticular hematocele, the hematocele should be extracted in time under aseptic manipulation. At the middle and late stages, the patient may take *Jiegu Pian*, *Jianbu Huqian Wan*, etc. After the removal of fixation, *Erhao Xiyao* should be used for local fumigation and bathing.

3. Dirigation

At the early and middle stages, relaxation-contraction exercises of the quadriceps muscle of the thigh may be practiced. Proper functional exercises of the knee joints may also be done on condition that redisplacement of the fracture will not be induced so as to benefit the molding of articular surface and prevent joint rigidity. Generally, traction will be removed in six weeks but splint fixation should remain. After clinical healing, the patient can get up and move about on crutches with the injured limb bearing no weight. It is only after bone union that the patient can practice weight-bearing walk and functional exercises.

● **Prognosis**

There is a good blood supply at the condyle of the femur so clinical healing may take place in 5—6 weeks. Since the fracture is of the intra-articular type, a poor reduction may leave over inversion or eversion of the knee joints which will impede the articular balancing, or rough articular surface. In either case traumatic arthritis may ensue. Therefore, in case of a fracture with poor reduction, open reduction and internal fixation should be taken into consideration. If the patient fails to take satisfactory functional exercises during splintage and after the removal of fixation, joint rigidity and restriction of movement of the knee joint may be left over.

Section V Fracture of the Patella

The patella is the largest sesamoid bone in the human body. It is a triangular flat bone with its basal side up and apex down. Behind the patella is the articular surface of cartilage and in front it is covered by the quadriceps muscle of the thigh. It is the supporting point for the quadriceps muscle of the thigh in its action of extending knee and thus becomes a part of the knee-extending apparatus.

● **Causes and Pathogenesis**

This injury can be produced by either an indirect force or a direct force but more commonly by the former. When one falls and the knee joint is in flexion position, in order to maintain articular position, the quadriceps muscle must contract strongly to cause collision and crush of the patella with trochlear surface of the femur, as a result, transverse fracture happens. Fracture of the patella may occur as a result of a fall from heights or jumping or slipping. Generally, the upper fragment of the fracture is larger and the lower, smaller. After the fracture faciae of the quadriceps muscle of the femur on both sides of the patella, the synovium and articular capsule are also lacerated. If severe laceration appears, there will be serious displacement of fragments. When the patella is injured by such direct forces as a blow or impact, the fracture is mostly comminuted or longitudinal, usually with only slight displacement of fragments.

● **Clinical Manifestations and Diagnosis**

After the injury, there are pain, swelling and subdermal ecchymosis. The patient is unable to stand and extend his knee actively. If there is separation of bone fragments, groove-like pitting can be touched before the patella. Bony crepitus and abnormal movements may appear. X-ray films of lateral and axial views may help ascertain the type and displacement of the fracture.

● **Treatment**

Before the reduction of fracture of the patella is done, intraarticular hematocele in the knee joints must be drawn up so as to facilitate reposition and fixation. It is required that after reduction the articular surface be intact and smooth so as to restore its functions as the knee-extending apparatus and prevent traumatic arthritis.

1. Manual reduction

On reducing a displaced fracture, the proximal end should be brought to meet the distal end, because the quadriceps muscle of the femur on the superior border of the proximal end has a greater elasticity while the tellar ligament of the inferior border of the distal end has very small malleability. After local anesthesia, the patient lies on his back with the knee in a slight flexion position. The operator holds the proximal fractured end with the thumb and the forefinger and middle finger of one hand, pushes it downwards and holds the distal end between the thumb and the index and middle fingers of the other hand to push it upward to bring the two ends close together. Then, he purposely makes the two ends move in the medial and lateral directions to release the fascia impacted between the fractured ends. When this movement is followed by perceivable crepitus, it is indicated that the two ends have come together. A temporary fixation may be applied. If the anterior aspect is not smooth to the touch, the operator may fix the depressed end with the thumb and forefinger of one hand and press the anteriorly protruding end with the thumb and forefinger of the other hand to make it level and try to keep them as close together as possible.

In cases of severe separation displacement which is difficult to restore by manual reduction, close pin reduction along with pressure fixation or open reduction and internal fixation may be carried out (Fig. 4—11).

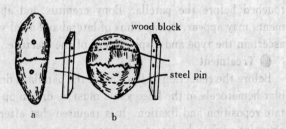

Fig. 4—11　Close pin reduction with pressure
fixation of fracture of patella
a. sites of pins on lateral view　b. two steel
pins plus pressure fixation with wood blocks

2. Fixation

For undisplaced fracture and fracture with separation displacement within 0.5cm, the reposition is easy and knee hoop fixation may be used. The knee hoop is made up of soft rattans or iron wires which are wound with layers of bandages. Four pieces of cloth strips or bandages 50cm in length are tied to the knee hoop in equal distances. Before fixation a thin cotton pad is placed on top of the anterior aspect of the patella followed by a thin cardboard disc, then the knee hoop is crowned to the patella. A long wooden board is laid at the posterior side of the limb extending from the

162

thigh to the ankle. The knee hoop is fastened to the board with four cloth strips or bandages tied to the hoop. Finally the leg is secured straight to the board with bandages (Fig. 4—12).

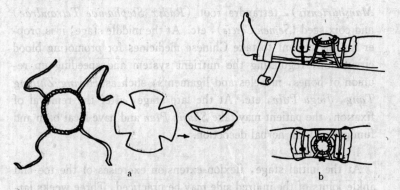

Fig. 4—12   Fixation of fracture of the patella
a. Knee hoop with 4 cloth straps and a cardboard disk
b. Anteroposterior and lateral views of fixation

In case of fracture with wide displacement of the fractured ends, manual reduction should be tried. If it is successful, elastic knee cap or knee cap with multiple elastic cloth straps may be used for fixation. Patella fixer, etc. may also be used for external fixation (Fig. 4—13).

3. Herbal therapy

The fracture is often accompanied with intraarticular hematocele, therefore, besides a thorough extraction of the hematocele, at the initial

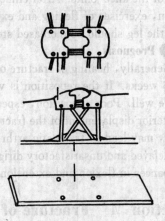

Fig. 4—13   Fixation with elastic knee cap

163

stage, the patient should take large dosage of Chinese medicines for promoting blood circulation to remove blood stasis and subduing swelling such as *Huoxue Quyu Tang* plus plantain seed (*Semen Plantaginis*), manshurian aristolochia stem (*Caulis Aristolochiae Manshuriensis*), tetrandra root (*Radix Stephaniae Tetrandrae*) and coix seed (*Semen Coicis*), etc. At the middle stage, it is proper for the patient to take Chinese medicines for promoting blood circulation, regulating the nutrient system and speeding up reunion of bones, muscles and ligaments, such as *Heying Zhitong Tang*, *Jiegu Pain*, etc. At the late stage, after the removal of fixation, the patient may take *Shujin Pian* and have local bath and fumigation with herbal decoction.

4. Dirigation

At the initial stage, flexion-extension exercises of the toe and ankle joints of the injured side may be practiced. Three weeks later when swelling diminishes gradually, the patient may walk on crutches with the injured limb bearing no weight. After 4 or 5 weeks, the patient may walk on one crutch but should avoid flexion of the knee joints. After clinical healing and the removal of fixation, exercises of flexing and extending the knee joints and raising the leg should be increased step by step.

● **Prognosis**

Generally, healing of fracture of the patella can be achieved in 4 to 6 weeks. If the reposition is well done, the functions will restore well. Poor apposition, especially when there is anterior and posterior displacement of the fracture ends and rough articular surface, may lead to traumatic arthritis. Prolonged external fixation or delayed and unsatisfactory dirigation may render functional disturbances in flexion and extension of the knee joints.

Section VI Fracture of the Shaft of Tibia and Fibula

The tibia and fibula are long tube-like bones of the shank. Of the two tibia is the main bone supporting the body weight. It is characterized by a thick superior part and a thin inferior part. Because the distal 3rd is very delicate with poor blood supply, it is most vulnerable to fracture, and moreover, fractures at this part tend to heal very slow. There is a strong interosseous membrane between the tibia and fibula.

Fracture of the tibia and fibula is common clinically, often seen in children, and fracture of the shaft of the tibia is more common.

● **Causes and Pathogenesis**

These injuries may be produced by direct forces such as crush, impact, etc. Transverse, oblique or comminuted types of fracture are common. The fracture lines of the two bones are usually at the same level. The injury can also be caused by indirect forces such as a fall from heights on a foot first or injury due to torsion of the shank. The fracture lines of this type are mostly oblique or spiral and the fracture line of the tibia is lower than that of the fibula. In a fracture of the upper-middle 3rd, the proximal fractured end of the tibia will be displaced toward the medioanterior direction because of the traction by the medial hamstring muscle and quadriceps muscle of the thigh. As a rule, in a fracture caused by a direct force, the soft tissues in the vicinity are more severely injured than in a fracture produced by an indirect force (Fig. 4—14).

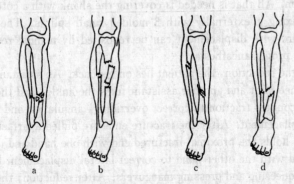

Fig. 4—14　Types of fracture in the shafts of tibia and fibula
a. comminuted　b. multiple　c. spiral　d. oblique

The external violent forces mentioned above may cause fracture in the shaft of only the tibia or fibula. Clinically, simple fracture of the tibia is more common than that of the fibula. The displacement in either of these fractures is not great.

● **Clinical Manifestations and Diagnosis**

After injury, local pain, tenderness, swelling, and ecchymosis are present. The affected limb is unable to bear any weight and has abnormal movement and bony crepitus. Angulation, shortening or rotatory deformity may occur in the cases with apparent displacement. When x-ray films are to be ordered, the total length of the tibia and fibula should be included so that nothing will be missed in making the diagnosis.

Attention should be paid to the pulsation condition of the dorsal artery of the foot and the posterior tibial artery of the affected limb so that judgment can be made about whether there are injuries of blood vessels. Symptoms of injury of the common peroneal nerve such as foot drop, etc. should also be noted. For open injury, pay more attention to the condition of the wound and preventing infection.

● **Treatment**

1. Manual reduction

The undisplaced fracture in children or adults doesn't need reduction. All that is needed is covering the shank with a cotton pad and fixing it externally with 5 molded small splints. The closed fracture with displacement can be reposited by manual reduction under proper anesthesia.

In the reduction, the patient lies on his back. An assistant holds the knee joint and another assistant fixes the ankle, and they perform counter traction to correct overriding, angulation and rotatory displacement. After the fracture ends are pulled apart, the operator holds the proximal fractured end with one hand and the distal end with the other hand to correct lateral displacement by lifting, squeezing and pressing maneuvers. After reduction, the operator should check the condition of reduction by moving the fingers along the crest and the medial aspect of the tibia and make the bro-

166

ken ends in close contact with each other by tapping longitudinally (Fig. 4—15).

In cases of unstable type of fractures, transcalcaneal traction may be done before manual reduction and splint fixation. The reduction for simple fractures of the tibia and fibula is similar to the reduction mentioned above.

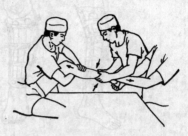

During the reduction not only good reposition of the tibia is necessary, but a good reposition of the fibula

Fig. 4—15 Reduction of fracture in the shafts of tibia and fibula

is also important, which will strengthen supplementary supporting force and stability of the leg and can stimulate the union.

2. Fixation

After successful reduction, according to the displaced condition, a proper compress covered with a cotton pad is applied properly to the fracture site and fixed with five molded splints or bamboo slips which are fastened with four laces. The anteromedial and antero-lateral splints should be narrow and placed at either side of the anterior crest of the tibia to help maintaining flux line of the tibia. The other three splints are placed respectively at the medial, lateral and posterior side of the shank. Generally the superior ends of the splints should not go beyond the knee joint and the inferior ends should not exceed the ankle. The lateral splint should not compress the head of the fibula. For fractures of upper-middle 3rd or lower-middle 3rd, however, the small splints should exceed the knee or ankle joints. For unstable type of fracture, a wooden board about 10cm wide is added to the lateral side of the shank and beyond the knee or ankle and wound up with bandages (Fig. 4—16).

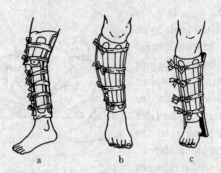

Fig. 4—16 Splinting of fracture in the shafts of tibia and fibula
a. fracture at the upper 3rd   b. fracture at the middle 3rd
c. fracture at the lower 3rd

In recent years, various external fixers developed in China have been used in the treatment of fracture of the tibia and fibula and good results have been obtained. Their advantages are:

(1) Closed nailing of the fracture plus fixing with fixation stand is simple and convenient.

(2) The reduction by traction serves at the same time the purpose of fixation.

(3) Early dirigation is made possible, which is beneficial to the union of fracture and maintenance of functions.

3. Herbal therapy

In most cases, medicaments are prescribed in the light of the principles of herbal therapy described in Section V, Chapter 2. For a fracture in the distal 3rd of the tibia, at the initial stage the patient should take Chinese medicines for promoting blood circulation to remove blood stasis in large dosages. At the late stage, the patient should take more Chinese medicines for nourishing the liver and the kidney, strengthening muscles and bones, such as *Zhuangjin Xugu Dan*, etc. For delayed union of fracture, *Guzhi Zengsheng Wan*, *Zuogui Wan*, *Yougui Wan*, etc. may be added.

4. Dirigation

For patients with splint fixation and skeletal traction, at the initial stage, flexion-extension exercises of the toe and ankle joints may be practiced. When the fracture becomes stable, relaxation-contraction exercises of the quadriceps muscle of the thigh may be done. For the stable type of fracture, after 2—3 weeks, the patient may gradually do flexion-extension exercises of the knee joint and leg-raising exercise under the doctor's guidance and 3 — 4 weeks later, the patient with the splint fixation on may get out of bed and move about on crutches with the injured limb bearing no weight. Exercises of the knee and ankle joints should be taken up as early as possible on condition that the stability of the fracture is not handicapped so the functions of joints can quickly and completely recover after union of the fracture.

● **Prognosis**

Since the blood supply at the middle and lower segments of the tibia is poor, delayed union or non-union often occurs after a fracture there. In other cases, clinical healing may be achieved generally in 6—8 weeks. Sometimes mild lateral displacement or angulation may remain due to poor reduction but if there is no apparent shortening of the limb or rotatory deformity, the functions of the limb are not affected. In case of malunion, operation should be taken into consideration.

Section VII   Fracture of the Ankle

The ankle joints consist of the inferior extremities of the tibia and fibula and the ankle bone or talus. The inferior extremities of the tibia and fibula form the inferior tibiofibular articulation. Between them is the tibiofibular ligament which connects them. The anterior and posterior borders of the inferior extremity of the tibia protrude out like a lip. The posterior protrusion is apparent and is called hind ankle. The inferior extremity of the fibula which is relatively narrow and long and forms the lateral lies somewhat behind the medial malleolus. The articular surface of the inferior extremity of the tibia together with the medial malleolus, lateral malleolus and the hind ankle constitutes the ankle burrow, which forms a joint with the superior articular surface of the ankle bone. The body of talus is broad in the front and narrow at the back, so when the foot makes dorsal extension, the broad part of the talus enters the ankle burrow. At the time, the ankle burrow is broader than in plantar flexion, the inferior tibiofibular ligament becomes tense and the articular surfaces are in close contact with one another so that the ankle is relatively stable and ankle sprain seldom happens. However, if a foreign force is too strong, a fracture may still be produced. When the ankle joints are in plantar flexion, the ankle bone is rather free in the ankle burrow, and therefore, during descends from doorsteps, stairs or from a slope, the ankle joints are easily subjected to injuries. The medial triangular ligament of the ankle joint is stronger than the talofibular ligament and fibulocalcaneal ligament on the lateral side, therefore, the force that can prevent eversion of the ankle is larger than that which can prevent an inversion.

● **Causes and Pathogenesis**
Although the articular surface of the ankle joint is small, the weight the joint bears is great and it moves a great deal, so it is vulnerable to injury. Fracture of the ankle is relatively complicated. By direction and degree of the external violent force acting on the ankle, the mechanism of injury and displacement condition of the ankle, it can be divided into three types:
1. Inversion type
This type of fracture is produced when the foot is forced into inversion by a strong violent force, for example, when one falls from heights with his foot in inversion position and the lateral aspect of the foot against the ground first, or when the medial aspect of the foot treads on a raised object, resulting in sudden strong inversion of the foot. A fracture occurs because the medial malleolus is compressed and squeezed. The fracture line may go obliquely from lateroinferior part to the mediosuperior part and the torn fragment may displace inwardly. Meanwhile, the lateral malleolus is avulsed by the traction of the lateral ligament, the fragment is

170

small and displaces inwardly and the fracture line is transverse. Thus fractures of both the medial and lateral malleoli occur. Sometimes the collateral fibular ligament and inferior tibiofibular ligament are lacerated or even the ankle bone is dislocated toward the medioposterior side (Fig. 4—17).

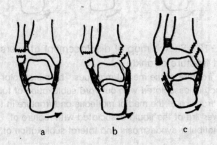

Fig. 4—17 Sketch map of inversion type of
fracture displacement of the ankle
    a. fracture of the medial malleous b. bimalleolar
fracture associated with inward subluxation of talus
c. fracture of the medial malleous accompanied by
rupture of lateral ligament and inward subluxation
of talus

2. Eversion type

This is produced by strong eversion of the foot caused by a great force. For instance, on a fall from heights, the patient's foot is in eversion position with the medial part of the foot against the ground first, a fracture arises from the compression of the lateral malleolus mostly with an oblique line. At the same time because the medial malleolus is tracted by great force, transverse avulsion fracture occurs, or the triangular ligament and inferior tibiofibular ligament are lacerated to result in displacement of the talus toward the lateral side (Fig. 4—18).

171

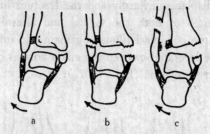

Fig. 4—18 Sketch map of displacement of eversion
type of fracture of ankle
  a. fracture of the medial malleous b. bimalleolar
  fracture associated with outward subluxation of talus
  c. fracture of the medial malleous and fracture in the
  lower 3rd of the fibula associated with rupture of
  tibiofibular syndesmosis and lateral subluxation of talus

3. Extorsion type

When the foot is in place but the shank is excessively intorted,
or when the shank keeps steady but a violent force makes the foot
overly extorted, the foot will be in extorsion and eversion resulting
in avulsion of the medial malleolus and drastic collision of the ankle bone against the lateral malleolus to produce a fracture with a
spiral or oblique fracture line. If the force is too great, a trimalleolar fracture may be produced with backward dislocation of the ankle bone (Fig. 4—19).

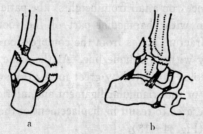

Fig. 4—19 Sketch map of displacement of extortion
type of fracture of the ankle
  a. bimalleolar fracture b. tri-malleolar fracture with
  posterior subluxation of the talus

172

Based on the above types of fracture and the severity of dislocation, the fracture can be divided into three degrees: The monomalleolar fracture is regarded as the first degree, the bimalleolar fracture with mild dislocation of the ankle bone, the second degree, and the trimalleolar fracture with dislocation of the ankle bone, the third degree.

● **Clinical Manifestations and Diagnosis**

After injury, there is blood stasis, swelling, pain and tenderness around the ankle, and functional disturbances and bony crepitus. Different forms of deformity may appear in different types of the fracture. Inversion deformity may occur at the foot and inward displacement of the medial malleolus may be touched in the inversion type; eversion deformity at the foot and slight pitting of the medial malleolus may occur in the eversion type; and when the extorsion fracture happens, foot extorsion and eversion may appear. In the fracture accompanied with dislocation of the ankle bone, there is more apparent deformity.

X-ray films of the ankle in anteroposterior and lateral views may show the fracture type and the degree of fracture dislocation.

● **Treatment**

1. Manual reduction

As ankle fracture is intraarticular nature, anatomic reduction is required. In manual reduction of the fracture, local anesthesia or peridural anesthesia should be given. Different types of fracture should be reposited with different methods, and in principle, manipulative correction should be taken contrary to the direction of the action of the external force.

(1) Inversion type

The patient lies on his side with the affected side on top. With an assistant holding the upper segment of the shank of the affected side, the operator holds the dorsum and pedis with one hand and the heel with the other, props both thumbs against the lateral malleolus, pulls the medial malleolus with forefingers and middle fingers and does countertraction with the assistant, and at the same time everts and extends dorsally the ankle joint to reposit the

173

fragments. Then the affected foot is kept in neutral position and is meanwhile made to do dorsiextension and plantar flexion several times to stabilize the fracture and restore the normal articular surface through the molding effect.

(2) Eversion type

The patient lies on the affected side. The assistant does the same upward traction but the operator props against the medial malleolus with both thumbs, pulls the lateral malleolus with the forefingers and middle fingers of both hands to make the foot invert on the basis of traction and reposit the fragments. Other maneuvers are the same as those for the inversion type.

(3) Extorsion type

The manual reduction is roughly the same as that for eversion fracture. But on the basis of traction and inversion, the foot should be intorted as well.

2. Fixation

After manual reduction, fixation with small splints or cardboard which should go beyond the ankle is conducted. The affected ankle should be fixed in the position opposite to the acting direction of the violent force. For instance, for the fracture of eversion and extorsion types, the ankle should be fixed in inversion and dorsiextension position while for the inversion type, the ankle should be fixed in eversion and dorsiextension position.

(1) Fixation with small splints

Five small splints similar to the splints for the shank are used. The medial, lateral and posterior splints should be so long that they can reach the proximal 3rd of the shank at the upper and level with the heel at the lower ends. The anteromedial and anterolateral splints should be narrower and they should start immediately from below the tubercle of the tibia and extend to the upper part of the ankle joint. The splints should be molded or used with the help of a compression pad so as to ensure that an inversion fracture is fixed at an inversion position while a fracture of eversion and extorsion type is fixed at an inversion position. Finally, the splints should be bound up with three laces. Sometimes an ambulatory

174

ankle joint splint may be added to fix the ankle joint at the neutral position or at slight dorsiextension position (Fig. 4—20).

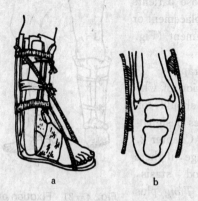

Fig. 4—20 Splinting of fracture in the ankle
a. lateral view b. anterior view; fixation at
eversion position for inversion type of injury

In case that the fracture fragments of the ankle show the tendency to displace, hollow or horse-shoe pads should be applied to the lower part of the medial or lateral malleolus to strengthen the fixation.

(2) Fixation with cardboard

The ankle should first be covered with cotton pads. Prepare two pieces of cardboard into trapezoid shape with a length extending from the proximal 3rd of the shank to the heel. The two pieces of cardboard are molded into arch shape and placed on the medial and lateral aspects respectively and overlapped in a cylinder shape. First, bind them up at the upper part with a lace, then apply a small cotton pad to the sole and cover it with a piece of cardboard slightly broader than the sole. Fasten the cardboard with a bandage whose two ends are pulled upwards tightly. Next, tie the cardboard with another lace above the ankle, to which the two ends of the bandage from the sole are attached. Finally, the two ends of the bandage should return to the sole to make a knot there

175

and be wrapped with a bandage. This method is applicable to those patients with a mild displacement or without displacement (Fig. 4—21).

3. Herbal therapy

The prescription of Chinese medicines should follow the principles designated in Section V, Chapter 2. At the initial stage, if there is severe blood stasis, *Fuyuan Huoxue Tang* plus burreed tuber (*Rhizoma Sparganii*), notoginseng

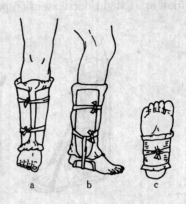

Fig. 4—21 Fixation of the ankle with arched cardboard

Radix Notoginseng) and chaenomeles fruit (*Fructus Chaenomelis*), or *Qili San* may be prescribed. At the middle stage, *Zhenggu Zijin Dan* may be taken. At the late stage, if local swelling is stubborn to subdue, Chinese medicines for promoting the flow of *qi* and blood circulation and invigorating spleen to remove dampness may be taken. *Shujin Tang* may also be used for local fumigation and bathing.

4. Dirigation

After reduction and fixation, active exercise of the toes can be practiced. Two weeks after the injury, flexion-extension exercises of ankle joints may be done gradually. In 4 weeks or so, removal of external fixation may be taken into consideration with regard to the actual condition. Flexion-extension and rotation exercises of the ankle should be strengthened. Early exercise of the ankle joints is of great significance in articular molding.

● **Prognosis**

The prognosis of fractures of the ankle has a close relationship with the degree and reduction of the injury. Quick union and satisfactory functions can be expected in patients with good reposition

176

and anatomic apposition. In cases of severe injury which are difficult to set, the prospects are not good, the swelling disappears very slow and the patient is vulnerable to traumatic arthritis. At the early and late stages, it is very important for patients to do exercise for functional disturbances of ankle joints of various degrees often remain in patients without enough or proper exercise.

Section Ⅷ   Fracture of the Talus

The talus which is divided into a head, a neck and a body lies at the top of the arch of the foot. The head and the neck are relatively narrow while the body lying at the back of the talus is broad in the front and narrow at the back. The talus has six articular surfaces: the tibia is above it, the calcaneus is below it, the medial and lateral malleoli are on its sides and the navicular bone is in front of it. Therefore, most of the surfaces of the talus are covered by articular cartilage. Its blood supply which comes from articular branch of the dorsal artery of the foot, articular ligament of the tibiotalar joint and interosseous ligament of talocalcaneus is rather poor, for which reason ischemic necrosis is likely to occur after a fracture there.

● **Causes and Pathogenesis**

Clinically, fracture of the talus is uncommon. It is mostly produced by a strong indirect force. For example, when a patient falls from heights on a foot first, the downward impact force of the tibia and the upward crush of the calcaneus work together on the talus to break it.

1. Fracture of the talar neck

When subjected to a violent force, the foot is in dorsiextension position and the anterior border of the inferior end of the tibia is embedded in the neck of the talus from above like a chisel, resulting in a fracture of the neck of the talus. If the external force is great and the foot is in excessive dorsiextension, the inferior extremity of the tibia together with the body of the talus may continue to displace backward, the posterior ligament of the subtalar joint will be broken and dislocation of the subtalar joint will happen at the same time. Sometimes because of the elasticity of Achilles tendon and the surrounding tendons, the huge force may make the foot contract backward but the sustentaculum of the talus often catches the medial tuber at the lower part of the talar body to render the entire fractured body of the talus to rotate outward with the fracture surface facing the laterosuperior side and the body of the talus out of the malleolar burrow, forming the fracture of the neck of the talus associated with posterior dislocation of the talar body.

2. Fracture of the posterior process of the talus

When the ankle joint is injured in an overly plantar flexion position, the protruding part of the posterior border of the body of the talus is impacted or pulled by the posterior talofibular ligament, this fracture will be produced (Fig. 4—22).

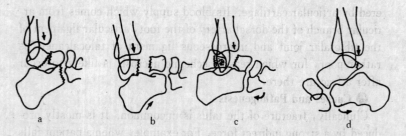

Fig. 4—22　Fracture and displacement of talus
a. fracture of the talar neck occurs when the foot is
in extreme dorsiextention　b. fracture of the talar neck
with anterior dislocation　c. fracture of the talar neck
with resupination of the talar body　d. fracture of the
posterior margin of talus

● **Clinical Manifestations and Diagnosis**

A definite history of trauma can be found. There is severe swelling, pain in the lower part of the ankle, blue ecchymosis and apparent bony crepitus. The patient is unable to stand and walk. Deformity will appear in a patient with apparent displacement and

178

fragments may be felt at the anterior and posterior areas of the ankle. When a fracture of the posterior process of the talus occurs, clinical manifestations are few. X-ray films of the ankle in anteroposterior and lateral views should be taken to help with the diagnosis.

● **Treatment**

1. Manual reduction

Undisplaced fracture does not need manual reduction Before the reduction of a simple fracture of the neck of the talus, lumbar anesthesia or local anesthesia is first given. The patient lies on his back and an assistant fixes the shank. The operator holds the front part of the foot to perform mild eversion, then pushes toward the posteroinferior part of the affected foot with one hand, holding the posterior part of the inferior extremity of the tibia with the other hand, he lifts and pushes it forward to make the fragment of the head and the body of the talus meet. For the fracture associated with subtalar articular dislocation, traction along the longitudinal axis of the shank should be carried out prior to the reduction mentioned above (Fig. 4—23).

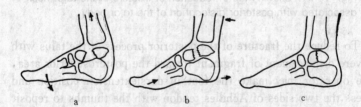

Fig. 4—23 Sketch map of reduction of fracture of the talar neck associated with dislocation of subtalar joints

In cases of fracture of the neck of the talus associated with posterior dislocation of the body of the talus, the patient takes the same position as mentioned above. Another assistant is needed to hold the front part of the foot and heel to perform countertraction with the other and in the course of traction, the ankle joint is made in extremely dorsiextension and slight eversion to remove the interlock of the talar body with sustentaculum of the talus. The operator presses the fragment in the superior part of the heel and pushes the body of talus toward the anterolateral part, at the same time the assistant holding the foot gently flexes, extends and shakes the ankle joint to help the talus enter the ankle burrow. Then while persisting in propping against the talar body with a thumb, the operator pushes the front part of the foot backward to render the foot in a slight plantar flexion position with the other hand so as to force the fragment to return to the normal place (Fig. 4—24).

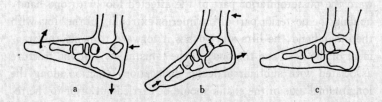

Fig. 4—24   Sketch map of reduction of fracture of the talar neck associated with posterior dislocation of the talar body

To reduce the fracture of the posterior process of the talus with severe displacement of fragment toward the posterosuperior area, the operator may make the foot in dorsiextension position and press the two sides of Achilles tendon with the thumbs to reposit it.

2. Fixation

Undisplaced fracture and fracture of the posterior process of the talus can be fixed with arch-shaped cardboard with the ankle joint at the neutral position for 5—6 weeks. Displaced fracture or fracture associated with dislocation should be fixed with five pieces of splints which go beyond the ankle plus an ambulatory splint of the ankle joint. The specifications of the splints and bandaging method are the same as those for fracture of the ankle. Fixation with tubular plaster is also applicable. Generally the ankle joint is fixed in a little eversion and plantar flexion position for 8 weeks.

After reduction and fixation, x-ray check should be ordered at times to prevent and rectify, if any, redisplacement of fracture. In case the fracture is too difficult to reposit and fix, open reduction and internal fixation should be practiced.

3. Herbal therapy

At the initial stage, for fracture of talus marked by severe swelling and ecchymosis, Chinese medicines for promoting blood circulation to remove blood stasis should be used adequately. As the fracture of the talus is vulnerable to ischemic necrosis, early at the middle stage, the patient should take Chinese medicines for tonifying the liver and the kidney, nourishing *qi* and blood, strengthening muscles and tendons to benefit union of the fracture.

4. Dirigation

After reduction and fixation, flexion-extension exercises of the knee joint and the toe may be practiced. Eight weeks later when the fixation is removed, decoction of herbal medicines should be used for local bath together with local massage. Flexion-extension exercises of the ankle and inversion-eversion exercise of the foot should be performed. The patient is encouraged to walk on crutches but the injured foot should not bear weight. Weight-bearing exercise must not be practiced until x-ray films confirm that the fractured ends have firmly knitted and no ischemic necrosis occurs.

● Prognosis

The prognosis of fracture of talus has a close relationship with the degree of injury and reduction. Fracture without displacement or with only mild displacement and with anatomic reduction can heal in time and have a good prognosis. The fracture with grave displacement, destruction of blood supply and poor reposition is easy to give rise to ischemic necrosis or traumatic arthritis, in which case surgery may be taken into consideration.

Section IX　Fracture of the Calcaneus

The calcaneus is the major load-bearing bone of the sole. It touches the ground during walking or standing. Its upper part articulates with the talus to form the calcaneotalar joint which enables the foot to make such movements as adduction, abduction, inversion and eversion. In the front it articulates with the cuboid bone to form the calcaneocuboid joint. At its medioanterior portion is the sustentaculum of talus which bears the neck of talus and at its posterior side is the tuberosity of calcaneus, to which the Achilles tendon is attached. The tie line of the upper margin of the tuberosity of calcaneus forms an included angle with the surface of calcaneotalar joint, known as tuber-joint angle, which is normally 30° — 45° and serves as a very important mark. If this angle narrows after injury, the function of the foot is usually hampered (Fig. 4 — 25).

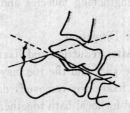

Fig. 4 — 25　The articular angle of tubercle formed by the articular surfaces of the calcaneus and talus

● **Causes and Pathogenesis**

Fracture of calcaneus is mostly caused by a violent transmitting force, e. g. when one falls from a high place vertically on the heel first, the downward force of the body gravity transmitting to the calcaneus via talus and the reacting force of the ground conveyed through the load-bearing point of the calcaneus compress the calcaneus hard and split it leading to longitudinal fracture of the tuberosity of calcaneus or sunken fracture of the calcaneus proper. If one falls from a high place on the heel which is in an inversion or eversion position, the downward force of the body gravity acting on the calcaneus via the medial or lateral side of the talus and the upward reacting force of the ground will jointly produce a shear force on the calcaneus resulting in different kinds of fracture

182

there, e. g. fracture of the sustentaculum of talus, longitudinal or transverse fracture of the tuberosity of calcaneus, comminuted and collapsed fracture of the articular surface, etc. (Fig. 4—26).

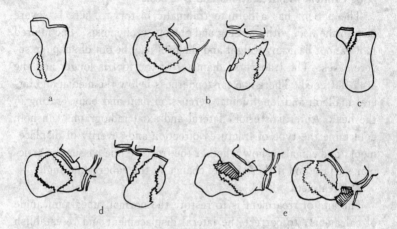

Fig. 4—26   Types of fracture of the calcaneus
a. longitudinal fracture of the tuberosity of calcaneus
b. transverse fracture of the tuberosity of calcaneus
c. fracture of the sustentaculum of talus   d. collapsed
fracture of the lateral of calcaneus   e. completely
collapsed fracture of calcaneus

In a few cases, fracture of calcaneus may be caused by an indirect violent force. For instance, when the gastrocnemius muscle makes violent contractions which will in turn tract the Achilles tendon, avulsion fracture of the tuberosity of calcaneus may result.

Fracture of the calcaneus can also be divided according to the site of fracture into two types: isolated fracture and fracture involving the surface of calcaneotalar joint. Comparatively, the former has a more favorable prognosis than the latter. After a fracture, the distal fragment is displaced upward by the combined action of the traction by the Achilles tendon and the foreign violent force, resulting in shallowness or even disappearance of the longitudinal arch of foot and narrowing of the tuber-joint angle, whereupon the strength of plantar flexion and the spring function of the longitudinal arch are decreased.

● Clinical Manifestations and Diagnosis

The patient has a definite traumatic history. There is severe pain in the heel with swelling and obvious ecchymosis. The injured foot cannot bear any weight and the heel may be out of shape in severe cases. The transverse diameter of the foot is longer and the arch flattened. There is clear tenderness below the medial and lateral malleoli and longitudinal percussion pain and bony grating in the heel. Anteroposterior, lateral and axial radiographs can help determine the type of fracture, direction and severity of displacement, and can also show whether the fracture line passes the articular surface and if there is any change in the tuber-joint angle.

● Treatment

The aim of treatment is to restore the normal tuber-joint angle of calcaneus, to correct the lateral displacement and re-establish the calcaneotalar articulation surface.

1. Manual reduction

Fracture of calcaneus with displacement should be reduced. The patient is given proper anesthesia and takes supine position. An assistant holds the patient's middle and upper parts of the shank and keeps the knee flexed to 90°. The operator cross-knits his fingers of the two hands and holds the injured heel from both sides in his palms and compresses in opposite directions. The lateral displacement and broadening of the calcaneus should be corrected first and the fragments of comminuted fracture can also be made compact together by the compression (Fig. 4—27). Then the operator holds the heel in one hand and the metatarsus in the other and performs countertraction with the assistant holding the leg to achieve utmost plantar flexion. In this way the fragment displaced upward can be corrected and the tuber-joint angle of the calcaneus be restored.

In case of unsuccessful manual reduction, reduction by traction of the calcaneus or reduction by prizing and poking with an osseous pin should be applied as follows: The patient lies on his stomach with the knee of the injured side flexed to 90°. One assistant holds tightly the middle and upper parts of the shank and another holds the metatarsus to keep the foot in a neutral or dorsiextension position. Under strict aseptic manipulation and fluorometry, the operator inserts an osseous pin from the posterior by lateral side of the heel in between the bone fragments of the tuberosity of calcaneus. Then the foot should be shifted into the plantar flexion position so as to relax the Achilles tendon. The operator holds the end of the pin to reposit the broken fragments and restore the tuber-joint angle. The pin can also be totally inserted in and left there, on the basis of the above manipulation, to fix the fragments internally (Fig. 4—28).

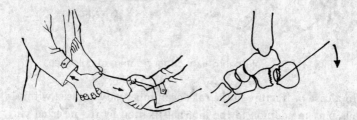

Fig. 4—27 Reduction of fracture of calcaneus

Fig. 4—28 Needle-poking reduction of fracture of calcaneus

In a case of comminuted fracture which is difficult to reduce and is accompanied by collapse or twisting of the surface of the calcaneotalar joint, surgical reduction is indicated, by which the collapsed bone fragments can be prized up or bone transplant can be performed to restore the level surface of the joint.

2. Fixation

For fracture without displacement and fracture that can be easily reposited with manual reduction, fixation with a piece of board under the sole is recommended. The board should be 1cm thick with a support for the plantar arch on one side in the middle part to keep the normal curve of the plantar arch. A cotton pad or a thin layer of cotton should be placed on the board. When the foot is in place, its dorsum should be first covered with a cotton pad and then with arched cardboard. The foot is first fastened to the board with straps and then fixed with bandage (Fig. 4-29). Alternatively, plaster support may be used to fix the foot in the functional position.

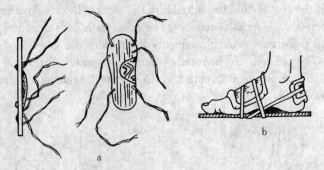

Fig. 4—29 Sole-board fixation for fracture of calcaneus

In a case of fracture in the calcanean tuberosity reduced with osseous pin, in addition to the internal fixation by the inserted pin, external fixation with plaster support can also be applied with the knee in semiflexion and the foot in plantar flexion.

3. Herbal therapy

At the early stage because of the local blood stasis with severe swelling and pain, *Fuyuan Huoxue Tang* should be prescribed along with achyranthes root (*Radix Achyranthis Bidentatae*), notoginseng (*Radix Notoginseng*) and bulgeweed (*Herba Lycopi*), or *Qili San* and *Huoxue Quyu Pian* should be given for oral administration. At the intermediate and late stages, *Jiegu Dan*, *Bali San* or *Zhuangyao Jianshen Wan* should be prescribed for internal use and *Jiegu Gao* for external application. Stiff joint, pain and discomfort may be present after removal of fixation so *Erhao Xiyao* or *Haitongpi Tang* should be prescribed for local fumigation and bathing.

4. Dirigation

When external fixation is applied, the injured leg should be properly raised. Gentle movement of the ankle and the toes is encouraged but vigorous plantar flexion and dorsiextension should be avoided. Some scholars uphold that functional therapy should be the principal treatment for fracture of calcaneus, i. e. for fracture with only slight displacement or with comminution, they think it unnecessary to perform reduction. Instead, the patient should do more functional exercises such as cycling activity, local rubbing, massage, etc. to achieve natural molding of the joint surface and prevent stiff joint. However, fracture with inversion deformity must be reduced manually and functional exercises cannot be done until the relief of pain. Six to seven weeks after reduction, the patient can get out of bed and take up walking exercise gradually in the specially prepared orthopedic shoe. Only in this way can good results be expected.

● **Prognosis**

Fracture of calcaneus can usually heal clinically in 6—8 weeks, but only after another 2—3 weeks can load-bearing movement begin. Malreduction or fracture involving the joint surface often leaves over flat foot, traumatic arthritis, eversion of the heel, deformity of broadened heel and pain in the heel during walking . If pain is rather serious and the dysfunction is obvious, surgical treatment should be considered.

Section X Fracture of Metatarsal Bones

Metatarsal bones are in fact a row of five short tube-like bones jointly constituting the transverse arch of a foot. The heads of the 1st and 5th metatarsal bones serve as the front load-bearing points of the longitudinal arch on the medial and lateral sides, and they together with the heel are the three load-bearing points of the whole foot. Fracture of metatarsal bones is most common among fractures in the foot.

● **Causes and Pathogenesis**

Fracture of metatarsal bones occurs as the result of either a direct or an indirect violent force.

1. Fracture caused by a direct force

When the front part of the foot is hit by a heavy object or crushed by a motor car, transverse, oblique or comminuted fracture may result. It may occur at the base, diaphysis or neck of a metatarsus, with that at the base being more common. The fracture may involve one or more metatarsal bones.

2. Fracture caused by an indirect force

Fracture caused by an indirect force is mainly due to the pulling by muscles, and often occurs at the base of the 5th metatarsus, e. g. when the foot is pulled by a powerful force into inversion position, avulsion fracture at the base of the 5th metatarsus will result from the violent contraction of the short peroneal muscle and the third peroneal muscle attached to the base of the metatarsus. The fractured fragment is usually not displaced much.

3. Fracture resulting from chronic strain

During a long military march, because of overfatigue of the muscles in the foot and the collapse of the arch of the foot, the metatarsal bones will bear more load than usual so that they are overstrained, gradually leading to fracture which is mostly found at the neck of the second metatarsal bone.

● **Clinical Manifestations and Diagnosis**

The fracture is characterized by local swelling, pain, tenderness, longitudinal impact pain and sometimes perceptible bony crepitus. Generally, there is no displacement for the metatarsal bones are arranged closely side by side. Fracture due to overfatigue of the metatarsal bones are manifested at the early stage as pain in the front part of the foot which is aggravated by walking and alleviated after rest. No obvious history of injury can be obtained. X-ray films of the foot in anteroposterior and lateral views are of value in making the diagnosis. The fracture at the base of the 5th metatarsal bone in children must be differentiated from the osteopiphyseal line and the sesamoid bone of the tendon of long peroneal muscle. The latter two on x-ray films are bilateral and the sesamoid bone is smooth and regular.

● **Treatment**

Fracture without displacement or fracture at the base of the fifth metatarsal bone is treated by applying medicinal plaster or paste externally and then fixed with arched cardboard or a plantar splinting board and bandage for 4—6 weeks.

1. Manual reduction and fixation

Fracture with displacement should be reduced under appropriate anesthesia. An assistant holds the lower leg firmly and the operator first tracts the toe corresponding to the fractured metatarsal bone to correct the angulation and overriding displacement. If up-down displacement is present, the operator should push with a thumb the fractured end from the sole to the dorsum. For lateral displacement, under traction of the corresponding toe with one hand, the operator can pinch the broken bone with thumb and index finger of the other hand from the dorsal side to force it back.

On the dorsal side, two bone-separating compresses are placed in the intermetatarsal spaces on both sides of the affected bone. On top of them cardboard should be placed. Then a plane compress is placed on the plantar aspect and topped by a sole board. In the end the foot is wrapped up with bandage in the same way as for fracture of the calcaneus.

2. Herbal therapy and dirigation

During fixation, exercises of the ankle and toes can be taken up. Although walking with the support of crutches is allowed at the early stage, the injured foot should not bear any weight. Drugs which can promote blood circulation and bone reunion, e. g. *Jiegu Dan*, may be prescribed for oral administration. Generally, fixation is removed in 4—6 weeks whereupon the decoction of *Shujin Tang* should be used to fumigate and bathe the injured foot so as to relieve the stiffness and pain in the joints.

● **Prognosis**

The prognosis of fracture of metatarsal bones is generally favorable without sequelae. However, bearing weight too early often results in slow healing, long-standing presence of the fracture line, pain on walking, etc., and it should, therefore, be avoided.

Section XI Phalangeal Fracture

● **Causes and Pathogenesis**
Phalangeal fracture is common, occurring mostly to the big toe. It is often produced by a direct violent force, such as crushing injury or kicking the toe against a hard object, and is divided into transverse, oblique and comminuted types. The fracture may occur at the head, shaft or base. Usually there is no displacement accompanying the fracture of a single phalanx while multiple fractures tend to be unstable. In fracture of a proximal phalanx due to the contraction of the interosseous muscle and the lumbrical muscle, the broken end often protrudes to the plantar aspect to form angular deformity which will give rise to permanent pain if not corrected.

● **Clinical Manifestations and Diagnosis**
There is a definite history of trauma and local swelling, pain, ecchymoses and hematoma beneath the nail. Load-bearing causes pain to the injured toe and bony crepitus can be felt. There can also be open injury and tearing-off of the nail. X-ray film can confirm the diagnosis.

● **Treatment**
For phalangeal fracture without displacement, it should be fixed with aluminum or bamboo splints, with adhesive tape or bandage around the injured toe, or with arched cardboard. In the case of fracture with displacement, manual reduction should be performed. Holding the proximal end between his thumb and index finger of one hand and the distal end between the thumb and index finger of the other, the operator first stretches the injured toe in opposite directions and then pushes the broken ends together to reduce the fracture. Fixation is the same as described in last section.

During fixation, drugs which can promote blood circulation and bone reunion should be prescribed for internal administration, e. g. *Qili San* or *Jiegu Dan*. After removal of the fixation, *Shujin*

190

Pian is recommended for internal use while *Erhao Xiyao* for external local bathing. In a case of fracture of the ungual phalanx, pain may sometimes last for a long time on account of injury to nerves, and fumigation and bathing with *Erhao Xiyao* is also applicable. In case of open injury, it should be well debrided and sutured and kept from infection.

● **Prognosis**

Phalangeal fracture usually recovers well. If the broken end of a fracture of the ungual phalanx protrudes towards the plantar aspect, pain will be felt during walking.

Chapter 5

Fractures in the Body Trunk

Section I Fracture of the Ribs

There are altogether 12 pairs of rib bones. They are symmetrically located on both sides of the chest and connected with the thoracic vertebrae and the sternum to form the thorax. At the back, all the 12 pairs of ribs are linked with the thoracic vertebrae but in the front only the first seven pairs are connected with the sternum by means of cartilage, and they are, therefore, called "true ribs". The 8th, 9th and 10th ribs are connected in the front by means of cartilage with the one above each of them, so they are known as "false ribs". The 11th and 12th ribs, the floating ribs, along with their cartilages are free and terminate amidst the muscles of the lateral abdominal wall.

Most rib fractures are found in the 4th to 7th ribs, for the first three ribs are rather short and are protected by the scapula and clavicle, and the 8h to the 12th ribs have good flexibility so fractures there are rather uncommon.

● **Causes and Pathogenesis**

A direct violent force, such as hitting by an automobile and blow by the fist or a stick, may cause fracture of the ribs involved. It is common to find that the broken ends displace inwardly or even pierce through the pleura. An indirect violent force such as that from a car accident, or collapse of earthwork or house, compresses the chest from both the ventral and dorsal sides may lead to fracture of ribs under the armpit with the severed ends protruding laterally. When elderly individuals with general debility and esteoporosis cough violently, they may occasionally sustain fracture of the ribs on account of the forceful contraction of the chest muscles.

Rib fracture may involve one or more ribs, or may be of double fractures. When double fractures take place simultaneously in several ribs, there will no longer be rigid support to the portion of the chest wall between the two fracture lines, and the chest wall there becomes flexible. When the victim attempts to inhale, the injured area of the chest wall sinks in due to the increased negative pressure in the thoracic cavity and when the victim tries to exhale, that part will bulge outward owing to the reduced negative pressure inside. Such abnormal movement of the chest wall is termed abnormal respiration, which affects the respiratory function gradually leading to oxygen deficit due to tachypnea and hypoventilation, or even disturbance of the respiratory and circulatory functions. If the fractures are complicated by opening wounds, pneumothorax, pneumohemothorax or tension pneumothorax may follow.

● Clinical Manifestations and Diagnosis

With a fractured rib, there will be pain and swelling at the site of injury. The pain is aggravated by deep breathing and coughing. On turning the upper body or coughing violently, the patient can hear bony grating. Tenderness or bony grating is present to the touch. The patient may feel severe pain at the site of fracture when the doctor compresses the chest vigorously with hands from the front and the back. This is said to be positive sign of thorax compression (Fig. 5−1). In a case of multiple fractures of ribs, the chest may cave in or become flattened. When the pleura and a lung are stabbed through, the injured part of the chest may sink in during inspiration and bulge out during expiration owing to the loss of rigid support to that part. This ab-

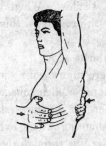

Fig. 5−1　Thorax compression test

193

ration may result in severe symptoms such as dyspnea, cyanosis and lung collapse.

If rib fractures are followed by closed pneumothorax, symptoms like chest distress, tachypnea, etc. may appear, respiratory movement in the injured side of the chest decreases and tympany is heard on percussion. In the case of fracture with open pneumothorox, dyspnea, cyanosis and lowering of blood pressure can be found, respiratory sound in the injured side of chest becomes weak and the sound of air entering and leaving the chest through the wound can be heard. When the fracture is complicated by tension pneumothorax, serious dyspnea, cyanosis and shock may develop and respiratory sound in the injured side of the chest becomes extremely weak or even disappears.

If the fractures are complicated by pneumohemothorax, there may be hematocele in the thoracic cavity, large amount of which can cause dyspnea, cyanosis and dullness on percussion. The blood of hematocele can be extracted with thoracentesis.

X-ray films are of help in locating the fractures and determining the type, but fissure fractures are likely to be overlooked and especially the fracture at the junction of the rib and cartilage is difficult to be detected. X-ray films can also reveal the severity of pneumothorax. When there is small amount of hematocele in the thoracic cavity, the costophrenic angle will disappear on the film and if the hematocele is in large quantity, the lungs will be overcast by a shadow. When both pneumothorax and pneumohemothorax are present, a fluid level will be produced on the film (Fig. 5—2).

● **Treatment**

For severe injury with such emergent symptoms and signs as pneumo-thorax, pneumohemothorax, abnormal respiration and shock, emergent measures should be taken promptly. In case of closed pneumothorax, air exhaustion should be performed on the midclavicular line through the second intercostal space. For pneumohemothorax and tension pneumo-thorax, closed drainage should be conducted. If chest wall of the injured area is floating, tentative treatment with local pressure dressing should be provided first followed by continual traction of the ribs or surgical internal fixation. As for simple fracture, reduction and fixation should be carried out.

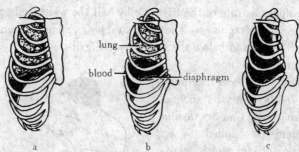

Fig. 5—2　Sketch map of pneumohemothorax
a. small quantity of blood　b. medium quantity
c. large quantity

1. Manual reduction

Non-displaced fractures of the ribs do not call for reduction whereas the displaced types should be reduced as properly as it could be. The patient takes the sitting or supine position. An assistant presses with his palms the patient's upper abdomen and tells the patient to breathe in as deeply as he can and cough with effort. While the patient coughs, the assistant presses the abdomen flat. In the meantime the operator pushes the protruding ends of the fractured ribs with both hands. If the fractures are of the collapsed type, the operator should place a hand on each side of the thorax level with the site of fractures to perform bilateral compression so as to force the sunken ribs to rise up.

2. Fixation

(1) Adhesive tape fixation

Several pieces of long adhesive tape strappings of 7—10cm in width should be prepared beforehand. The patient sits upright after reduction, exhales to minimize the circumference of the chest and then holds up his breath for fixation which should be per-

195

formed as follows: The first tape is stuck starting on the back from the median line of the scapula of the normal side, passing the fractures and ending on the median line of the clavicle of the unaffected side. The second tape is placed in the same way but overlapping the upper margin of the first one by half the width and so are the succeeding strappings. The tape strappings should reach the sites both above and below the injury by 1—2 ribs.

(2) Bandage fixation

In cases with local swelling, prior to fixation, plaster such as *Quyu Xiaozhong Gao* or *Shenjin Gao* should be applied. Then cover the plaster with cardboard, which is stuck to the chest with adhesive tape and wrapped up with bandages encircling the thorax for several thicknesses, or fastened with a many-tailed bandage. The plaster should be replaced every 4— 5 days (Fig. 5—3).

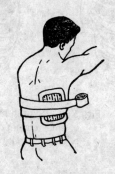

Fig. 5—3 Fixation of fracture of ribs with cardboard and bandage

3. Herbal therapy

At the initial stage, drugs for promoting blood circulation to remove blood stasis and invigorating the flow of *qi* to alleviate pain should be prescribed. If the fractures are accompanied by symptoms mainly due to impairment of *qi*, *Liqi Zhitong Tang* or *Chaihu Shugan San* can be selected for use, to which bitter apricot kernel (*Semen Armeniacae Amarum*), trichosanthes fruit (*Fructus Trichosanthis*), bitter orange (*Fructus Aurantii*), etc. may be added accordingly if cough and dyspnea are present. When the fractures are associated with symptoms chiefly due to blood disorder, it is proper to prescribe *Xuefu Zhuyu Tang* or *Heying Zhitong Tang*, to which Hairy vein agrimony (*Herba Agrimoniae*), hyacinth bletilla (*Rhizoma Bletillae*), node of lotus root (*Nodus Nelumbinis Rhizomatis*), etc. should be added accordingly if hemoptysis is present. At the intermediate stage, the principle of treatment is promoting reunion of bones and muscles and replenishing *qi* and blood. *Jiegu Dan* and *Jiegu Zhijin Dan* are of choice. At the late stage, if vague pain in the thoracic and costal regions exists, medicaments for promoting the flow of *qi* to ease pain and removing blood stasis to heal wounds should be given. *Sanleng Heshang Tang*, *Lidong Wan* are recommended. If the patient manifests symptoms due to deficiency of both *qi* and blood, *Shiquan Dabu Wan and Chaihu Shugan San* are advisable recipes.

Drugs for external use may also be given. *Shuangbai San*, *Xiaozhong San*, *Xiaozhong Zhitong Gao* or *Dingtong Gao* may be selected at the initial stage; for the intermediate stage, *Jiegu Gao* or *Jiegu Xujin Gao*, and for the late stage, *Wanying Gao*, *Zhenjiang Gao* or *Wanling Gao*.

4. Dirigation

Patients with simple fracture of the rib can walk shortly after reduction and immobilization. In severe cases, the patient should be confined to bed in the recumbent position and practice abdominal breathing. As soon as the symptoms are remitted, he can get out of bed and walk on foot.

● **Prognosis**

Generally, the fractured ribs can be knitted after fixation for 3 —4 weeks. Most of the early complications and the injuries to the lung and pleurae will recover after prompt and proper treatment, but any delay in treatment of the severe cases may endanger the patient's life.

Section Ⅱ　Fracture of the Cervical Spine

The cervical vertebrae, seven in all, comprises part of the spinal column, joining to the occipital bone at the upper and connecting with the thoracic vertebrae at the lower. The first two cervical vertebrae are of a different structure: The first one, looking like a ring, has no vertebral body and spinous process and is appropriately named the atlas. The second one is called the axis because it has a tooth-like upward process to form a pivot around which the atlas bearing the skull may rotate. The movement range of cervical vertebrae is fairly wide. The rotary movements take place chiefly between the atlas and the pivot. The third to the seventh vertebrae can make anteflexion, retroextension and lateral curvature movements. The foramina of the cervical vertebrae together with the foramina of the other types of vertebrae form the vertebral canal within which is the spinal cord. Eight pairs of cervical nerves arise from the spinal cord in the cervical part. The spinal cord has two enlargements, one of which is located between the 3rd and 7th cervical vertebrae known as cervical enlargement; the other is between the 10th thoracic vertebra and first lumber vertebra. Motor and sensory nerve centers of the limbs converge here and therefore, when vertebral fracture occurs in the parts where the enlargements are located, paraplegia may accompany.

● **Causes and Pathogenesis**

Both direct and indirect violent forces can bring about fracture of the cervical spine. For example, when the top of the head is hit by a violent force, the force may act on the atlas through the occiputal condyle, causing fracture of the atlas, single or multiple, usually occurring at the anterior or posterior arc of the atlas where the atlas is thin and insolid, especially at the posterior arc. When the neck is subjected to an injury in hyperflexion, fracture of the dentate process of the pivot may arise, more commonly found at the base of the process. If the fracture is associated with atlas dislocation, the medullary bulb may also be injured (Fig. 5—4).

When the head is subjected to violent force with the neck in flexion position, or when the neck suffers from a "whip-wielding" injury, flexion fracture or dislocation of the cervical vertebrae may be rendered. For instance, when one is bending at work and the head is struck by a heavy object, or when one is traveling in a very fast car which brakes abruptly and the head and neck are still moving forward in an extreme ante-flexion due to the inertia, compression fracture of the cervical spine or dislocation may occur between the 3rd and 7th cervical vertebrae, especially between the 5th and

198

7th vertebrae.

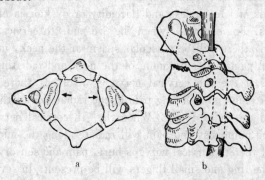

Fig. 5—4 Fracture of the cervical spine
a. fracture. of atlas   b. fracture of the pivot
associated with dislocation of atlas

When the neck is subjected to a violent force in the overextension position, e. g. when one falls down from a high place on the
upper part of the back with the face upward and the neck and head
suspending in midair, the cervical spine will incur an injury due to
the overextension of the neck and head. Elderly people and individuals with cervical spondylopathy in particular will incur cervical
injury when they fall down on the ground supinely owing to the
poor mobility and slow protective flexibility of the neck. As a result, fractures at the anteroinferior margin of the vertebrae, the
vertebral body, lamina or arc, or fractures of the articular process
associated with posterior dislocation of the vertebral body may ensue. Any type of fracture of the cervical spine complicated by severe dislocation can bring about injury to the spinal cord.

● **Clinical Manifestations and Diagnosis**

A definite injury history of the head and neck is available with
such symptoms as local pain, stiff neck and inability to turn
about. The patient often supports the chin with both hands so as
to fix the head and avoid any attempt to move it. There is obvious
tenderness and muscular spasm at the injured area.

When a fracture of the cervical spine is complicated by displace-

199

ment or dislocation, it may, in mild cases, cause numbness of the upper limbs and feebleness and flaccidity or dyskinesia of all the extremities. For example, when the 3rd and 4th cervical nerves are injured, there will be muscular spasm at the neck, unilateral or bilateral pain in the trigonum of the neck and radiating to the shoulders. If the 5th cervical nerve is involved, there will be numbness, pain and radiating pain in the radial side of the hand, thumb and the index finger. When the 7th cervical nerve is involved, the numbness and pain will radiate along the middle finger, and if the 8th cervical nerve is hurt, pain and sensory disturbance in the ring and small fingers will be present. In severe cases, paralysis or hypoesthenia of the limbs or pain in the innervation area of the greater occipital nerve may occur. In very severe cases, high paraplegia or even death may ensue.

The location, type and displacement of the fracture may be shown in x-ray films of anteroposterior and lateral views, or sometimes when necessary, in mouth-open anteroposterior view.

● **Treatment**

1. Reduction and fixation

Undisplaced stable fractures without evident symptoms of spinal injury can be treated with jaw-occiput strap traction for 1 — 2 weeks (Fig. 5 — 5), and then followed by immobilization with a hard frame collar for 4 — 6 weeks. When the fracture of cervical spine is complicated by obvious displacement, injury of the spinal cord, or fracture of the base of dentate process of the pivot or dislocation, skull traction or jaw-occiput strap traction should be applied for 2 — 6 weeks in line with the condition. After reduction or after the fracture becomes stable, plaster helmet or hard frame collar should be

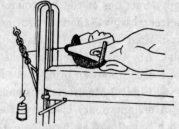

Fig. 5 — 5　Jaw-occiput strap traction for fracture of cervical spine

used instead for external fixation until the fracture heals.

2. Herbal therapy

At the early stage after reduction, *Huoxue Wan* or *Bujin Wan* are recommended for internal use. One to two weeks later, *Zhenggu Zhijin Dan* or *Jiegu Wan* may be prescribed for oral use. At the natural cure stage, *Qiangjin Wan*, etc. is suitable.

3. Dirigation

After the fixation is removed, gentle massage on the neck and proper functional exercise of the neck are advisable, and the range of movement should be enlarged progressively.

● **Prognosis**

Patients with fracture of cervical spine without displacement or dislocation will recover well, but it is common that slight discomfort in the neck may remain. The possible dysfunction and sensory disturbance of the upper limbs from the fracture of dentate process can usually recover naturally. The prospects of cases with high paraplegia are not optimistic. In some cases of fracture of dentate process associated with dislocation of atlas, the spinal cord may be constricted leading to hemiparalysis or paraplegia 2—3 months or even decades later. Usually, the constriction to the spinal cord develops gradually but it may also come on abruptly, frequently induced by mild injuries. At the early stage, it is often paroxymal but if not treated promptly, the constriction may become persistent.

Section Ⅲ Fracture of the Thoracolumbar Vertebrae

Because the first to the tenth thoracic vertebrae are connected with ribs on both sides and their range of movement is very small, their chances of injury are slight, whereas the vertebrae from the 12th thoracic vertebra down to the 5th lumbar vertebra have a large range of movement, so they are susceptible to injuries, especially the 12th thoracic vertebra and the first lumbar vertebra, which are the turning point between the thoracic curve and lumbar curve and are the border of the thoracic vertebrae that move very little and lumbar vertebrae which move a great deal, are the most common site of compressive fracture of thoracolumbar vertebrae.

● **Causes and Pathogenesis**

Fracture of the thoracolumbar vertebrae can be produced by a direct or an indirect violent force, e. g. when one falls down from heights on the feet or buttocks with the small of the back in a bending posture, forces from both the upper and lower vertebrae act mainly on the front part of the thoracolumbar vertebrae and compress the vertebrae into wedge shape, often resulting in fracture of the 11th and 12th thoracic vertebrae and the 1st and 2nd lumbar vertebrae, known as flexion fracture. If the vertebra bodies are compressed too much, fractures of the vertebra appendices such as articular process, transverse process and spinous process are also likely to be produced. The former is of a stable type and the latter unstable type. In severe cases, injury of the spinal cord of various degrees may also develop.

When one falls with the small of the back striking against a solid projecting object on the ground, the vertebral column is rendered in a sudden overextension, fracture or displacement of the thoracolumbar vertebrae will occur, known as extension fracture.

● **Clinical Manifestations and Diagnosis**

There is a definite history of trauma. Pain and swelling in the small of the back, muscular tone on both sides of the fractured site, inability to stand and dyskinesia are typical of the condition. In the case of flexion fracture, local protrusion to the back and evident tenderness in the fractured region can be found. Fracture of lumbar vertebrae may also produce such symptoms as distending pain in the abdomen, anorexia, constipation, etc. due to the stimulation to the sympathetic nerve by retroperitoneal hematoma. Severe fracture with injury to the spinal cord may give rise to paraplegia and changes below the injury level such as numbness of the limbs, anesthesia, dyskinesia, loss of control in defecation and urination, etc.

Study of the x-ray films in anteroposterior and lateral views may provide evidences as to whether there is fracture of the spinal column, the type of fracture and any displacement. Deformity, comminuted fracture or dislocation of vertebral body should be observed. Information about fractures of transverse process, spinous process and articular process or vertebral lamina can also be obtained by study of the x-ray films. When doubt exists as to whether the pedicle of vertebral arch has been fractured, oblique x-ray film should be ordered.

● **Treatment**

1. Reduction and fixation

(1) Stable type

Reduction is unnecessary for ordinary stable thoracolumbar fracture. However, in a case with compression of the vertebral body over 1/2 of its height, proper skills should be adopted to fulfill the reduction.

① Ankle-suspending traction: Prior to reduction local anaesthesia should be given. The patient takes the prone position on a bed with the ankles covered with cotton pads, securely tied with strong strings and then slowly pulled up so as to make the portion below the loin at an angle of 45° to the bed (Fig. 5—6). Then, the operator presses down with his palms the highly protruding deformity at the injured part. After reduction the patient should lie on his back on a rigid wooden bed. This method was described in

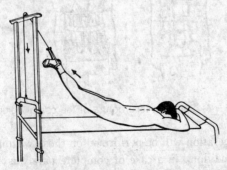

Fig. 5—6 Overextension traction by suspension of both ankles

Effective Formulas Handed Down for Generations by Wei Yilin of the Yuan Dynasty.

② Bolstering: In the case of compressive fracture, the patient should lie dorsally on a board bed with the fractured part supported by a soft bolster, which can be gradually heightened to produce hyperextension of the vertebral column so that the compressed vertebral body can recover gradually.

(2) Unstable type

Transportation of the patient and reduction must be performed with great care, otherwise complete or incomplete paralysis may result.

Reduction by traction: The patient lies in prone position. Persistent upward and downward traction with a specially made traction belt should be conducted and the appropriate tracting weight should be such as is just enough to tract the compressed vertebrae apart and restore the normal intervertebral spaces. In a case of incomplete paralysis, if there is improvement after traction for 2 weeks, the traction should last 5 — 6 weeks and there are good chances of recovery. After reduction, the spinal column should be fixed with splints or a metal supporting frame (Fig. 5—7). An

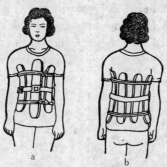

a   b

Fig. 5—7   Splinting for fracture of the spinal column

exploratory operation will be performed on those with increasingly aggravated condition. In a case of complete paralysis, if there is improvement after traction for 4 — 5 weeks, chances of recovery are very slight. In such cases, the traction should be discontinued and stress should be placed on a good nursing care or an explorative operation be performed.

2. Herbal therapy

At the initial stage, in view of the severe pain and swelling, the principle for treatment should be promoting circulation of *qi* and blood to relieve swelling and pain. Modified *Gexia Zhuyu Tang* and *Fuyuan Huoxue Tang* can be prescribed. If abdominal distension with distending pain and constipation is present, modified *Dacheng Tang* can be prescribed for it has a purgative action and can eliminate stagnancy. If the fracture is complicated by dysuria, recipes which can promote blood circulation to remove blood stasis and invigorate *qi* to induce diuresis should be prescribed. For instance, *Gexia Zhuyu Tang* together with *Wuling San* should be prescribed for internal use and *Xiaoyu Gao* for external application. At the intermediate stage, it is recommended to use medicaments which can promote circulation of blood, regulate the nutrient system, and promote reunion of bones and muscles. *Dieda Yangying Tang* is a proper internal medicine and *Jiegu Dan* is suitable for external application. At the late stage, on account of the aching, feebleness and flaccidity in the small of the back and the four extremities, tonifying recipes should be used to tonify and invigorate *qi*, blood, liver and kidney. *Bazhen Tang* and *Liuwei Dihuang Wan* are of choice for internal use and *Goupi Gao* for external application.

If a thoracolumbar fracture is accompanied by paraplegia, medical treat-ment at the early stage should concentrate on promoting circulation of blood, removing blood stasis and dredging the *Du* channel. *Huoxue Quyu Tang* reinforced with pangolin scale (*Aquama Manitis*), earthworm (*Lumbricus*), Red Sage root (*Radix Salviae Miltorrhizae*), vaccaria seed (*Semen vaccariae*), etc., or modified *Buyang Huanwu Tang* should be prescribed. After 2—3 months, medical treatment should lay stress on tonifying the kidney-*yang* and warming and clearing the channels and collaterals. The recipe *Bushen Zhuangyang Tang* supplemented with pangolin scale (*Aquama Manitis*) and psoralea fruit (*Fructus Psoraleae*) should be prescribed. At the late stage, nourishing the blood and liver, calming down the endopathic wind and relieving spasm are the principles of medication. The recipe *Siwu Tang* with supplement of uncaria stem with hooks (*Ramulus Uncariae cum Uncis*), ground beetle (*Eupolyphaga seu Steleophaga*), scorpion (*Scorpio*), centipede (*Scolopendra*), common clubmoss (*Herba Lycopodii*), etc. is usually prescribed for internal use. If deficiency of both *qi* and blood is manifested, *Bazhen Tang*, *Buzhong Yiqi Tang* or *Guipi Tang* should be prescribed to the patient. In case of complication of insufficiency of the liver and kidney, in addition to other recipes, *Bushen Huoxue Tang* should also be prescribed.

3. Dirigation

Exercise should be commenced on the third day after reduction of stable compressive fracture and after 4−5 weeks, the patient may get out of bed and move about with splint-fixation, but back bending movement is not allowed during exercise. In a case of an unstable fracture, exercise may start from the 4th week after injury and 8 weeks later the patient may get out of bed and move about with splint fixation. However, waist bending action should be avoided within 3−4 months. Proper exercise can help the injured part recover to keep the stability of the spinal column. Moreover, exercise beginning at the early stage can increase the myodynamia of the back, prevent muscular atrophy (myophagism) and osteoporosis and reduce or eliminate the possibility of consequential chronic lumbago. For example patients with compressive flexion fracture can do the following exercises:

(1) Five fulcra exercise

The patient lies supinely on a rigid board bed, supports the body with the head, elbows and heels and raises the lumbar region as high as possible to make hyperextension exercise (Fig. 5−8).

(2) Three fulcra exercise

This method is similar to the five fulcra exercise except that the elbows are no longer used as two fulcra. Instead, the arms should

206

be placed on the chest (Fig. 5—9).

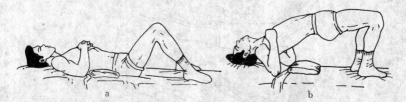

Fig. 5—8   Five-fulcra exercise

(3) Four-fulcra exercise

The patient also takes the supine position and then supports the body with the hands and feet, lifts the body trunk as high as he can to form a bridge-like arch (Fig. 5—10).

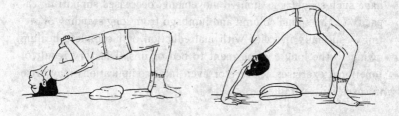

Fig. 5—9   Three-fulcra exercise   Fig. 5—10   Four-fulcra exercise

(4) Flying swallow exercise

The patient lies in prone position on a rigid board bed and with the abdomen as the fulcrum he stretches and lifts the four extremities up as high as possible (Fig. 5—11).

Patients are encouraged to do these exercises as early as possible and step by step. The times and intensity of exercises should be based on the patient's injury condition, constitute and psychological state.

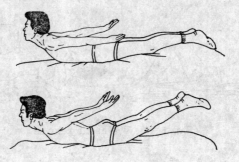

Fig. 5—11 Flying swallow exercise

● **Prognosis**

It is not uncommon for fracture of thoracolumbar vertebrae to have such sequelae as limited movement, decreased supporting capacity of the spinal column and lumbago from long standing or sitting, especially in cases with malreduction or incomplete healing owing to the long confine ment to bed or unsatisfactory result of functional exercises. Severe or even fatal complications may arise in cases with paraplegia.

Section Ⅳ   Fracture of the Pelvis

The pelvis is a funnel-shaped ring structure consisting of the sacral bone, the coccyx, the hip bone, the pubis and the ischium and is the bridging section of the trunk and lower limbs. The pelvis can be divided into two parts, anterior and posterior. The former is the connecting arch whose function is supporting and stabilizing the body, while the latter, the main arch of the pelvis, is the weight-bearing arch which bears the body weight. The sacrofemoral arch of the posterior part bears the body weight during standing while the sacrosciatic arch bears the body weight on sitting. Within the pelvis are the urinary and reproductive organs and plenty of nerves and blood vessels, and therefore when the pelvis is fractured, it is likely that organ injury, internal hemorrhage and peritonitis may accompany.

● **Causes and Pathogenesis**

Fracture of pelvis is mostly caused by violent indirect or direct forces which come from, for example, traffic accidents, collapse of houses, and earthquake, and compress the pelvis from both the front and back or from the two sides to produce pelvic fractures, such as bilateral fractures of the superior and inferior rami of pubis associated with separation of pubic symphysis or with dislocation of the sacro-iliac joint, unilateral fracture of the superior and inferior rami of pubis companied by dislocation of the sacroiliac joint or by fracture of the wing of the ilium. A direct force may give rise to fractures of the sacrum, the wing of the ilium, the pubis and the coccyx. Clinically, fracture of pelvis is often divided into stable and unstable types. The former usually has fewer complications and a favorable prognosis whereas the latter usually involves two or more sites in the pelvic ring, often leading to fracture dislocation and deformity of the pelvis.

● **Clinical Manifestations and Diagnosis**

The victim has a definite traumatic history. Local pain, swelling and tenderness are typical. The victim can't sit or stand. Separation test of pelvis (with a hand on each side of the anterior superior iliac spine, the doctor presses the pelvis posterolaterally) or compress test of pelvis (with a hand on each wing of the ilium, the doctor presses the pelvis inwardly) will bring on pain in the fractured site. Fracture of the coccyx will be manifested by local pain when the patient attempts to sit. Sometimes shock may occur.

Radiographs of anteroposterior and lateral views should be taken and, if necessary, oblique film of the sacro-iliac joint should also be ordered to locate the site and find out the type of fracture.

On clinical examination, attention should be paid as to whether there is injury of blood vessels, nerves, urethra or rectum.

● **Treatment**

In case of hemorrhagic shock due to profuse bleeding or traumatic shock, the cause of the shock must first be removed and organ injuries in the pelvis, if any, must be managed promptly, otherwise they may endanger the patient's life.

1. Manual reduction

Reduction is usually unnecessary for fracture which does not damage the integrity of the pelvis such as fracture of wing of ilium, fracture of unilateral superior or inferior ramus of pubis, transverse fracture of the sacrum or fracture of only one pelvic arch. Fracture of pelvis with displacement, especially fracture of both arches of the pelvic ring, should be reduced by manual manipulation if the condition allows. The reduction methods to be adopted vary on account of the actual condition of fracture displacement. For example, in case of fracture of pubis with displacement of overriding broken ends and intorsion of the wing of ilium, the patient should take the supine position and the operator should first make longitudinal traction of the leg on the affected side to correct the upward translocation of the pelvis. Then, placing a hand on the anterior superior iliac spine of each side, he presses laterally to push the broken pelvis apart to the two sides and bring about the reduction. In the reduction of separation of the pubic symphysis with extorsion of the wing of ilium, the patient should lie on the back and the operator should first do longitudinal traction on the leg of the affected side to correct the upward displacement of the pelvis in the affected side. Then with a hand on each wing of the ilium, he compresses in opposite directions the wings of the ilium to accomplish the reduction. Alternatively, the patient may take the lateral recumbent position, with the affected side on top and with the help of an assistant making traction of the leg of the affected side, the operator presses the pelvis from the top to force the separated pelvis to be reposited (Fig. 5—12).

In the reduction of fracture of coccyx with evident displacement, the operator should insert his index finger in rubber glove into the patient's anus to press the distal end of the fracture backwards to realize reduction (Fig. 5—13).

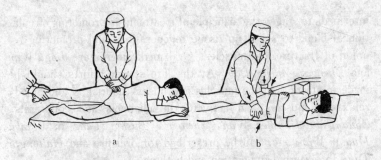

Fig. 5—12 Reduction of facture of the pelvis

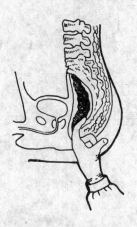

Fig. 5—13 Reduction of fracture of the coccyx

2. Fixation

Fixation is not needed for pelvic fracture without displacement and bed rest for 4—6 weeks is all that is necessary. For fracture with inward displacement, skin traction by the lower limb on the affected side is advisable. If the upward displacement is over 2cm, skeletal traction through tibial tubercle or through supracondyle of femur of the injured side should be performed with a tracting weight being 1/6 — 1/7 of the body weight and a duration of 6 —8 weeks. For fracture of symphysis pubis with separation and displacement and extorsion of the wing of the ilium, multi-tailed bandage fixation or pelvic hammock should be considered after manual reduction (Fig. 5—14).

3. Herbal therapy

At the early stage, it is important to promote blood circulation, remove blood stasis, promote subsidence of swelling and alleviate pain, so *Fuyuan Huoxue Tang* and modified *Taohong Siwu Tang* should be prescribed to the patient for oral administration. At the

211

intermediate stage, the principle of treatment is promoting circulation of blood to speed up tissue regeneration, and promoting reunion of fracture and muscles. Oral medicaments are *Jiegu Wan* and *Zhenggu Zhijin Dan*. At the late stage, efforts should be made to strengthen the muscles and bones, nourish *qi* and blood, relax the muscles and activate the channels and collaterals. *Zhuangyao Jianshen Wan*, *Shengxue Bushui Tang* or *Jianbu Huqian Wan*, etc. can be prescribed for oral use and *Haitongpi Tang* for external fumigation and bathing.

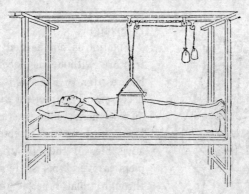

Fig. 5—14 Fixation with pelvic hammock suspension

4. Dirigation

Fracture of pelvis is usually stable after reduction because of the plump muscles around the pelvis so that functional exercises should be taken up early on condition that they will not affect the stability of the fracture. Early exercises include various exercises of the upper limbs, flexion and extension exercises of the foot, ankle and knee joints, and relaxation and contraction movements of the quadriceps muscle of thigh. Six to eight weeks later, with his injury condition and healing of the fracture taken into consideration, the patient may get out of bed, walk on crutches on a gradual basis and do functional training. Massage and physical therapy can also be given to speed up the restoration of functions.

💮 Prognosis

Bone union will take place in 6 — 8 weeks for stable fracture of pelvis. Unstable fracture e. g. two or more fractures in the pelvic ring and fracture with malreduction may render the pelvis out of shape and weight carrying capacity decreased. Many of the complications of pelvic fracture improperly managed can leave adverse sequelae, or even cause death. The statistics show that the mortality rate is 10% — 20%.

Chapter 6

Articular Dislocations
in the Upper Limbs

Section I   Dislocation of the Shoulder Joint

The shoulder joint (scapula-humerus joint) is composed of the scapula glenoid cavity and the head of the humerus. It is unstable because the former is shallow and small and the latter is big. As the joint capsule and the ligaments around it are thin and loose without ligament or muscle covering it on the anteroinferior portion, and as the range of articular movement is quite wide, the joint is liable to dislocation, which occurs most frequently in men of 20—50 years old.

●**Causes and Pathogenesis**

Dislocation of the shoulder joint is produced by either a direct or an indirect sudden force. By the location of the dislocated humeral head, it can be divided into anterior and posterior types. The former can be subdivided into subcoracoid, infraglenoid and subclavicular dislocations. Clinically anterior dislocation is more common and most of the cases are of subcoracoid type (Fig. 6 — 1). In terms of duration, it can be further divided into fresh, old and habitual.

1. Dislocation caused by a direct force

When the shoulder is subjected to a sudden external force, such as an impact force from the back, anterior dislocation will happen. If the force comes from the front, which is rather rare in clinic, posterior dislocation may be produced.

214

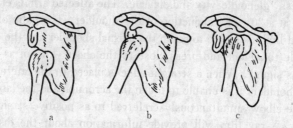

Fig. 6—1   Types of anterior dislocation of the shoulder joint
a. infraglenoid   b. subcoracoid   c. subclavicular

2. Dislocation caused by an indirect force

If one falls down laterally on his palm or elbow with the limb in
an abducent and extorsive position, the external force will pass a-
long the disphysis to the humeral head, which will break the anterior wall of the articular capsule to bring forth a subcoracoid dislocation. If the force cannot be checked, subclavicular dislocation
will occur. If one falls with his arm raised very high in an abducent
and extorsive rotatory position, his greater tuberosity of humerus
will contact the acromion to form a lever fulcrum, the external
force will compel the humeral head to slide anteroinferiorly, causing infraglenoid dislocation first; and thereafter subcoracoid dislocation will be produced by the joint traction of greater pectoral
muscle and subscapular muscle.

Apart from the soft tissue injuries around the joint, dislocation
of the shoulder joint may be complicated by avulsion fracture of
the greater tuberosity of humerus, fracture of the humeral head
and lesson of the axillary nerve.

● **Clinical Manifestations and Diagnosis**

The patient has a definite history of traumatic injury. (As far
as those with habitual dislocation are concerned, the dislocation
might be induced by only a slight injury). There is local pain and
swelling with limited movement. The acromion projects evidently
to produce a "square shoulder" deformity instead of the original
bulged arc shape. The humeral head is palpable under the coracoid

215

process, glenoid cavity and clavicle. The affected arm is elastically fixed at a 20°—30° abduction of the shoulder. The palm of the affected limb is unable to reach the normal shoulder and the elbow is unable to adduct and press close to the chest (known as positive Dugas signs). When a straight edge is placed to the lateral side of the shoulder, it is unable to touch the acromion and the lateral side of the elbow simultaneously (referred to as positive straight edge test). X-ray film will provide information about the dislocation and fracture, if any.

If the axillary nerve is also injured, deltoid muscle paralysis and hypo-esthesia at the side of the shoulder will develop.

● **Treatment**

1. Manual reduction

(1) Reduction of fresh dislocation

At the early stage of a fresh dislocation, there is only slight local swelling, pain and muscular spasm, for which reason manual reduction should be applied as early as possible and can be performed without anesthesia within 24 hours after injury. For dislocation of longer time, intra-hematoma anesthesia or anesthesia with traditional Chinese drugs should be considered in accordance with the patient's condition. Brachial plus cervical nerve plexus block is suitable for muscular patients or patients, with mental stress or spasm of shoulder muscles.

The method of manual reduction for habitual dislocation is much the same as that for fresh dislocation.

① Reduction with the aid of a chair-back:The patient sits on a chair, placing his arm of the injured side behind the back of the chair with a cotton pad or clothes under his armpit so that the axillary and costal regions are close to the back of the chair. An assistant is commissioned to hold the patient and the chair back steady. Grasping the arm of the injured side, the operator first abducts the arm and performs countertraction and rotates it laterally. At the same time of countertraction, he slowly adducts the arm and keeps it in ptosis, finally rotates medially and flexes the patient's elbow, and the reduction is achieved. The method is first described in *Se-*

216

crets of *Wound-healing and Bone-setting Handed Down by Immortals* written by Lin, a Taoist of the Tang Dynasty. The method makes clever use of the chair back as a lever fulcrum to reduce dislocation of the shoulder joint (Fig. 6—2).

② Sole-supporting reduction: The patient, who is supposed to have joint dislocation on the right shoulder, lies on his back on an examining couch. Standing beside the bed on the patient's affected side, the operator holds the wrist of the dislocated arm with both hands to abduct it slightly and places his right bare foot against the armpit of the affected side. Then the operator stretches his foot against the armpit and pulls the patient's arm to exercise countertraction for 1 — 2 minutes. When the

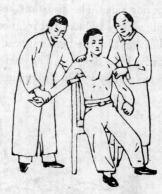

Fig. 6—2 Reduction with the aid of chair back.

humeral head comes to be level with the glenoid cavity, the operator should slowly adducts and rotates the dislocated arm medially. Meanwhile he turns his foot slightly into a "talipes varus" posture. The lateral margin of his foot will serve as a lever fulcrum to achieve a leverage which forces the humeral head to slip into the glenoid cavity. When a click-like sound is heard, the reduction is completed. This method is recorded in *Prescriptions for Universal Relief* by Zhu Su of the Ming Dynasty. Because of the desirable effect, the method is still in wide use up to date (Fig. 6—3).

③ Pulling-propping reduction: The patient takes the sitting position. An assistant stands on the patient's normal side, holding the patient firmly in place in his arms. Another assistant, holding the patient's wrist and elbow of the affected side respectively with his hands, abducts and rotates the arm laterally and pulls it at the same time. The operator stands on the patient's affected side with both thumbs resting on the patient's acromion and the rest fingers

217

girdling the armpit (or the operator puts one of his forearms under the patient's armpit to prop the humeral head) while the assistant is pulling the arm, the operator's thumbs press the acromion and the rest fingers forcibly raise the humeral head toward the latero-superior side. The assistant keeps on pulling the arm and meanwhile slowly adducts and rotates it medially until a click-like sound indicating that the humeral head has returned to its normal place is heard (Fig. 6 — 4). The method is recorded in *Compilation of Traumatology* by Hu Tingguang of the Qing Dynasty.

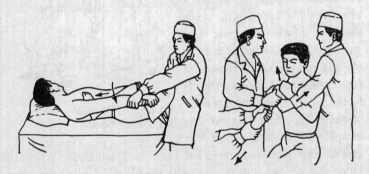

Fig. 6—3 Reduction with sole-supporting method

Fig. 6—4 Reduction with pulling-propping method

④ Knee-pushing and wrist-pulling method: The patient is seated on a bench. Standing by the injured side (left for instance) of the patient and facing the same direction as the patient, the operator puts his right foot on the bench, supports the patient's armpit with the flexed knee, puts his right palm on the injured shoulder and grasps the wrist of the injured limb with the other hand from behind his own back. When this posture is ready, the operator elevates his knee, pulls the patient's arm by the wrist, pushes the shoulder with his palm, and at the same time turns his body slowly but with force. The humeral head will be propped up by the knee to return to its original position (Fig. 6—5).

218

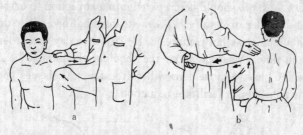

Fig. 6—5　Reduction with knee-pushing and wrist-pulling method

⑤ Traction and rotation method : The patient takes a sitting or lying position and the operator stands beside the patient's injured side. Take the right side for example. The operator holds the patient's elbow of the injured side with the right hand and grasps the wrist in the other. First the operator should apply a downward continual traction, lateral abduction and extorsion to the upper arm with his right hand to move the humeral head to the anterosuperior edge of the glenoid cavity. While the upper arm is under traction and extorsion, the patient's elbow should be adducted to press tightly to his chest. By now the humeral head has been moved outwardly from the anterosuperior edge of the glenoid cavity, the rupture of the articular capsule gradually opens. When the upper arm is adducted to the utmost, the operator quickly rotates it inwardly and the humeral head will slip into the glenoid through the enlarged rupture of the articular capsule, possibly with a sound indicating reposition. Because of great stress of this method, the neck of humerus bears a great twisting force, so the maneuver should be gentle, firm and careful, otherwise, fracture of the neck of humerus might be induced, especially with old patients, who often suffer from osteoporosis. This method is adopted only after other methods fail (Fig. 6—6).

(2) Old dislocation of the shoulder joint

Manual reduction may be tried if the dislocation is less than 3 months old without osteoporosis in the upper part of the humerus and calcification around the joint. One to two weeks before reduction, *Erhao Xiyao* should be prepared into a hot lotion to bathe the affected shoulder or distiller's dregs steamed hot be applied on the affected shoulder as hot compress, 1—2 times a day and at least 1 hour each time. Massage about the shoulder should also be given because the passive movement will soften the scar tissues and relieve the adhesion to facilitate reduction.

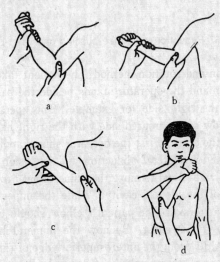

Fig. 6—6 Reduction with traction and rotation method
a. traction and abduction of the upper arm b. traction and extortion of the upper arm c. adduction of the upper arm under traction d. intortion of the upper arm under traction

Anesthesia by brachial and cervical plexus block for reduction is necessary. The patient lies on his back. With the help of a broad cloth strap round the patient's chest, the first assistant tracts the affected side towards the healthy side. A second assistant holds the affected arm and wrist and pulls towards the affected side. A third assistant holds a wooden rod which stands in the armpit of the injured side. The operator grips the upper end of the arm with both hands. The first and the second assistants perform counter-traction, and in the process, the second assistant slowly adducts the arm. With the rod as a lever fulcrum and the cooperation of the main operator, the humeral head will be forced to return to its normal position (Fig. 6—7).

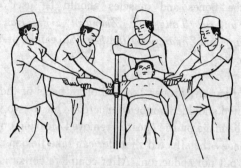

Fig. 6—7 Reduction of old dislocation of the shoulder joint

The patient may also take the sitting position when this method is used. On examination after the reduction, "square shoulder" should disappear and x-ray film should be ordered to show whether the reduction is successful.

2. Fixation

Proper fixation after reduction should be performed with the affected arm in the adduction and intorsion position. Clinically, fixation with bandage and triangular bandage is often employed (Fig. 6—8). The fixation usually lasts 2—3 weeks for fresh dislocations so that the injured soft tissues may be repaired to prevent redislocation. Old or habitual dislocation must be fixed for another 1—2 weeks.

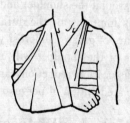

Fig. 6—8 Fixation of dislocation of the shoulder joint

3. Herbal therapy

Promoting blood circulation to remove blood stasis, subduing swelling and alleviating pain are the principles for early treatment.

221

Shujin Huoxue Tang, *Taohong Siwu Tang*, etc. can be prescribed to the patient for oral use. At the middle and later stages, drugs which can clear and activate the channels and collaterals, strengthen the bones and muscles should be used, such as *Zhuangjin Yangxue Tang* and *Zhenggu zijin Dan*. *Bushen Zhuangjin Tang* and *Zhuangyao Jianshen Wan* can be prescriped to the habitual cases.

4. Dirigation

Soon after fixation, proper exercise of all parts of the body except the affected shoulder can be conducted. One to two weeks later when the bandage on the chest is removed, leaving only the triangular bandage, the affected shoulder can take flexion and extension exercise but not abduction. After complete defixation, shoulder exercise in all directions can be done gradually, and massage therapy and physiotherapy can be given as well to prevent adhesion of the soft tissues around the shoulder.

● **Prognosis**

Fresh dislocation of the shoulder joint may recover completely if reduction is in time and fixation proper. Adhesion of some soft tissues around the shoulder and limited movement often occur if exercise is improper or the duration of fixation is too long. Avulsion fracture of greater tuberosity of humerus accompanying joint dislocation of the shoulder will usually be reduced at the same time of the dislocation reduction, and it will take about 3 months for the associated sprain of nerves to recover.

Section Ⅱ   Dislocation of the Elbow Joint

The elbow joint is composed of humeroradial articulation, upper radioulnar articulation and humeroulnar articulation which is the main joint. The walls of the joint capsule is thin and loose in the front and back but the brachiocubital ligaments and brachioradial ligaments at the two sides are strong. There are three osseous markers on the back of the elbow: internal and external epicondyles of humerus and olecranon process. The three points form an equilateral triangle on flexion of elbow and are in a line on extension of elbow. The elbow joint is the pivot of movement of the upper limb and its dislocation is most common of all dislocations of the larger joints in the body, especially in the young and middle aged adults.

● **Causes and Pathogenesis**

The dislocation of elbow joint usually refers to that of the humeroulnar joint which is often caused by an indirect force and rarely by a direct force. The dislocation of the elbow joint is divided into anterior type and posterior type which are frequently accompanied by lateral dislocation.

Anterior dislocation: it happens when one falls on a flexed elbow. Posterior dislocation: it is often induced by an indirect force. For instance, when one falls on the palm with the elbow joint straight and the forearm in supination, the olecranon process will prop against the olecranon fossa to form a lever fulcrum, the external force makes the elbow joint in overextension and the lower end of the ulna slips over the corchid process, causing posterior dislocation accompanied by laceration of brachial muscle and anterior wall of the articular capsule. Because of the link of the orbicular ligament and interosseous membrane, posterior dislocation of both the ulna and the radius is produced. With the variation of the external violent force in terms of strength and direction, the brachiocubital and brachioradial ligaments may also be injured, and as a result, a posterior dislocation may be complicated by a radial or ulnar dislocation. Sometimes, after a dislocation, the lower end of the humerus may set in between the ulna and radius, which is called a separate dislocation and is very rare. Damage to the blood vessels and the nerves may also arise from serious displacement.

● **Clinical Manifestations and Diagnosis**

An evident traumatic history can be related to. Swelling and pain are present at the elbow in association with dysfunction.

In a case of a posterior dislocation, it is full in front of the cubital fossa and the lower end of the humerus is palpable. The olecranon projects posterosuperiorly. The posterior cubital region is

223

void and the elbow assumes a "boot-shaped" deformity. The elbow joint is elastically fixed at a semi-flexion position with anteroposterior diameter longer than usual but a normal left-right diameter. The relationship of the three osseous markers at the back of the elbow is changed. If lateral dislocation is also present, cubitus varus and cubitus vulgus may occur.

In a case of an anterior dislocation, the antecubital region becomes bulged and the upper ends of the radius and ulna can be felt there. The lower end of the humerus and the displaced fragments of the olecranon can be felt in the posterior cubital region. The elbow joint is elastically fixed at the hyperextension position.

Radiographic examination can confirm the types and severity of the dislocation and presence or absence of fracture.

● **Treatment**

1. Manual reduction

(1) Elbow-traction and flexion method

The patient takes the sitting (or dorsally lying) position. An assistant stands behind the patient and firmly fixes the patient's upper arm with both hands. Standing in front of the patient, the operator grips the wrist of the affected side with one hand, and performs countertraction with the assistant (in a semi-flexion position); the thumb of the other hand rests on the anteriorly displaced lower end of the humerus and the rest fingers pull the olecranon; at the same time of traction, the thumb pushes backward, other fingers pull the olecranon forward and the elbow joint is flexed till a reduction sound is heard (Fig. 6－9). If the patient takes the lying position, the operator presses with one hand the middle and lower segment of the affected upper arm, and tracts the forearm and flexes the elbow joint with the other hand (Fig. 6－10).

(2) Pulling and knee-pushing method

The patient sits upright on a bench. The operator stands by the patient's affected side with one hand holding the affected upper arm and the other holding the wrist to make the elbow flexed at 90°. With one foot on the bench, the operator supports the

224

patient's cubital fossa with his knee, tracts the arm with the hand holding the wrist in the direction of the longitudinal axis of the forearm and meanwhile props up the elbow with the knee. When a sound of the end of a bone slipping into a cotyle is heard, reduction is completed (Fig. 6—11).

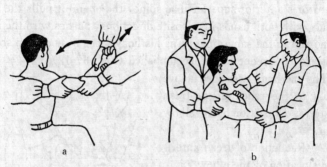

Fig. 6—9　Elbow traction and flexion at sedentary posture

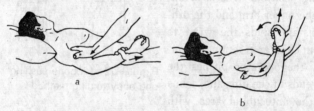

Fig. 6—10　Elbow traction and flexion at supine posture

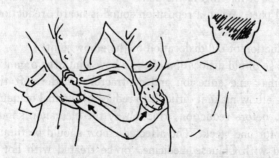

Fig. 6—11　Pulling and knee-pushing method

(3) Hipbone-pushing and body-turning method

The patient takes the sitting position. The operator stands by the patient's affected elbow with one hand gripping the upper arm and the other holding the wrist and abducting the elbow to the semiflexion position. With the cubital fossa resting on the operator's anterior superior iliac spine, the operator pulls the arm firmly with both hands in opposite directions, pushes with the iliac spine and at the same time turns his body when a reposition sound is heard, the reduction is accomplished (Fig. 6—12).

The methods described above apply to the reduction of fresh posterior dislocation of the elbow joint.

(4) Reduction of fresh anterior dislocation of the elbow joint

The patient takes the sitting or lying position. One assistant fixes the upper arm and the other assistant holds the wrist to perform counter-traction. Meanwhile, the operator pushes the upper ends of the ulna and radius from the antecubital area with

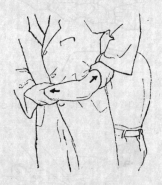

Fig. 6—12　Hipbone pushing and body-turning method

both thumbs towards the posterointerior side and pulls forward with the rest of his fingers the distal end of the humerus from the postcubital part. When a reposition sound is heard, reduction is a success.

(5) Reduction of old dislocation of the elbow joint

In the case of old dislocation of the elbow joint, the organization of hematoma, and adhesion and contracture of the soft tissues around the elbow make it difficult to reduce by manual maneuvers. Therefore, before reduction, traction by the olecranon should be performed for one week. The affected elbow should be fumigated and bathed with Chinese medicine, or be treated with hot compress with hot distiller's dregs. Flexion and extension exercise of

226

the elbow joint and other swinging exercise should be done to loosen the joint. If the attempt of manual reduction fails, surgical treatment should be considered.

2. Fixation

After successful reduction, the elbow joint should be fixed at an angle less than 90° in a posterior dislocation and well wrapped with cubital ∞-shape bandaging. The forearm should be suspended in front of the chest with a triangular bandage for 2—3 weeks.

3. Herbal therapy

At the early stage, herbal therapy should concentrate on promoting blood flow, removing blood stasis, subduing swelling and relieving pain. Internal medicine such as *Qili San* and modified *Fuyaun Huoxue Tang* should be taken orally. At the middle and late stages, traditional Chinese drugs which can relax muscles and tendons, activate collaterals, nourish the blood, activate vital energy and strengthen bones and muscles, such as *Heying Zhitong Tang*, *Liuwei Dihuang Tang* and *Shujin Pian*, should be taken orally. *Erhao Xiyao* should be used for external bathing.

4. Dirigation

During fixation exercises such as clenching the fist and shrugging the shoulder are encouraged. When fixation is removed, active flexion and extension of the elbow joint, and more exercise of the shoulder joint should be done but the range of movement should be enlarged gradually.

● **Prognosis**

A perfect recovery can be expected for a fresh dislocation after a successful reduction. But as for old dislocation, the result is poor. Movement disturbance of the elbow joint of varying degrees may be left and traumatic arthritis may be found in isolated cases.

Section Ⅲ   Subluxation of the Capitulum Radii

Since the capitulum radii in the children under five is not fully developed, the diameter of the capitulum is practically equal to that of the neck and the orbicular ligament is loose, subluxation of the capitulum radii is easily produced by the action of an external force. The condition is common in children of 2—5 years old.

● **Causes and Pathogenesis**

When a parent leads a child by the hand on a walk or stair-climbing or pulls up a child's hand to dress it, the elbow is tracted by a sudden force, the space of the humeroradial articulation broadens with an increased negative pressure in it, the antecubital wall of the joint capsule and the orbicular ligament will be drawn in by the pressure and the capitulum radii is stuck. It is also held by some doctors that when the elbow is straight and pulled, the capitulum radii slips away downward from the orbicular ligament and because of the contraction of brachial biceps, the capitulum radii is tracted forward resulting in the subluxation of the capitulum radii to the anteromedial aspect.

● **Clinical Manifestations and Diagnosis**

There is a typical history of sudden passive traction of the affected limb. Local pain is present. The elbow joint fixes at the semiflexion position with the forearm in pronation. The child dreads to raise up the affected limb, make supine movement or flex the elbow. The capitulum radii is tender to the touch but no obvious swelling can be observed. Abnormality cannot be found in x-ray films.

● **Treatment**

The reduction of subluxation of the capitulum radii is fairly simple. The child sits on the lap of its parent who holds it in one arm and grips the child's affected upper arm with the other hand (or by an assistant). Take the right arm for example. the operator gets hold of the child's affected wrist with the right hand and the elbow in the left with the thumb resting on the lateral aspect of the capitulum radii. Then he pulls the wrist while the parent's holding the upper arm and meanwhile extorts the forearm. When the arm is extorted to the utmost, the elbow joint should be flexed. At the same time the operator presses the capitulum radii hard with the

228

thumb of the left hand. Generally, a faint reposition sound is perceivable, which indicates that the reduction is finished. The child may soon feel relieved of the symptoms and is able to move the elbow at will and raise the arm to reach things. The treatment can be repeated if the first attempt fails. In most cases, the condition can be set right (Fig. 6—13). Usually, it is unnecessary to fix the elbow or prescribe medication after manual reduction. If there is local swelling, a triangular sling or ordinary bandage can be used to suspend the forearm in front of the chest at a 90° flex position for 2—3 days.

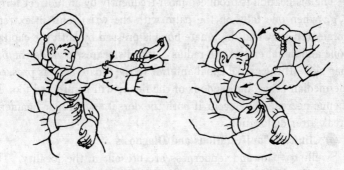

Fig. 6—13　Reduction of subluxation of the capitulum radii

● **Prognosis**

The subluxation of the capitulum radii is very common clinically but is easy to treat with an immediate result and very good prognosis. However, quite a few children are apt to have it recurrently, and therefore, sudden and forceful pulling of the arm should be avoided after the first reduction so as to prevent habitual subluxation.

Section Ⅳ　Dislocation of the Lunate Bone

The lunate bone presents a semilunar appearance and is located in the proximal row of the carpal bones. It is broad at the palmar side as a tetragonal and pointed at the dorsal side. Its proximal end presents a convex shape and forms a joint with the lower end of the radius. Its distal end assumes an umbilicate shape and constitutes a joint with the capitate bone. On the medial side it forms a joint with the triangonal bone and on the lateral side, with the scaphoid bone. There are articular surfaces all around it and tiny vasa vasorum going to the lunate bone via the posterior and anterior radiocarpal ligaments to maintain normal blood supply.

● **Causes and Pathogenesis**

The dislocation is produced most frequently by an indirect force, e. g. when one falls on the palm with the wrist joint in extreme dorsiextension, and the lunate bone is pressed by both the capitate bone and distal end of the radius, so it dislocates towards the palmar side. If the carpal canal anterior to the lunate bone is pressed, the median nerve and tendons of the flexor will be pressed too. Ischemic necrosis may occur if both the dorsal and palmar ligaments break after dislocation.

● **Clinical Manifestations and Diagnosis**

Swelling, pain and tenderness are present in the locality. The wrist is in slight dorsiextension with difficulties in both active and passive flexion and extension. The middle finger is unable to stretch straight. Sensory disturbance of three fingers and a half at the radial side may occur if the median nerve is compressed. The third metacarpal bone may be sunken when the patient clenches the fist. There is remarkable pain on percussion of the metacarpal bone. The process of the dislocated lunate bone can be felt at the palmar side of the wrist.

In the anteroposterior radiograph, instead of the quadrilateral shape, the bone presents a triangular profile. In the lateral radiograph, the cup of the lunate bone turns to the palmar side, no longer forming a joint with the capitate, and the bone lies in the anterior side of the wrist joint (Fig. 6—14).

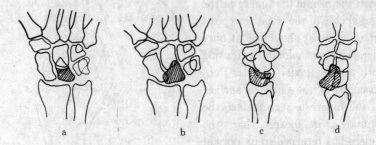

Fig. 6—14 Sketch map of x-ray films of dislocation of the lunate bone

● Treatment

1. Manual reduction

(1) Fresh dislocation of the lunate bone

Reduction of fresh dislocation of the lunate bone is performed under brachial plexus block or local anesthesia. The patient takes the sitting position. An assistant grasps the elbow of the affected side and another holds the fingers. With the elbow flexed to 90°, the two assistants perform countertraction and at the same time let the wrist extend dorsally to 80° so as to enlarge the space between the capitate and the radius. The operator, holding the wrist with both hands, presses with force the distal end of the concave side of the lunate bone to force it to rotate and go back into the space between the capitate and the radius in the same route as it has dislocated. Then the assistant who is holding the fingers is asked to gradually flex the wrist to the palmar side and the reduction will be over (Fig. 6—15).

(2) Needle-poking method

The method should be adopted when the attempt of simple manual reduction fails. Under anesthesia and aseptic manipulation and with the help of fluoroscopy, a round thin osseous bone needle is poked in from the palmar side of the wrist and the needle tip should touch the distal end of the concavity of the lunare. While the wrist is countertracted by the assistants, the operator pushes

231

with the needle the lunare to the dorsal side of the wrist to reposit it. The wrist should be at once changed from dorsal extension into palmar flexion. Under fluoroscopy, if the concave surface of the lunare is seen to face the capitate, it means that the lunare has returned to its normal position (Fig. 6—16).

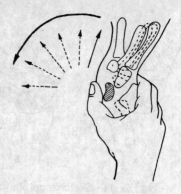

Fig. 6—15 Sketch map of the reduction of lunate bone

2. Fixation

After successful reduction, two poroplastic splints or plaster supports should be applied to the wrist joint to fix it at palmar flexion of $30° - 40°$ (Fig. 6 — 17). In $1 - 2$ weeks the fixation should be changed into neutral position and kept for another two weeks.

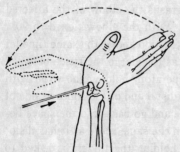

Fig. 6—16 Sketch map of the needlepoking reduction of the lunate bone

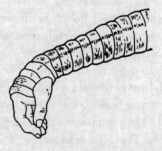

Fig. 6—17 Dorsal plaster fixation with the wrist at palmar flexion of 30°

3. Herbal therapy

See "Dislocation of the Shoulder Joint" in Section I of this chapter.

4. Dirigation

During external fixation, flexion-extension exercise of the finger joints and metacarpophalangeal joints can be done. When the fixation is removed 3−4 weeks later, active flexion-extension exercise of the wrist joint can be gradually performed, but care should be taken that any attempt to make excessive dorsal extension of the wrist should be avoided.

● **Prognosis**

If the reduction is successful, good results can be expected. But in some cases, the serious damage to blood supply may lead to necrosis of the lunate bone, in which case, the lunare may be extracted by surgery. In case the manual reduction fails, or an old dislocation has lasted for over three weeks with oppressive symptoms of the median nerve and flexor digitorum, surgical reduction may be taken into account.

Section V Dislocation of the Metacarpophalangeal Joints

The joints under discussion are composed of the heads of all the metacarpal bones and the bases of the proximal phalanxes of the fingers. Most of their movements are flexion and extension. At full extension position the joints can move 20°−30° laterally, but the flexion position allows little lateral movement, therefore, dislocation is apt to occur under the action of an unexpected foreign force with the joints in full extension. Of all the dislocations of the metacarpophalangeal joints, dislocation of the thumb is commonest in clinic, and that of the metacarpophalangeal joint of the index finger comes the second. Dislocations of the metacarpophalangeal joints of the rest fingers are by far uncommon.

● **Causes and Pathogenesis**

Dislocation of the metacarpophalangeal joints is most commonly caused by a sudden foreign force acting on the finger tips or on the palmar side of fingers to result in excessive dorsal extension of the fingers.

Take the dislocation of the metacarpophalangeal joint of the thumb for example. Attached to both sides of the palmar wall of the articular capsule is the short flexor muscle (Flexor brevis), which prevents dislocation at the base of the proximal phalanx of the thumb or the metacarpal neck, whereas because the palmar wall of the articular capsule is not strong at its median line, where vertical split is liable to occur, the metacarpal head is mostly dislocated to the palmar side from this crevice. The head of the metacarpal bone is like a coat button stuck in between the split walls and the two short flexor. Moreover, when the head of the metacarpal bone is dislocated towards the palmar side, the tendons of the long flexor muscles of the thumb may be clamped in between the base of the phalangeal bone and the head of the metacarpal bone. These physiological changes render great difficulties to manual reduction. Another example is dislocations of the metacarpophalangeal joints of the 2nd to 5th fingers. They are also commonly induced by overextension force which makes the heads of the metacarpal bones break up the articular capsules, be dislocated to the palmar side, and be stuck by the surrounding walls of the capsules, ligaments and tendons so that they are prevented from repositing.

● **Clinical Manifestations and Diagnosis**

A history of trauma can be obtained and local pain, swelling and dysfunction develop. Overextention of metacarpophalangeal articulation, flexion deformity of interphalangeal joints and elastic fixation may also be present. The heads of the metacarpal bones are palpable at the palm. The dislocation and fracture, if any, can be clearly observed in x-ray films.

● **Treatment**

Generally, anesthesia is unnecessary. With the help of an assistant holding the forearm affected, the operator holds the phalanx with one hand (or by means of tying one end of a bandage to the proximal end of the phalanx and the other end round the operator's hand) to perform traction and gradually pulls the finger to excessive dorsiextension. His thumb of the other hand should press the base of the first phalanx and push toward the palmar side while the

234

index finger pulls up the distal end of the phalanx to the dorsal side. In the meantime of the traction by one hand and the pushing and pulling by the other hand, the metacarpophalangeal joint is slowly flexed and the dislocation can be corrected (Fig. 6—18). If the head of the metacarpal bone is stuck by the tendon of flexor muscles and the ruptured capsule, it is very difficult to accomplish the reduction, in which case it is improper to push and pull with too much force. Instead, gentle massage, shaking

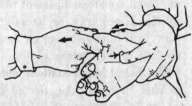

Fig. 6—18 Reduction of dislocation of the 1st metacarpophalangeal articulation

and swaying may be applied to relieve the incarceration. After reduction, the affected joint should be bandaged in flexion position for 2 — 3 weeks. When bandage fixation is removed, the joint should be fumigated and bathed with *Erhao Xiyao* and active flexion-extension exercise should begin but should be done gradually. At the early stage, *Dieda Wan* or *Huoxue Quyu Pian* may be taken orally, and *Shujin Pian* at the intermediate and late stages.

● **Prognosis**

Generally a good prognosis can be expected after a successful reduction. In case of dislocation with impaction of soft tissues into the joint which has not been successfully reduced, early surgical reduction is necessary.

Section VI Dislocation of the Interphalangeal Joints of the Hand

An interphalangeal joint of the hand is made up of a proximal phalanx and middle phalanx or a middle phalanx and a distal phalanx. The joint allows flexion-extension movement. Dislocation of interphalangeal joints is a common injury which may occur at both the proximal and the distal joints.

● **Causes and Pathogenesis**

235

When the anterior or lateral part of a finger is subjected to a violent force, hyperextension or lateral deviation of the finger, or rupture of the articular capsule in the palmar side or laceration of the distal collateral ligament of the finger may be produced, resulting in posterior or lateral dislocation of an interphalangeal joint, which may sometimes be associated with fragment torn off the base of the phalanx.

● **Clinical Manifestations and Diagnosis**

After an injury, the affected joint is swollen like a shuttle with local pain, deformity of digital hyperextension or lateral deviation, tenderness, elastic fixation and dysfunction in voluntary flexion and extension. X-ray film can reveal the condition of dislocation and presence or absence of avulsion fracture.

● **Treatment**

The reduction maneuvers are rather simple and anesthesia is unnecessary. The operator holds respectively the distal end and the proximal end of the injured finger with the thumb and finger of either hand and makes countertraction with appropriate force, then corrects the lateral deviation and flexes the affected finger, and reduction can be achieved. If avulsion fracture is present, the fragment should be pinched to its original position by the thumb and finger. After reduction, the finger is fixed with adhesive tape or aluminum plate for 1—2 weeks, or 2—3 weeks if accompanied by fracture.

When fixation is removed, active flexion and extension exercises of the affected finger should begin and the range of movement should be enlarged gradually.

During fixation, drugs for promoting blood circulation, removing blood stasis, and relieving swelling and pain should be used, such as *Dieda Wan* and *Huoxue Quyu Pian* for oral administration. At the late stage, drugs for relaxing muscles and tendons, activating channels and collaterals are recommended. Fomentation are also encouraged for local external use.

● **Prognosis**

If dislocation is accompanied by injury of ligament, the function of the finger will recover slowly in about three months, and sometimes such sequelae as arthrocele, pain and dysfunction of flexion and extension may be left.

Chapter 7

Articular Dislocations
in the Lower Limbs

Section I   Dislocation of the Hip Joint

The hip joint, an important part connecting the body trunk with the lower limb, is composed of the head of the femur and acetabulum. Apart from its main function of carrying heavy loads, it possesses an important motor function. Because of the large and deep acetabulum and the strong joint capsule, ligaments and thick muscles all around, the hip joint is stable with a large mobility, so dislocation here can only be incurred by a very strong violent force in certain postures. Most victims are young and robust adults.

● **Causes and Pathogenesis**

Dislocation of hip joint is commonly induced by an indirect force, and is clinically divided, according to the position of dislocated head of femur, into three types: posterior, anterior and central (Fig. 7—1).

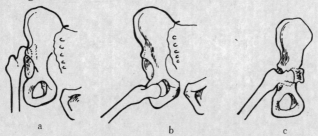

Fig. 7—1   Common types of dislocation of the hip joint
a. posterior type   b. anterior type   c. central type

1. Posterior type

Posterior dislocation mostly occurs when a person is in a bending posture and a heavy object or collapsed earthwork falls on his lumbar region, or when he jumps down from a high place, or falls down on a foot or knee from a horse with the hip in flexion, for in the hip-flexion posture, the shaft of the femur is overly adducted and rotated inwardly, most part of the femoral head is not in the acetabulum but moves to the posteroinferior part where the wall of the articular capsule is rather weak, the anterior margin of the femoral neck rests on the anterior margin of the acetabulum to form a lever fulcrum and the force from the back of the loin or from the front of the knee forces by means of the lever action the femoral head to break the wall of joint sac and get out of the acetabulum. The dislocation may be complicated by fracture of the posterior margin of the acetabulum or injury to the sciatic nerve due to the oppression and traction by the displaced femoral head.

2. Anterior type

If the hip joint is forced to abduct and rotate outwards by a foreign force, the top of the greater tuberosity of the femur will meet with the superior margin of the acetabulum to form a lever fulcrum and the femoral head is forced by the leverage to break the wall of the joint sac and protrude to the anteroinferior part of the acetabulum leading to anterior dislocation of hip joint. The femoral artery and vein are sometimes oppressed to result in circulatory disorder in the whole leg.

3. Central type

If a foreign force comes from the lateral and acts on the lateral tuberosity of the femur, or when one falls on a foot from a high place with the thigh slightly abducted, the force will transmit along the neck of the femur to the femoral head which is forced to ram the acetabulum leading to fracture of the acetabulum, and at the same time the femoral head along with the bone fragments further advances inwardly resulting in central dislocation of the hip joint.

● **Clinical Manifestations and Diagnosis**

A definite history of injury by a violent force can be found. There is pain at the injured hip and total dysfunction. Since the joint is deep in the muscles, local swelling may be unremarkable. Signs of hip dislocation vary with types.

1. Posterior type

The limb of the injured side looks shorter than the other and presents a typical deformity of flexion, adduction and intortion (Fig. 7 — 2). The greater tuberosity displaces upward and the buttock rises high with the femoral head palpable. The knee of the affected side also flexes, often pressing close to the medial part of the thigh above the knee of the normal side. The limb of the injured side is unable to move voluntarily but remains elastically fixed. Displacement of the femoral head to the posterosuperior of the acetabulum can be found in x-ray films.

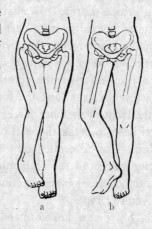

Fig. 7—2 Deformity during dislocation of the hip joint
a. posterior dislocation
b. anterior dislocation

2. Anterior type

The limb of the injured side is longer than the other, presenting an abducent, externally rotatory and slightly flexional deformity. The limb of the injured side can neither make active movement. The knee of the injured side cannot press close to the thigh of the normal side. The highly protruding femoral head is palpable in the groin and x-ray examination shows that the femoral head has moved to the anteroinferior part of the acetabulum.

3. Central type

In a case of mild dislocation of the femoral head, there may not be obvious signs; in severe cases, the limb of the injured side may be shorter but there is no deformity. Local swelling, pain and mild dysfunction are present. X-ray examination can reveal the fracture of the acetabulum and the protrusion of the femoral head into the pelvis.

● **Treatment**

1. Manual reduction

Epidural or general anesthesia may be necessary for the performance of manual reduction because of the thickness of the muscles around the hip.

(1) Posterior type

① Pulling and lifting flexed hip：The patient lies in dorsal position on a flat plank on the ground and an assistant fixes the patient's pelvis by pressing the two iliac crests with both hands. Facing the patient, the operator squats astride the leg of the injured side and raises the leg from beneath the popliteal fossa with the part of his cubital fossa so that both the knee joint and the hip joint of the affected limb are flexed to 90°. Then he pulls the thigh with force so as to let the femoral head come close to the rupture of the joint capsule. Simultaneously he rotates and shakes the affected limb slightly to help the femoral head slip into the acetabulum. When a click-like sound indicating the return of the femoral head into the acetabulum is heard, the affected limb should be put down slowly and let to extend straight (Fig. 7－3).

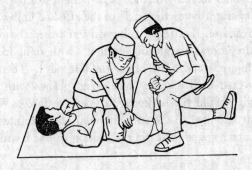

Fig. 7－3 Pulling and lifting the flexed hip

② Rotation method: The patient lies dorsally and the assistant fixes the patient's pelvis in the same way as described above. Standing on the patient's affected side, the operator holds the ankle of the affected limb with one hand and lifts the leg from beneath the popliteal fossa with the part of cubital fossa of the other arm until both the knee joint and the hip joint are in a 90° flexion. Then the operator adducts and intorts the thigh and in the meantime flexes the hip joint to such a degree that the knee presses close to the abdominal wall. Then, he abducts the limb, extorts it and puts it down straight. All of the above acts should be performed firmly and coherently and can be symbolized by a question mark ("?") with the knee as the sign. (The acts of reduction of dislocation on the left side can be symbolized by a "? " and on the right side by a " "). Hence the reduction method is also known as "Question Mark" method (Fig. 7 — 4), which is recorded in *Supplement to Traumatology* written by Qian Xiuchang of the Qing Dynasty. The method utilizes the lever principle to force the femoral head to move from the posterior upper margin to the lower margin and then slip into the acetabulum. During the reduction, the manipulative maneuvers should be gentle because the leverage is great, and strong force must be avoided; otherwise, fracture may be induced.

③ Tracting and treading method: The patient lies dorsally on a bed and the operator holds the ankle of the affected limb with both hands and treads on the ischial tuberosity and medial side of the groin with the lateral margin of one foot (with right foot if the right hip is injured, and left foot for the left side). The operator pulls the affected limb with his hands and pushes with his foot while his body should tilt backward to increase force. When the head of femur is pulled to the subacetabular edge, rotates the leg with hands, and a sound indicating reposition will be heard (Fig. 7 — 5).

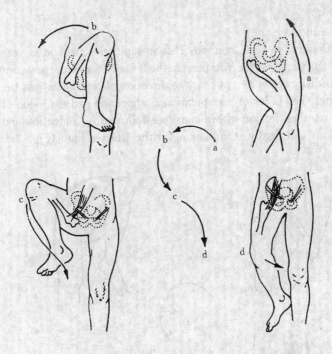

Fig. 7—4 Reduction of posterior dislocation
of the hip joint by rotation method

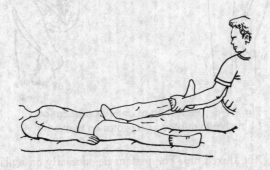

Fig. 7—5 Tracting and treading method

(2) Anterior type

① Counter-rotation method: This manipulative method is very much the same as the rotation method used to reduce posterior type of dislocations except that the direction of rotation is just the opposite. The order of manipulation is abduction and extorsion of hip first, then flexion of hip and knee followed by adduction and intorsion, and finally straightening of the affected limb (Fig. 7—6).

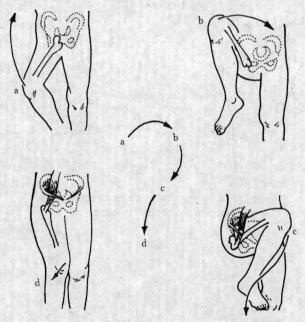

Fig. 7—6 Reduction of anterior dislocation of the hip joint by counter-rotation method

② Pulling the flexed hip: The patient lies dorsally on a plank on the ground. One of the two assistants fixes the patient's pelvis and the other holds the ankle and the upper part of the lower leg of the affected limb, and tracts after abduction and extorsion. Then he

244

slowly flexes both the knee and the hip to 90° and tracts upward. The operator holds the patient's distal end of the thigh with both hands and pulls to the posterolateral side until a click sound indicating that the femoral head has entered the acetabulum is heard.

③ Tracting and treading method: This method is similar to that for reduction of the posterior dislocations. The patient lies on his back. The operator holds the ankle with both hands, treads with the sole on the ischial tuberosity and groin and pushes the head of femur with the sole. By pulling and treading, the hip joint is rendered loose. Then the operator adducts the affected limb with both hands, pushing the head of femur laterally with the sole at the same time and reduction will be completed.

(3) Central type

The patient lies on his back. An assistant grasps both armpits firmly while another holds the ankle of the injured limb with both hands, puts the foot upright and abducts the hip to about 30°. Then the two assistants perform countertraction. Standing by the side of the affected limb, the operator grasps with one hand a wide cloth strap around the base of the patient's thigh and pulls the strap laterally while the other hand pushes the iliac bone medially so that the femoral bone displaced inwardly can be pulled out. When the greater tuberosity is felt symmetrical on both sides, the reduction is a success (Fig. 7—7).

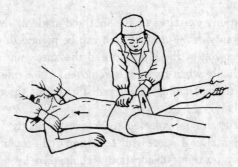

Fig. 7—7 Reduction of central type of dislocation of the hip joint

2. Fixation

After successful reduction, skin traction or long board splinting should be applied. In the case of posterior dislocation, the hip should be kept in a 20°—30° abduction position with the foot being upright. In the case of anterior dislocation, the affected hip should maintain an adduction, intorsion and extension position but not abduction. As for a central dislocation, skin traction or skeletal traction for serious cases at an abducent neutral position should be conducted for 3—4 weeks, and 6—8 weeks for a dislocation associated with fracture.

3. Herbal therapy

At the initial stage severe local swelling and pain may be present, so drugs for promoting circulation of blood and removing blood stasis to subdue swelling should be prescribed. *Shujin Huoxue Tang* may be prescribed for internal use and *Quyu Xiaozhong Gao* can be applied externally. If constipation is also present, *Dacheng Tang* can be taken to remove blood stasis, relieve constipation, invigorate the flow of *qi* and relieve pain. During the intermediate and natural cure stages, *Buzhong Yiqi Tang*, *Jianbu Huqian Wan* or *Shenjin Pian* is applicable for promoting blood circulation and regulating the flow of *qi*, strengthening the bones and muscles and tonifying blood and *qi*.

4. Dirigation

During fixation, exercises of the foot and ankle of the affected side and the joints in the normal limb can be practiced. Exercises of flexion-extension of the hip joint and the knee joint should be practiced gradually when fixation is removed. As a rule, walking and weight-carrying training should not start within three months.

● **Prognosis**

The affected joint is expected to recover perfectly for simple fresh dislocation after a successful reduction and proper exercise. In most cases, posterior dislocation accompanied by acetabulum fracture can recover after reduction whereas central dislocation may leave over traumatic arthritis owing to the complicated frac-

246

ture of acetabulum. Operation is necessary if the dislocation of the hip joint associated with bone fracture can not be reduced manually or in case an old dislocation with a history of more than three months.

Section II Juvenile Semiluxation of the Hip Joint

Juvenile semiluxation of the hip joint refers to a slight displacement of the head of the femur from acetabulum. However, owing to the lack of identical understanding to the pathogenesis, it is sometimes referred to as juvenile malposition of acetabulum, juvenile transient synovitis or dolichocnemia. Dysfunction of the affected joint may follow the disease but manual reduction may restore the function of the hip immediately. The semiluxation is mostly found in children of 2—15 years old and more frequently in the age group of 5—10.

● **Causes and Pathogenesis**

The semiluxation of the hip joint may occur as a result of extreme abduction or adduction position of the lower limbs which is the case often seen when a child exercises, plays, slips or falls accidentally. It is possible that the adductor and abductor muscles may be injured causing muscle spasm which in turn will press or pull the round ligament, and therefore, ischemic necrosis of femoral head may occur unless a prompt treatment is given.

● **Manifestations and Diagnosis**

Usually the child complains of pain in its hip the second day after an injury and the pain is aggravated by hip-flexion. On examination, the pelvis is inclined and the two legs are not equally long. In more cases the leg of the injured side looks longer than the other while only in a few cases, shorter. The gluteal creases at the two sides may not be symmetrical and there is tenderness in the middle part of the groin. Adductor tension develops in the cases with affected leg longer, and muscle tension of the buttock can be

247

found in the cases with the affected leg shorter. Nothing abnormal will be found on x-ray film.

● **Treatment**

Semiluxation of the hip can be treated with manual reduction. The child should take a supine position. An assistant holds the two shoulders and another presses the knee of the normal leg with one hand and the anterior superior iliac spine of the normal side with the other hand. The operator stands by the affected side, holds the lower segment of the affected leg with one hand and holds the knee part with the other. The manipulation should start with gentle repeated genuflex and hip-flexion to minimize the pain. Then the operator should flex swiftly and suddenly the knee and hip to the maximum limit. After a short while when the pain is relieved, he straightens the limb. In case that the affected limb is longer, it should be adducted and intorted with the hip flexed while the leg is being straightened. On the contrary, if the leg is shorter, it should be abducted and extorted with the hip flexed.

After reduction, the muscles can be completely relaxed and the two legs are equally long. In very few cases, the two legs of the sick child may still be unequally long and the sick child fears to flex the knee and hip by himself. In this case, the child should lie in bed for rest and usually his symptoms will disappear on the second day. As for fresh semiluxation, fixation is usually unnecessary after reduction, but the child must be told not to abduct the affected limb, and any recurrent semiluxation should be treated promptly. For old semiluxation with a history of over one month, fixation is necessary after manual reduction. The two thighs should be bound together with a cloth band for 2—3 weeks so as to prevent wide separation of legs and abduction of the hip.

After reduction, *Huoxue Quyu Pian* should be prescribed to those with fresh semiluxation and *Shujin Pian* as well to those with old semiluxation for 1—3 weeks.

● **Prognosis**

A few patients of juvenile semiluxation can recover spontaneously while most patients recover after treatment. If the recov-

248

ery is delayed over six months, ischemic necrosis of femoral head may occur.

Section III   Dislocation of the Knee Joint

The knee joint is made up of the lower end of the femur, the upper end of the tibia and the articular surface of the patella. They are joined together by the strong collateral ligaments, the intracapsular cruciate ligaments and the joint capsule. Between the condyle of femur and tibial plateau is the pad for semilunar plate and all around them are the quadriceps muscle of the thigh, gastrocnemius muscle and the hamstring muscles so the knee joint is very firm and dislocation there occurs only when it is subjected to a very violent force. The disease is mostly found in young and robust adults.

● **Causes and Pathogenesis**

The disease occurs mostly due to a violent force from the front, back or sides of the knee acting on the upper end of the tibia or the lower end of the femur. In terms of directions, it may be divided into anterior type, posterior type and lateral type. And an indirect violent twisting force may cause rotatory dislocation. Anterior and posterior types of dislocation are by far more common (Fig. 7 — 8). If the force is too violent, a complete dislocation may be theresult and if the force is less violent, semiluxation may occur. In either case, rupture or laceration of the collateral ligaments, cruciate ligaments and joint capsule, and break of the meniscus may develop, or even avulsion fracture of the spine of tibia, tubercle of tibia or condyle of femur in serious cases. In some cases dislocation may cause oppression or laceration of tibial nerve, common peroneal nerve and popliteal blood vessels.

● **Clinical Manifestations and Diagnosis**

There is sharp pain, swelling and obvious tenderness after trauma. In the case of complete dislocation, dysfunction and deformity of the knee with elastic fixation can be observed. The upper end of the tibia or the lower end of the femur can be felt at the anterior, posterior or lateral sides of the knee. In the case of semiluxation, spontaneous reduction may happen without any deformity left over. If the dislocation is accompanied by injury of cruciate ligaments, drawer test will be positive and when there is injury of collateral ligaments, lateral test will be positive. In cases that are complicated by the vascular or nervous injury, there may be abnormal pulsation of the dorsal artery of foot or paresthenia and dyskinesia of the leg and foot.

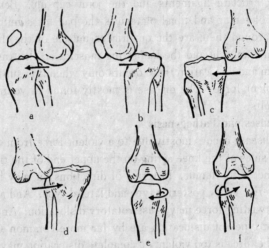

Fig. 7—8   Types of dislocation of the knee joint
a. anterior   b. posterior   c. lateral   d. medial
e. rotary   f. rotary

● **Treatment**
1. Manual reduction
In case of serious swelling of the knee, the hematocele or hydrops in the articular cavity should be drawn out first. The reduction is performed under anesthesia. The patient lies in dorsal position. One assistant holds the lower segment of the affected thigh with both hands and another holds the leg. With the knee in semiflexion they perform countertraction but attention should be paid

250

to avoid violent pulling and to protect the nerves and blood vessels in the popliteal fossa. The operator presses and pushes the upper end of the tibia and the lower end of the femur with both hands in opposite direction to the dislocation, and it is usually not difficult to accomplish reduction. When there is impaction of folding wall of the joint capsule or malposed semilunar plate that hinders the reduction, move the joint gently before reduction (Fig. 7—9).

2. Fixation

After reduction, the knee is usually fixed in flexion at 15°— 20° for 6—8 weeks with wooden or plaster support. The condition of the blood circulation in the affected leg must be observed closely at the early stage of fixation.

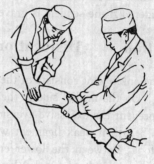

3. Herbal therapy

Since dislocation of the knee joint is usually complicated by severe injury to the soft tissues, during the initial stage, it is

Fig. 7—9 Reduction of posterior dislocation of the knee joint

preferable to invigorate circulation of the blood so as to eliminate blood stasis, relax muscles and tendons, and activate the flow of qi and blood in the channels and collaterals. Modified Shujin Huoxue Tang can be prescribed for internal use and Xiaoyu Gao for external application. During the intermediate stage and late stage, tonifying the liver and kidney and strengthening muscles and bones are the principles of medication. Bushen Zhuangjin Tang should be prescribed for internal use and Xiazhi Sunshang Xifang for external local fumigation and bathing.

4. Dirigation

During immobilization, the patient should do flexion and extension movement of his/her ankle joint and systolic movement of the quadriceps muscle of the thigh. After the removal of fixation, the range of movement of the knee should be gradually extended. During the entire course of treatment, exercise of muscles and functional activities should be done to help restore the stability and function of flexion and extension of the knee joint.

● **Prognosis**

The prospect of a simple dislocation of the knee joint with prompt treatment is bright. In some cases the serious ligament injury will result in unstable knee. Improper exercise may also cause limitation in the functions of the knee. Surgical treatment can be considered if the sequele is grave.

Section Ⅳ　Dislocation of the Ankle

The ankle joint consists of the lower ends of tibia and fibula and talus. On the medial side is the strong triangular ligament which can prevent the excessive eversion of the foot while on the lateral side, a rather weak ligament which prevents overly inversion of the foot. Between the lower ends of the tibia and fibula is the tibiofibular syndesmosis that binds the two bones closely together.

● **Causes and Pathogenesis**

The dislocation of the ankle joint is often the result of an indirect violent force. When one falls down from a high place on the medial margin of one foot, or when one walks with a foot accidentally and excessively everted and abducted, medial dislocation may be produced often complicated by fracture of the medial or lateral malleolus; if one falls down from a high place on the lateral margin of a foot or when one walks along an uneven or bumpy road with a foot accidentally made in excessive inversion and intorsion, lateral dislocation will happen possibly companied by fracture of the medial or lateral malleolus; if one falls from a high place with the back part of the sole touching the ground first and the body anteverted, anterior dislocation can be produced; or when one falls down from heights with the fore part of the foot touching the ground and the whole body retroverted, posterior dislocation may be caused, frequently associated with fracture of the posterior malleolus (Fig. 7 —10). Of all types of dislocations of the ankle joint, medial dislocation is far more common in clinic while the lateral type comes the second. Anterior and posterior dislocations are rather uncommon.

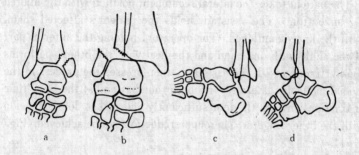

Fig. 7—10 Types of dislocation of the ankle joint
a. medial b. lateral c. anterior d. posterior

● Clinical Manifestations and Diagnosis

There is swelling, ecchymosis and pain in the ankle region after injury. If fracture is also present, swelling and pain are more severe and dysfunction develops. In medial dislocation, the foot exhibits an eversion and extorsion with a high process beneath the medial malleolus, a void beneath the lateral malleolus and an obvious deformity. Lateral dislocation is characterized by inversion, intorsion, a process beneath the lateral malleolus and avoid beneath the medial malleolus. In the case of anterior dislocation, the affected foot is in extreme dorsiextension. There are bony processes of the distal end of the tibia and fibula on both sides of the Achilles tendon and the forward displacement of the calcaneus. The posterior dislocation is marked by plantar flexion of the foot, backward protrusion of calcaneus, a void in front of Achilles tendon, the protruding distal end of the tibia palpable in front of the ankle joint and a void below the distal end of the tibia. X-ray examination can ascertain the type of dislocation and provide information as to whether there is fracture or not.

● Treatment

1. Manual reduction

Reduction should be carried out under appropriate anesthesia.

(1) Medial dislocation

The patient takes the lateral recumbent position with the injured leg on bottom. The assistant holds the patient's affected shank with the knee semiflexed. The operator, holding the anterior part of the ankle with one hand and the heel with the other, performs countertraction with the assistant, then presses the process of the medial malleolus laterally with both thumbs, and at the same time of traction, inverts the foot sufficiently and makes dorsiextension with the other fingers. Thereupon reduction can be achieved (Fig. 7−11.)

(2) Lateral dislocation

The patient lies on the normal side and the assistant fixes the leg of the injured side. Holding the anterior part of the ankle with one hand and the heel with the other, the operator performs countertraction with the assistant, presses the projecting part below the lateral malleolus with both thumbs, and at the same time of traction, makes the foot in extreme eversion with other fingers, and the reduction will be completed (Fig. 7−12).

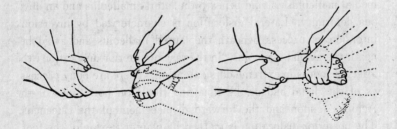

Fig. 7−11 Reduction of medial dislocation of the ankle

Fig. 7−12 Reduction of latera dislocation of the lankle

(3) Anterior dislocation

254

The patient lies on his back and the assistant holds the injured leg ringwise with both hands. The operator holds the upper part of the ankle with one hand and performs countertraction with the assistant. Meanwhile his other hand pulls the lower part of the tibia and fibula forwards, bends the foot in plantar flexion and pushes the foot backwards with the other hand. The coordinated maneuvers will bring about the reduction (Fig. 7—13).

(4) Posterior dislocation

The patient takes the dorsal position. One of the two assistants holds the leg of the injured side with both hands and the other holds the metatarsus with one hand and the heel with the other. While they do countertraction, the operator presses the lower ends of the tibia and fibula backwards. The assistant holding the foot keeps on the countertraction and simultaneously pulls the foot anteroinferiorly first and then only anteriorly with slight dorsal extension of the foot and the reduction can be achieved (Fig. 7—14).

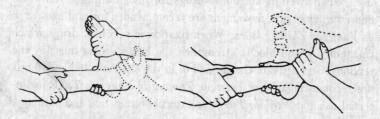

Fig. 7—13 Reduction of anterior dislocation of the ankle   Fig. 7—14 Reduction of posterior dislocation of the ankle

Fracture of the medial or lateral malleolus associated with the dislocation should be reduced at the same time.

2. Fixation

After reduction, molded beyond-ankle leg splints or plaster support should be used to fix the affected ankle for 3—4 weeks. For medial dislocation, the ankle joint should be fixed in inversion po-

255

sition (Fig. 7－15), and in eversion position for lateral dislocation. In the case of anterior dislocation, the ankle should be fixed
in neutral position with slight plantar flexion while the ankle
should be fixed in neutral position with dorsiextension in a case of
posterior dislocation. If joint dislocation is complicated by fracture, the fixation should last 5－6 weeks.

3. Herbal therapy

Owing to the grave swelling or
blister at the injured ankle at the
initial stage of ankle injury,
drugs for promoting blood circulation, removing blood stasis,
excreting dampness and inducing
subsidence of swelling should be
prescribed in heavy dosages.
Modified *Huoxue Shujin Tang*
should be prescribed for internal

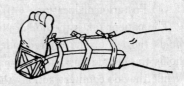

Fig. 7－15 Fixation of
medial dislocation of
the ankle joint in inve-
rsion position with beyond
-ankle leg splints

use. When swelling subsides, drugs for invigorating *qi* and blood
and improving joint movement are recommended for oral use, such
as *Yangxue Zhitong Wan*. When fixation is relieved, drugs which
can tonify *qi* and blood, strengthen the bones, relax muscles and
tendons, and activate the flow of *qi* in the channels and collaterals
are recommended. For example *Zhuangjin Yangxue Tang* for internal use and *Wujiapi Tang* for external fumigation and bathing .

4. Dirigation

During immobilization stage, the toes of the affected foot can do
flexion-extension movement, when fixation is off, flexion-extension exercise of the ankle should be intensified progressively in
combination with massage therapy. (Prognosis Because dislocation
of the ankle joint involves laceration of joint capsule and ligaments
or is complicated by fracture, secondary dislocation is liable to occur if the fixation molding is not well done.

Section V. Dislocation of the Tarsometatarsal Joint

Tarsometatarsal joints consist of the bases of five metatarsal bones, and the articular surfaces of some tarsal bones (three cuneiform bones, and one cuboid bone).

⚫ **Causes and Pathogenesis**

The injury is usually produced when the dorsum of the foot is squashed by heavy objects, or run over by motor vehicles, or when the fore part of the foot is subjected to a very violent twisting force. The base of metatarsal bones may displace medially, laterally, metatarsally or dorsally, and one or more metatarsal bones may be involved in the dislocation. Clinically, most cases of tarsometatarsal dislocation are medial dislocation of the first metatarsal bone or dorsolateral dislocation of the second to the fifth ones, or worse still, the two types occur at the same time, leading to the separation of the first metatarsal bone from the second one (Fig. 7—16). The soft tissues are usually severely injured in tarsometatarsal dislocation, and in a very severe case the dorsal artery of foot may be injured causing necrosis of the fore part of the foot.

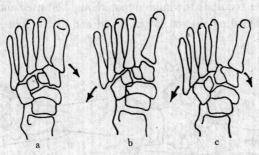

Fig. 7—16　Common types of dislocation of the tarsometatarsal joints

● **Clinical Manifestation and Diagnosis**

After injury swelling of the dorsum of the foot and pain will appear. There is decurtation of the fore part of the foot with broadening of the transverse diameter. The foot arch is flattened associated with foot dysfunction. Sometimes deformity of lateral process is present. Careful examination of the pulsation of dorsal artery of foot is necessary. X-ray films of anteroposterior, lateral or oblique views should be taken to make sure the position and direction of dislocation and whether there is fracture.

● **Treatment**

After local anesthesia or extradural anesthesia, an assistant holds the affected leg with both hands and another assistant holds the injured toes to perform countertraction. The operator presses, with his palms or thumbs from the opposite sides to force the displaced metatarsal bone to return to its original position (Fig. 7—17). After reduction, place cotton pads on and beneath the fore part of the foot and cover them with two pieces of arched cardboard, the medial piece overlapped by the lateral one, then tie them up for two rounds with straps and finally bind them up with bandages. In the case of unstability of tarsometatarsal joint or fallen plantar arch, the foot fixed in the above way should be placed on a wooden slipper bearing a plantar arch supporter and bandaged to it. After fixation, the injured foot should be raised and the condition of blood circulation in the distal end of the foot should be watched.

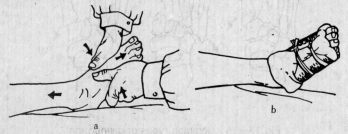

Fig. 7—17 Reduction and fixation of
dislocation of the tarsometatarsal joints

At the initial stage, drugs for promoting blood circulation and subsidence of swelling, activating qi and easing pain should be prescribed for patients, such as *Fuyuan Huoxue Tang* and *Dieda Wan* for oral administration. After 4—5 weeks when the fixation is removed, *Shujin Pian* can be prescribed for oral use and *Erhao Xiyao* for external fumigation and bathing to help relax the rigidity of muscles and activate the collaterals. At the late stage, flexion-extension exercises of the foot should be practiced gradually and weight-bearing exercise shouldn't start until 8 weeks later.

● **Prognosis**

A serious dislocation or malreduction may cause traumatic arthritis with the sequele of local pain. Surgical operation is usually necessary for a joint which is unstable after manual reduction and for old dislocation.

Section Ⅵ Dislocation of the Metatarsophalangeal Joint

Metatarsophalangeal joints are composed of the heads of metatarsus and proximal phalanx. Clinically, the dislocation is mostly found at the first metatarsophalangeal joint.

● **Causes and Pathogenesis**

The injury is often produced as the result of squashing of the toes by heavy objects or kicking a hard object with the toes, or overextension of the toes due to a foreign force, e. g. on a fall from heights with the toes touching the ground first, causing the basal segment of the proximal phalanx to move to the dorsal side of the metatarsal head. The first phalanx is most liable to injury for it is longer than others.

● **Clinical Manifestations and Diagnosis**

A history of injury can be obtained. Local swelling, pain, and dysfunction are present. The injured toe is shortened with deformity of overextension of metatarsophalangeal joint and flexion of interphalangeal articulation (Fig. 7 — 18). Displaced metatarsal

heads are palpable at the sole.
X-ray film should be ordered to
establish the diagnosis of dislocation and ascertain whether
there is fracture.

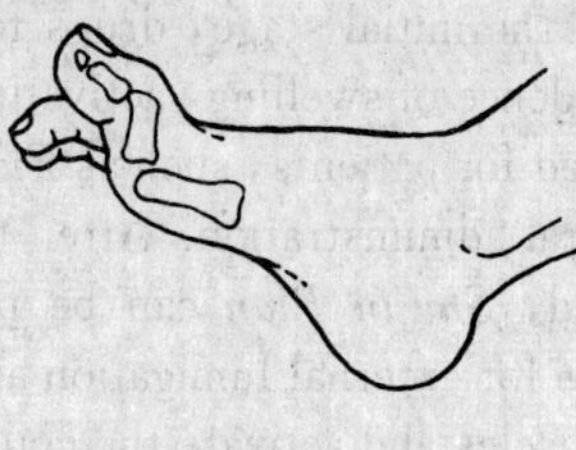

● **Treatment**

Generally, anesthesia is unnecessary for manual reduction.
With an assistant holding the
lower segment of the leg, the
operator holds the dislocated toe between his thumb and forefinger
of one hand (or fastens the toe-tip with a bandage loop so as to facilitate traction) and tracts the toe steadily along the direction of
the longitudinal axis of the proximal phalanx. His thumb of the
other hand presses the base of the phalanx and pushes to the sole.
Simultaneously, he pulls the distal ends of the phalanx dorsally
with the forefinger and middle finger and slowly flexes the
metatarsophalangeal joint. A sensation of the toe entering a cotyle
indicates that the reduction is completed (Fig. 7—19).

Fig. 7—18 Deformity due
to dislocation of the 1st
metatarsophal-angeal joint

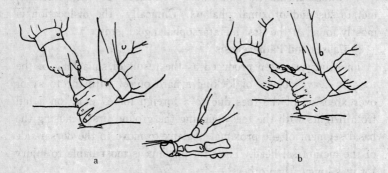

a   b

Fig. 7—19 Reduction of dislocation of
the 1st metatarsophalangeal joint
a. traction by counter-pulling   b. correction
of plantar flexion by pulling-lifting

After reduction, coil the affected toe with bandage for several

thick-nesses and fix it with
arched cardboard or small splints
and bind them up with several
layers of bandage (Fig. 7—20).

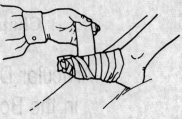

During the initial stage,
Huoxue Quyu Pian, and *Dieda
Wan* are recommended for oral
use. Drugs for local bath and fumigation can be prescribed.
Three weeks later, when the
fixation is removed and more

Fig. 7—20 Fixation of dislocation of a metatarsopha-
langeal joint

functional exercise of the affected foot should be done.

Chapter 8

Articular Dislocations
in the Body Trunk

Section I Dislocation of the
Temporomandibular Joint

The temporomandibular joints which consist of the mandibular condyloid process and temporal fossa are movable joints located symmetrically on both sides of the face. The dislocation here is clinically very common.

● **Causes and Pathogenesis**

A person may suffer dislocation of the jaw from opening his mouth too widely, as in yawning, laughing and tooth extraction, from biting hard food, opening mouth by a mouth-gag under anesthesia, or from being struck on the chin with his mouth open. Because when the mouth is wide pen, the mandibular condyloid process will slip excessively forward, and because the anterior wall of the capsule of mandibular joint is relatively thin and weak and lacking support by any ligament, the condyloid process will slip in front of the tubercle of the joint. After dislocation, the condyloid process is stuck under zygomatic arch before the temporomandibular joint due to the spasm of the chewing muscles.

In old age or after a protracted disease, a person tends to be weak or debilitated and deficient of *qi* and blood, his liver and kidney are deficient and his blood is unable to nourish the muscles and tendons, which may lead to looseness of the ligaments and articular capsules so that he is more vulnerable to jaw dislocation or even suffers from habitual jaw dislocations.

● **Clinical Manifestations and Diagnosis**

Experiences of yawning, laughing or biting a big piece of hard food or history of injury can be related to. The victim always opens his mouth halfway with inability to close the mouth, to stop salivation and to speak clearly. In the case of bilateral dislocations, the jaw bone is misplaced forwards, there are pitting voids in front of both antilobia and the condyloid processes are palpable at the acupoint *Xiaguan*. Unilateral dislocation is marked by the chin slanting toward the normal side and pitting void only in front of the antilobium of the affected side. On the basis of the above symptoms and signs, diagnosis usually presents no difficulty.

● **Treatment**

1. Manual reduction

Generally, anesthesia is unnecessary.

(1) Intraoral reduction

This method was described for the first time in the *Prescriptions Worth A Thousand Gold for Emergencies* by Sun Simiao of the Tang Dynasty. The victim sits on a stool with the head against a wall (or fixed by an assistant). The operator stands facing the patient, puts both of his thumbs which are wrapped beforehand with several thicknesses of clean gauze into the mouth and rests them on the patient's lower molar teeth, one thumb on each side. His index fingers hold the mandibular angles and the other fingers support the mandibular body from outside. The operator starts reduction by exerting steady and vigorous pressure on the molars, and at the same time, lifting the chin with other fingers. With the help of the leverage, the spasm of the chewing muscles is overcome so that the condyloid process will lower down and the fingers outside simultaneously push the jaw bone anterosuperiorly (Fig. 8—1). When the jaw bone snaps back into normal position, the operator should quickly slip his thumbs sideways into the space between the patient's teeth and cheeks to avoid being bitten. As soon as the reduction is successful, all the symptoms and deformity disappear automatically.

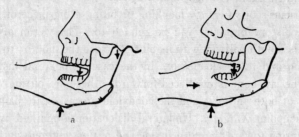

Fig. 8−1 Intraoral reduction of temporomandibular joint

In the reduction of unilateral dislocation, the operator's thumb resting on the normal side need not exert pressure on the molar teeth and push backward but rather keep the position. Other maneuvers are just the same as in the reduction of bilateral dislocation.

(2) Extraoral reduction

The patient sits on a stool and the operator stands facing the patient with his thumbs resting on the border of the mandibular body and the anterior margin of the ramus of the mandible on both sides and with other four fingers supporting the mandibular body. When the reduction begins, the two thumbs exert pressure on the mandibular body first gently and by and by vigorously, then the rest fingers lift and push the mandibular body backward, and the snap of reposition can be heard. This method is simple and applicable to patients in old age and without teeth or with muscular relaxation and patients with habitual dislocations.

2. Fixation

Once the jaw returns to its normal position, fixation should follow with a four-tailed bandage, that is, a wide bandage which is cut into two on both ends to give four tails, and which is applied with the middle part supporting the chin and the homologous tails tied respectively at the vertex and occiput of the head and then linked together (Fig. 8−2). The fixation should be kept usually for 3 − 5 days, and with habitual dislocations, about 2 weeks.

During fixation, the mouth should not open wide and hard food should be avoided.

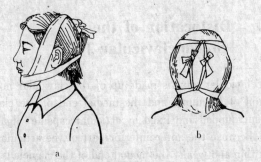

Fig. 8—2   Fixation of dislocation of temporomandibular joint with four-tailed bandage

3. Herbal therapy

For fresh jaw dislocation, herbal treatment is not absolutely necessary. In cases with severe local swelling, *Huoxue Quyu Pian* or *Sanqi Pian* should be taken orally. After removal of fixation, if there is local pain when the jaw is moved, *Kanlisha* or *Huoxue Zhitong San* decocted and wrapped while hot in a piece of cloth can be used as hot compress.

For patients with habitual dislocation, Chinese medicines which tonify *qi* and blood, reinforce the liver and kidney, and strengthen bones and muscles should be prescribed. For example, *Bushen Zhuangjin Tang*, *Shiquan Dabu Tang*, etc. can be administered orally.

4. Dirigation

During fixation, the patient should not open mouth wide and should be on liquid or semi-liquid diet. After removal of fixation, the movement range of the jaw should be gradually enlarged.

● **Prognosis**

Desirable prognosis can be expected after the reduction of a fresh jaw dislocation. However, if the period of fixation is too short or the mouth opens too wide during fixation, redislocation

265

may develop, especially in aged or weak patients, and habitual dislocation may follow in some cases.

Section II Dislocation of the Sternoclavicular Joint

The sternoclavicular joint is made up of the clavicular notch of the manubrium of sternum, and the medial end of the clavicle. The joint is surrounded and fixed by articular capsule, ligaments and muscles. Because the anteroinferior part of the articular capsule is rather thin and weak, the medial end of the clavicle is liable to dislocate forward on the action of an external violent force.

● **Causes and Pathogenesis**

This condition may be produced either by a direct violent force or an indirect force. For instance, when a direct violent force blows on the medial end of the clavicle causing laceration or rupture of the sternoclavicular ligaments and costoclavicular ligaments, the medial end of the clavicle displaces toward the posteroinferior part, resulting in its posterior dislocation. If an external violent force acts on the shoulder to force it to move downward and backward, the medial end of the clavicle and the superior margin of the first rib form the lever fulcrum to compel the medial end of the clavicle to displace forward and upward, leading to anterior dislocation. If one often makes abducent movements of the clavicle, the sternoclavicular ligaments may suffer from forced chronic sprain or strain, in which case an external force, sometimes even a small one, may cause this dislocation.

● **Clinical Manifestations and Diagnosis**

After injury, there is local swelling, pain, evident tenderness and sometimes ecchymosis. Protrusive or depressed deformity may be found in the injured spot. Shoulder drops and movement limitation of the affected side may develop. In serious cases of posterior dislocation, the dislocated part may constrict the trachea, esophagus or cervical blood vessels, giving rise to dyspnea or dysphagia.

266

Radiographs should be ordered to help make a definite diagnosis and find out if there is fracture.

● **Treatment**

1. Manual reduction

The manual reduction should be carried out under local anesthesia and the patient sits with the same posture as in the reduction of clavicle fracture. An assistant props up the middle part of the patient's back with a knee and pulls both shoulders backwards with two hands or two bandage rings round the patient's shoulders. In the reduction of anterior dislocation, the operator stands in front of the patient, exerts a steady pressure on the highly protruding medial end of the clavicle with the back part of his palm or both thumbs to push it backwards. In the case of posterior dislocation, the operator should grip the clavicle with the thumb and other fingers to lift and pull it forward until the injured part is smooth to the touch, which indicates reposition is achieved (Fig. 8－3).

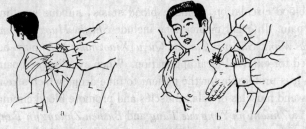

Fig. 8－3　Reduction of dislocation of the sternoclavicular joint

2. Fixation

The fixation for this dislocation is rather difficult. After reduction the two bandage rings round the two shoulders should be pulled tight and tied to each other (in the same way as in the fixation of fracture of clavicle) to keep the shoulders in retro-extension. As for anterior dislocation, the joint is first covered with a cotton pad and cardboard and then fixed up with bandages round the chest and shoulder. The fixation should be kept for about 4 weeks or so (Fig. 8－4).

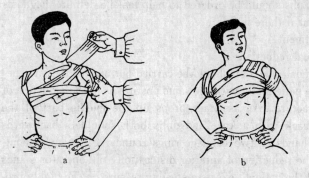

Fig. 8—4 Bandaging of dislocation of
the sternoclavicular joint

3. Herbal therapy

At the early stage, because of the presence of swelling and
pain, it is preferable for the patient to take drugs which can stimulate blood circulation, remove blood stasis, subdue swelling and
ease pain. Internal medications include *Shujin Huoxue Tang* and
Dieda Wan. *Shenjin Gao* or *Quyu Xiaozhong Gao* may be prescribed for external local application. When swelling and pain sub-
side, it is preferable for the patient to take drugs which strengthen
bones and muscles or relax muscles and promote blood circulation,
such as *Zhuangjin Yangxue Tang* and *Bushen Zhuangjin Tang*. At
the late stage, weak patients may take drugs which tonify the
blood and *qi* or warm and invigorate channels and collaterals, such
as *Buzhong Yiqi Tang* and *Bazhen Tang*.

4. Dirigation

During fixation, much exercise of the elbow and wrist should be
done and after removal of fixation, functional exercise of the
shoulder should be increased gradually.

● **Prognosis**

Fairly good prognosis can be anticipated in cases of anterior dislocation; even if there is mild displacement, usually no apparent
sequele is left. For posterior dislocation which is difficult to set by

268

manual reduction and old dislocation with remarkable local pain, open reduction and steel-pin internal fixation or resection of the medial end of the clavicle should be considered.

Section Ⅲ Dislocation of the Acromioclavicular Joint

The acromioclavicular joint is composed of the medial acromial extremity and the lateral end of clavicle connected and held in place by means of the surrounding articular capsule, acromioclavicular ligament, corococlavicular ligament, deltoid muscle and trapezius muscle, etc. Clinically, this is a very common dislocation mostly seen in young and middle-aged adults.

● **Causes and Pathogenesis**

When the acromion is blown by a direct external force in a laterosuperior—medioinferior direction, or when the shoulder joint is overstretched downward by an indirect force, dislocation of acromioclavicular joint may be induced. When there is only damage to the articular capsule and acromioclavicular ligament with mild displacement, subluxation of the acromioclavicular joint is evolved but when the injury is severe leading to tearing of the coracoclavicular ligament, complete dislocation will occur (Fig. 8 — 5).

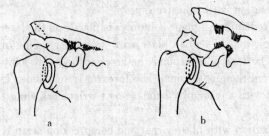

Fig. 8—5 Dislocation of acromioclavicular joint
a. subluxation b. complete dislocation

269

● **Clinical Manifestations and Diagnosis**

A history of trauma can be obtained. There is pain, swelling, and local tenderness in the vicinity of injury and mild disturbance in the movement of shoulder joint. In a case of subluxation, the lateral end of clavicle sticks up slightly, while in a case of complete dislocation, the lateral end of clavicle shows a highly protruding deformity and is elastic to the touch.

On x-ray examination, it can be found that the acromioclavicular space is enlarged and the lateral end of the clavicle protrudes upward. If the condition is a mild one, comparative observations should be made with the other side.

● **Treatment**

1. Manual reduction

The patient is given local anesthesia and takes sitting position with the elbow flexed at 90°. Standing by the patient's injured side and using one hand, the operator presses down the highly protruding lateral end of the clavicle firmly and pushes up the arm from below the elbow with the other hand. Thereupon the dislocation is corrected.

2. Fixation

While the dislocation being discussed is easy to set, effective fixation is difficult to maintain. Here are two common fixation methods:

(1) Fixation with adhesive tape

After reduction, a plane compress is placed on the lateral end of the clavicle and is kept in place with an adhesive tape of 10cm in width. The tape goes around the acromioclavicular joint and also to and from the elbow joint. The forearm is suspended in front of the chest with a triangular bandage or a wrist-neck sling (Fig. 8—6).

(2) Fixation with plaster cast and compression strap

A plaster cast is first made around the patient's waist with the upper margin reaching the nipples and the lower margin level with the anterior superior iliac spine. An iron ring is then embedded both in the front and at the back in the upper-middle part of the cast. When the plaster becomes thoroughly dry, a cotton pad is placed on top of the lateral end of the clavicle, covered with the middle part of a cloth strap or a bandage which is 4—5 cm in width and whose ends go through the rings in the front and at the back. The cloth strap is pulled tight and fastened to the rings. The fixation pressure should be just enough to keep the up-sticking lateral end of clavicle down to its original position (Fig. 8—7).

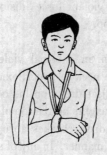 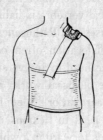

Fig. 8—6 Fixation of dislo- cation of acromioclavicular joint with adhesive tape

Fig. 8 — 7 Fixation of the acromioclavicular joint with plas- ter cast and compression strap

3. Herbal therapy
See "Dislocation of the Sternoclavicular Joint".
● **Prognosis**
The reduction of dislocation of the acromioclavicular joint at the early stage is easy; however, the fixation is difficult to keep. The results of the treatment of subluxation are generally good but in the case of complete dislocation, if the fixation is not effectively maintained, redislocation tends to happen, and therefore the fixation should be frequently checked for displacement, which should be dealt with promptly if it occurs. In case of unsuccessful reduc- tion and fixation, steel-pin fixation or open reduction can be con- sidered.

271

Section IV Dislocation of the Cervical Vertebrae

A joint between two cervical vertebrae consists of the lower vertebral process of the upper vertebra and the upper vertebral process of the lower vertebra. The articular surface, short and almost at a horizontal position, is covered with transparent cartilage. The articular capsule is attached to the edges of the cartilage and is rather loose, so under the action of a violent force, dislocation of the cervical vertebra is liable to develop.

● Causes and Pathogenesis

The dislocation often occurs when an external violent force makes the head in anteversion and the neck in hyperflexion, e. g. when one bends at work, a heavy object drops on his occiput or when an acrobat or athlete falls from heights on the top of his head with the neck in flexion, or when a driver brakes abruptly, his head bends forward in a whip-wielding manner. In any of such cases, the articular capsule may be torn and the lower vertebral process of the upper vertebra may slide forward, get over and is misplaced in front of the upper vertebral process of the lower vertebra to form complete dislocation of a cervical vertebra. If the displacement is slight and the articular surfaces of the two processes are still partly in contact, subluxation of the cervical vertebra is the result. When one's head is subjected to a twisting as well as flexion external violent force, unilateral dislocation may occur, which is much less common than the bilateral type.

● Clinical Manifestations and Diagnosis

A history of trauma can be obtained and there is always pain in the neck. In a case of complete dislocation, there is local tenderness and loss of functions with relation to movement. In a case of bilateral dislocation, the victim's head bends forward with the spinous process of the lower vertebra remarkably protruding backward while the spinous process of the injured vertebra caved in. Unilateral dislocation is characterized by tilt of the jaw to the nor-

272

mal side, wryness of the spinous process of the injured vertebra to the injured side and forward depression, and slight backward projection of the lower vertebra.

In a case of complete dislocation, the spinal cord may possibly be compressed to result in various degrees of high paraplegia or even endanger the victim's life. Subluxation of cervical vertebra may give rise to irritative symptoms of the cervical nerve roots, such as numbness and radiating pain in the shoulder and upper limbs.

X-ray films of the cervical vertebrae in anteroposterior and lateral views should be ordered to help make a clear diagnosis.

● **Treatment**

When a person is suspected to be suffering from dislocation of cervical vertebra, precautions should be taken to prevent further injury. In the course of handling such a patient, a person should be commissioned to hold the head and neck at all times so that they will not turn from right or left, nor extend backward or bend forward. When the patient needs to be turned over to one side, the head must be moved in line with the body. On transportation of such patient, suitable bolsters or clothes should be put under or beside the head and neck to keep them from moving aside. During x-ray examination, the patient must also be attended to by a specially assigned person. In a very serious case, preparation for first-aid work should be made to prevent life danger. If both the patient's conditions and treatment circumstances allow, immediate reduction should be carried out.

1. Manual reduction

(1) Reduction under countertraction

The patient lies on his stomach with the shoulders level with the end of the bed. An assistant holds the patient's occiput with one hand and jaw with the other hand to perform countertraction with another assistant who grasps the two shoulders with both of his hands. Standing on one side, the operator presses the spinous process of the vertebra below the injured one with both thumbs and pulls the upper part of the neck from front with the rest of his fingers. While performing steady traction, the assistant holding the patient's head should make the cephalocervical part into dorsal extension position. At the same time, the operator presses down his thumbs firmly until low snaps indicating reposition are heard or a sense of reposition is felt and the deformity disappears. Thereupon the dislocation is set right (Fig. 8—8).

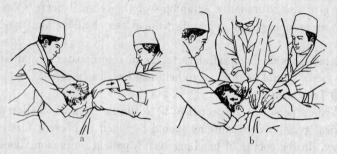

Fig. 8—8 Reduction of dislocation of cervical spine under countertraction

(2) Reduction under traction

The patient lies on his back on a bed with a small bolster under the neck and is given continual jaw-occiput strap traction with a weight of 1.5—2kg for 4—5 days prior to manual reduction. In the reduction of bilateral dislocations, with the help of continual traction, the operator presses both his thumbs on the spinous process of the vertebra below the injured one and holds the upper part of the neck from the front with his other fingers. While the cephalocervical part is made in dorsal extension, the operator presses with his thumbs firmly and usually the sound characteristic of the reduction can be heard. In the reduction of a unilateral dislocation, the operator presses the thumb of one hand on the wry spinous process of the injured vertebra and holds the opposite side of the spinous processes of the vertebrae lower than the injured one with other fingers of the hand. His other hand holds the patient's head and makes the cephalocervical part extend slightly backward and rotate to the injured side. Meanwhile, his thumb pressing on the wry process pushes steadily and firmly until a sound characteristic of reduction is heard. X-ray films should be taken to verify the reduction.

In severe cases of complete dislocation, reduction should be performed under skull traction.

2. Fixation

A successful reduction should be followed by jaw-occiput strap traction with the patient lying on his back on a bed. The traction weight is 1.5−2 kg. A small bolster should be placed under the neck to maintain the neck in dorsal extension. The traction usually lasts 3 weeks or so (Fig. 5−5).

3. Herbal therapy

See "Dislocation of the Sternoclavicular Joint" in Section II of this chapter.

4. Dirigation

See "Fracture of the Cervical Spine" in Section II, Chapter 5.

● **Prognosis**

Good result can be expected of a subluxation of cervical vertebra after proper treatment. In a severe case of complete dislocation of the vertebra above the 4th one, patient's life may be endangered at any time; severe complete dislocation of the vertebra below the 4th one may constrict the spinal cord resulting in high paraplegia. If the dislocation which has not yet caused damages to spinal cord is properly set and the constriction of the spinal cord is relieved , the functions of the vertebra can be restored.

Section V Subluxation of the Sacro-iliac Joint

The sacro-iliac joint, consisting of the sacrum and the auricular surface of the ilium, is connected and protected by strong ligaments all around it, and therefore, only when it is affected by a very strong violent force can subluxation or transposition of the joint occur.

● Causes and Pathogenesis

The condition is commonly caused by a transmitting violent force. For instance, when one falls from heights on one foot or hip, the downward body gravity and impaction meet with the upward reacting force from the foot or hip at the sacro-iliac joint to force the two bones to transposit there. In high jumping and basket-ball games, the body gravity on a descent together with the twisting violent force of the pelvis may also lead to sacro-iliac subluxation. A direct force acting on the posterosuperior margin of the ilium may also lead the ilium to an inward, upward or downward displacement.

In the late stage of pregnancy or shortly after child delivery, a woman's ligaments around the joint are rather loose because of the endocrine changes, whereupon a wrong body posture or a sudden turning of the upper body may also incur subluxation of the joint. People who bend a lot in their work or lift and carry heavy weight for many years may suffer from articular retrograde degeneration in the sacro-iliac joint, which is very likely to give rise to traumatic transposition.

● Clinical Manifestations and Diagnosis

After injury, there is local pain which worsens on standing, walking or bending the body, and tenderness in the sacro-iliac joint. The Petrick Test is positive, and there is remarkable local pain on pelvic compression and separation test.

In x-ray film of anteroposterior view, it can be found that the sacro-iliac joints on the two sides are asymmetrical and the ilium of the injured side displaces upward and inward (Fig. 8—9).

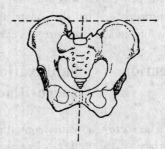

Fig. 8—9 Sketch map of subluxation of the sacro-iliac joint

● Treatment

The condition can be corrected

276

by manual reduction. The patient lies on his stomach. While an assistant grips the ankle of the injured side to perform downward traction and another assistant vigorously pushes the ischial tuberosity of the normal side upward with both hands overlapped, the operator presses the posterior superior iliac spine of the injured side forward and downward with both hands overlapped. The manipulations of the three should be well coordinated. Sometimes the sound characteristic of reposition may be heard. Finally the operator should press the sacro-iliac joint 3—4 times with a palm to stabilize it.

After the subluxation is corrected, the patient should confine himself to bed for 3 weeks.

At the early stage, the patient may take *Dieda Wan* or modified *Shujin Huoxue Tang* and apply *Quyu Xiaozhong Gao* externally. At the middle and late stages, *Bushen Zhuangjin Tang* and *Zhuangyao Jianshen Wan* should be prescribed to the patient for oral use and *Huoluo Gao* for external application.

● **Prognosis**

If corrected in time and treated with proper medicaments, the disease recovers well, but if it is not completely corrected, vague pain in the sacro-iliac joint may be the sequele.

Appendix

Index of Recipes

* All the recipes are arranged in the following way: (1) Name of the recipe in Chinese *pinyin*; (2) Name of the recipe in English; (3) Title of the book where the recipe was recorded, or other notes, in brackets. Take the first recipe for example:

(1)"*Angong Niuhuang Wan*" — Name of the recipe in Chinese *Pinyin*;

(2) "Cow-bezoar Bolus for Resurrection" — name of the recipe in English;

(3) "*Detailed Analysis of Epidemic Febrile Diseases*" — Title of the book where the recipe was recorded.

* * Each drug in a recipe is listed in English followed by its Latin name in brackets and often its exact or proportional dosage in the recipe.

Angong Niuhuang Wan — Cow-bezoar Bolus for Resurrection (from *Detailed Analysis of Epidemic Febrile Diseases*)

Ingredients:

cow-bezoar (*Calculus Bovis*)	4 portions
curcuma root (*Radix Curcumae*)	4 portions
coptis rhizome (*Rhizoma Coptidis*)	4 portions
scutellaria root (*Radix Scutellariae*)	4 portions
capejasmine fruit (*Fructus Gardeniae*)	4 portions
rhinoceros's horn (*Cornu Rhinocerotis*)	4 portions
realgar (*Realgar*)	4 portions
cinnabar (*Cinnabaris*)	4 portions
musk (*Moschus*)	1 portion
borneol (*Borneolum*)	1 portion
pearl (*Margarita*)	2 portions
honey (*Mel*)	proper amount

278

Efficacy and indications: Clearing away the heart fire, removing toxic substances, inducing resuscitation and tranquilizing the mind; used to treat unconsciousness, delirium, fever, mania, convulsion and syncope, and unconsciousness from intracerebral injury.

Preparation and administration: All the drugs are ground together into a very fine powder which is mixed with boiled honey to make boluses, 3g each; take 1 bolus a time, 1—3 times a day.

Baijiang Dan—White Sublimate Powder (from *The Golden Mirror of Medicine*)

Ingredients:

cinnabar (*Cinnabaris*)	6g
realgar (*Realgar*)	6g
mercury (*Hydragyrum*)	30g
borax (*Borax*)	15g
niter (*Natrii Nitras*)	45g
table salt (*Natrii Chloridum*)	45g
alum (*Alumen*)	45g
melanterite (*Melanteritum*)	45g

Efficacy and indications: Inducing erosion and removing pterygium, used for ruptured sores with difficulty in discharging pus and necrotic tissues, or fistula, pyogenic swollen sores resistant to rupture, warts, scrofula, etc. which have been treated with other drugs applied externally but without much effect.

Preparation and administration: Grind all the drugs into a fine powder. For a larger sore, 2g of the powder is mixed with water to paint the center of the sore, and for a smaller one, 0.6g. The powder can also be mixed with rice flour paste and rolled into very thin suppository which will be inserted into the ulcerative hole and then covered with a plaster.

Bali San—*Ba Li* Antibruise Powder (from *The Golden Mirror of Medicine*)
Ingredients:

279

pyrite (*Pyritum*)   (calcined) 10g
myrrh (*Myrrha*)   10g
frankincense (*Resina Olibani*)   10g
dragon's blood (*Resina Draconis*)   10g
safflower (*Flos Carthami*)   3g
sappan wood (*Lignum Sappan*)   3g
ancient copper coin   3g
clove (*Flos Garyophylli*)   1. 5g
musk (*Moschus*)   0. 3g
nux vomica (*Semen Strychni*)
                   (deep-fried and rid of the hairs) 3g

Efficacy and indications: Promoting the flow of *qi* to relieve pain and removing blood stasis to promote the reunion of broken bones; used for traumatic injuries.

Preparation and administration: All the drugs are ground together into a very fine powder, 0. 2—0. 3g (eight *li*) a time, taken orally with rice wine, 1—2 times a day.

Bazhen Tang — Decoction of Eight Precious Ingredients (from *Classification and Treatment of Traumatic Diseases*)

Ingredients:
dangshen (*Radix Codonopsis Pilosulae*)   10g
white atractylodes rhizome
        (*Rhizoma Atractylodis Macrocephalae*)   12g
poria (*Poria*)   12g
licorice root (*Radix Glycyrrhizae*) (*stir-fried*) 5g
Chinese angelica root (*Radix Angelicae Sinensis*) 10g
chuanxiong rhizome (*Rhizoma Ligustici Chuanxiong*) 6g
rehmannia root (*Radix Rehmanniae*) (Prepared)   12g
white peony root (*Radix Paeoniae Alba*)   12g
fresh ginger (*Rhizoma Zingiberis*)   3 slices
Chinese date (*Fructus Ziziphi Jujubae*)   2 pieces

Efficacy and indications: Invigorating *qi* and enriching blood; used at the middle and late stages of a traumatic injury with such signs and symptoms as deficiency of both *qi* and blood, watery and thin pus from the wound and protracted wound resistant to heal.

Preparation and administration: The drugs are decocted in water for an oral decoction, a dose a day.

Bujin Wan — Bolus for Strengthening Muscles (from *The Golden Mirror of Medicine*)

Ingredients:

eagle wood (*Lignum Aquilariae Resinatum*	30g
cloves (*Flos Caryophylli*)	30g
cyathula root	
(*Radix Cyathulae*)	30g
acanthopanax bark (*Cortex Acanthopanacis*)	30g
cnidium fruit (*Fructus Cnidii*)	30g
poria (*Poria*)	30g
lotus stamen (*Stamen Nelumbinis*)	30g
desertliving cistanche (*Herba Cistanches*)	30g
Chinese angelica root (*Radix Angelicae Sinensis*)	30g
prepared rehmannia root	
(*Radix Rehmanniae Praeparata*)	30g
moutan bark (*Cortex Moutan Radicis*)	30g
chaenomeles fruit (*Fructus Chaenomelis*)	30g
ginseng (*Radix Ginseng*)	9g
costus root (*Radix Aucklandiae*)	9g

Efficacy and indications: Strengthening the kidney and muscles, nourishing *qi* and blood and activating collaterals to relieve pain; used for traumatic injury and injury to muscles and tendons marked by cyanosis, swelling and pain due to blood stasis.

Bushen Huoxue Tang — Decoction Invigorating Kidney and Promoting Blood Circulation (from *A Great Collection on Traumatology*)

Ingredients:

prepared rehmannia root	
(*Radix Rehmanniae Praeparata*)	10g
eucommia bark (*Cortex Eucommiae*)	3g

wolfberry fruit (*Fructus Lycii*)	3g
malaytea scurfpea (*Flos Psoraleae*)	10g
dodder seed (*Semen Cuscutae*)	10g
Chinese angelica root (*Radix Angelicae Sinensis*)	3g
myrrh (*Myrrha*)	3g
dogwood fruit (*Flos Corni*)	3g
safflower (*Flos Carthami*)	2g
pubescent angelica root (*Radix Angelicae Pubescentis*)	3g
desertliving cistanche (*Herba Cistanchis*)	3g

Efficacy and indications: Invigorating kidney, strengthening muscles, promoting blood circulation and relieving pain; used in the treatment of various kinds of muscular distress and flaccidity at the late stage of an injury, especially the injury in the lumbar region.

Preparation and administration: Boil the drugs in water for an oral decoction.

Bushen Zhuangjin Tang (*Wan*) — Decoction or Pill for Strengthening Kidney and Muscles (from *Supplement to Traumatology*)

Ingredients:

prepared rehmannia root	
(*Radix Rehmanniae Praeparata*)	12g
Chinese angelica root (*Radix Angelicae Sinensis*)	12g
achyranthes root (*Radix Achyranthis Bidentatae*)	10g
dogwood fruit (*Flos Corni*)	12g
poria (*Poria*)	12g
teasel root (*Radix Dipsaci*)	12g
eucommia bark (*Cortex Eucommiae*)	10g
white peony root (*Radix Paeoniae Alba*)	10g
green tangerine peel	
(*Pericarpium Citri Reticulatae Viride*)	5g
acanthopanax bark (*Cortex Acathopanacis*)	10g

Efficacy and indications: Nourishing and invigorating kidney and liver, and strengthening muscles and bones; used to treat habitual articular dislocation due to insufficiency and impairment of kidney-

qi.

Preparation and administration: Boil all the drugs in water for an oral decoction, a dose a day; or prepare the drugs into pill for oral use.

Bushen Zhuangyang Tang—Decoction Reinforcing the Kidney and *Yang* (A proved recipe)

Ingredients:

prepared rehmannia root	
(*Radix Rehmanniae Praeparata*)	15g
ephedra (*Herba Ephedrae*)	3g
white mustard seed (*Semen Sinapis*)	3g
baked ginger (*Rhizoma Zingiberis Recens*)	6g
eucommia bark (*Cortex Eucommiae*)	12g
cibot rhizome (*Rhizoma Cibotii*)	12g
cinnamon bark (*Cortex Cinnamomi*)	6g
dodder seed (*Semen Cuscutae*)	12g
achyranthes root (*Radix Achyranthis Bidentatae*)	9g
teasel root (*Radix Dipsaci*)	9g
luffa (*Retinervus Luffae Fructus*)	6g

Efficacy and indications: Warming and clearing channels and collaterals and invigorating the liver and kidney; used for lumbar injury at the middle and late stages.

Preparation and administration: Boil the drugs in water for an oral decoction.

Bushun Xujin Wan—Bolus Promoting Reunion of Bone Fracture and Muscular Lesion (from *The Golden Mirror of Medicine*)

Ingredients:

Chinese angelica root (*Radix Angelicae Sinensis*)	25g
chuanxiong rhizome (*Rhizoma Ligustici Chuanxiong*)	15g
white peony root (*Radix Paeoniae Alba*) (*prepared*)	15g
prepared rehmannia root	
(*Radix Rehmanniae Praeparata*)	15g
costus root (*Radix Aucklandiae*)	25g

283

moutan bark (*Cortex Moutan Radicis*)	25g
frankincense (*Resina Olibani*)	25g
myrrh (*Myrrha*)	25g
drynaria rhizome (*Rhizoma Drynariae*)	15g
pyrite (*Pyritum*) (calcined)	15g
safflower (*Flos Carthami*)	15g
dragon's blood (*Resina Draconis*)	15g
cinnabar (*Cinnabaris*)	5g
clove (*Flos Caryophylli*)	5g
ginseng (*Radix Gingeng*)	50g
tiger bone (*Os Tigris*)	100g
ancient copper coin (tempered in vinegar)	3 pieces

Efficacy and indications: Promoting reunion of broken bones, injured muscles, ligaments and tendons, subduing swelling to relieve pain, increasing body resistance and tranquilizing the mind; used for traumatic injury with bone fracture, muscular lesion, opening wound with bleeding, persistent pain, etc.

Preparation and administration: All the drugs are ground together into fine powder which is mixed with boiled honey to make boluses, 10g each. Adults should take 10g (1 bolus) a time, 2—3 times a day.

Buyang Huanwu Tang—Decoction Invigorating *Yang* for Recuperation (from *Correction on Errors of Medical Works*)

Ingredients:

astragalus root (*Radix Astragali seu Hedysari*)	30g
Chinese angelica root (*Radix Angelicae Sinensis*)	6g
red peony root (*Radix Paeoniae Rubra*)	4.5g
earthworm (*Lumbricus*)	3g
chuanxiong rhizome (*Rhizoma Ligustici Chuanxion*)	3g
peach kernel (*Semen Persicae*)	3g
safflower (*Flos Carthami*)	3g

Efficacy and indications: Promoting blood circulation, replenishing *qi* and dredging the channels and collaterals; used for apoplexy and facial hemiparalysis caused by blood stagnation due to deficien-

cy of *qi*, and for traumatic paraplegia.
Preparation and administration: Boil all the drugs in water for an oral decoction.

Buzhong Yiqi Tang — Decoction for Reinforcing Middle-*jiao* and Replenishing *Qi* (from *Dongyuan's Ten Books*)
Ingredients:

astragalus root (*Radix Astragali seu Hedysari*)	15g
dangshen (*Radix Codonopsis Pilosulae*)	12g
white atractylodes rhizome	
(*Rhizoma Atractylodis Macrocephalae*)	12g
tangerine peel (*Pericarpium Citri Reticulatae*)	3g
licorice root (*Radix Glycyrrhizae*) (*prepared*)	5g
Chinese angelica root (*Radix Angelicae Sinensis*)	10g
cimicifuga rhizome (*Rhizoma Cimicifugae*)	5g
bupleurum root (*Radix Bupleuri*)	5g

Efficacy and indications: Invigorating the spleen and replenishing *qi*; used to treat morbid conditions due to deficiency of primordial *qi* resulting from chronic sores, or due to deficiency of *qi* of the middle-jiao resulting from consumption of *qi* and blood after injury.

Chaihu Shugan San — Bupleurum Powder for Relieving Liver-*qi* (from *Jingyue's Complete Works*)
Ingredients:
bupleurum root (*Radix Bupleuri*)
white peony root (*Radix Paeoniae Alba*)
bitter orange (*Fructus Aurantii*)
licorice root (*Radix Glycyrrhizae*)
chuanxiong rhizome (*Rhizoma Ligustici Chuanxiong*)
cyperus tuber (*Rhizoma Cyperi*)
Efficacy and indications: Soothing the liver and regulating the flow of *qi* and to ease pain; used in the treatment of injuries in the sternocostal region.
Preparation and administration: The dosage of the drugs in the

recipe should be fixed and the recipe itself may be modified according to the patient's actual condition. Boil the drugs in water for an oral decoction.

Da Chengqi Tang — Major Drastic Purgative Decoction (from *Treatise on Febrile Diseases*)
Ingredients:
  rhubarb (*Radix et Rhizoma Rhei*)
                    (decocted later than other drugs) 20g
  magnolia bark (*Cortex Magnoliae officinalis*)   15g
  immature bitter orange (*Fructus Aurantii Immaturus*) 15g
  mirabilite (*Natrii Sulphas*)
          (to be infused with the decoction of other drugs) 15g
Efficacy and indications: Eliminating the retained fluid by its drastic purgation; used in the treatment of abdominal distension with severe tenderness, tidal fever, inability to lie down due to dyspnea, constipation, etc. after traumatic injury.
Preparation and administration: The drugs are boiled in water for oral decoction and should be discontinued as soon as the symptoms are relieved.

Dacheng Tang — Decoction of Great Achievement (from *Secret Recipes of Treating Wound and Bone-setting Taught by Celestials*)
Ingredients:
  rhubarb (*Radix et Rhizoma Rhei*)   20g
  mirabilite (*Natrii Sulphas*) (*to be infused*)   10g
  Chinese angelica root (*Radix Angelicae Sinensis*)   10g
  manshurian aristolochia stem
          (*Caulis Aristolochiae Manshuriensis*)   10g
  bitter orange (*Fructus Aurantii*)   20g
  magnolia bark (*Cortex Magnoliae Officinalis*)   10g
  sappan wood (*Lignum Sappan*)   10g
  safflower (*Flos Carthami*)   10g
  tangerine peel (*Pericarpium Citri Reticulatae*)   10g
  licorice root (*Radix Glycyrrhizae*)   10g

Efficacy and indications: Removing blood stasis by catharsis; used in the treatment of accumulation of blood stasis in the interior, marked by soporous state, dysuria and constipation after a traumatic injury, or intestinal paralysis and abdominal distension after injury of the lumbar vertebrae.

Preparation and administration: The drugs are decocted for an oral dose. It should be discontinued as soon as dysuria and constipation are relieved.

Da Huoluo Dan—Major Bolus for Activating Energy Flow in the Channels and Collaterals (from *General Collection for Holly Relief*)

Ingredients:
white-spotted snake (*Agkistrodon Acustus*)
black-tailed snake (*Zaocys*)
clematis root (*Radix Clematidis*)
rhizome of radde anemone
        (*Rhizoma Anemones Raddeanae*)
wild aconite root (*Radix Aconiti Kusnezoffii*)
gastrodia tuber (*Rhizoma Gastrodiae*)
scorpion (*Scorpio*)
fleece flower root (*Radix Polygoni Multiflori*)
tortoise plastron (*Plastrum Testudinis*)
ephedra (*Herba Ephedrae*)
basket fern (*Rhizoma Dryopteris Crassirhizomae*)
licorice root (*Radix Glycyrrhizae*) (*stir-fried*)
notopterygium root (*Rhizoma seu Radix Notopterygii*)
cinnamon bark (*Cortex Cinnamomi*)
agastache (*Herba Agastachis*)
lindera root (*Radix Linderae*)
coptis rhizome (*Rhizoma Coptidis*)
rehmannia root (*Radix Rehmanniae*)
rhubarb (*Radix et Rhizoma Rhei*)
costus root (*Radix Aucklandiae*)
eaglewood(*Lignum Aquilariae Resinatum*)

asarum herb (*Herba Asari*)

red peony root (*Radix Paeoniae Rubra*)

myrrh (*Myrrha*)

clove (*Flos Caryophylli*)

frankincense (*Resina Olibani*)

batryticated silkworm (*Bombyx Batryticatus*)

arisaema tuber (*Rhizoma Arisaematis*)

green tangerine peel (*Pericarpium Citri Reticulatae Viride*)

drynaria rhizome (*Rhizoma Drynariae*)

round cardamon seed (*Semen Cardamoni Rotundi*)

benzoine (*Benzoinum*)

prepared daughter root of common monkshood

 (*Radix Aconiti lateralis Praeparata*)

scutellaria root (*Radix Scutellariae*)

poria (*Poria*)

cyperus tuber (*Rhizoma Cyperi*)

scrophulari root (*Radix Scrophulariae*)

white atractylodes rhizome

      (*Rhizoma Atractylodis Macrocephalae*)

Each of the above drugs 50g

ledebouriella root (*Radix Ledebouriellae*)	125g
pueraria root (*Radix Puerariae*)	75g
tiger's tibia (*Os Tigris*)	75g
Chinese angelica root (*Radix Angelicae Sinensis*)	75g
dragon's blood (*Resina Draconis*)	25g
earthworm (*Lumbricus*)	25g
rhinoceros horn (*Cornu Rhinocerotis*)	25g
musk (*Moschus*)	25g
rosin (*Colophonium*)	25g
cow bezoar (*Calculus Bovis*)	7.5g
borneo-camphor (*Borneo-camphora*)	7.5g
ginseng (*Radix Ginseng*)	150g
honey (*Mel*)	proper amount

Efficacy and indications: Promoting the flow of *qi* and circulation of blood and clearing and activating the channels and collaterals; used in the treatment of apoplexy with paralysis, flaccidity with cold limbs, spasm and pain, and muscular constricture and pain at the late stage of a traumatic injury.

Preparation and administration: All the drugs are ground into fine powder which is made into pellets by mixing it with boiled honey. Take 3g of the pellets each time with old rice wine, twice a day.

Daizhang Dan — Stick-replacing Bolus (from *Standards of Sore Medicine*)

Ingredients:
pyrolusite (*Pyrolusitum*)
myrrh (*Myrrha*)
frankincense (*Resina Olibani*)
earthworm (*Lumbricus*)
pyrite (*Pyritum*)
cochinchina memordica seed (*Semen Momordicae*)
                                                 All in equal amounts

Efficacy and indications: Removing blood stasis, promoting regeneration of tissues and alleviating pain; used in the treatment of various kinds of injuries.

Preparation and administration: Grind all the drugs into a fine powder; 1—3g of which is taken with warm boiled water or rice wine, 1—3 times a day; or the powder can also be mixed with boiled honey to make honeyed boluses, 5g each, one bolus a time, 1—2 times a day.

Danggui Buxue Tang—Chinese Angelica Decoction for Nourishing Blood (from *On Differentiation of Internal and Traumatic Diseases*)

Ingredients:
astragalus root (*Radix Astragali seu Hedysari*)   15—30g
Chinese angelica root (*Radix Angelicae Sinensis*)   3—6g

Efficacy and indications: Replenishing *qi* and benefiting hematopoiesis; used for fever due to deficiency of blood or syndrome of deficiency of both *qi* and blood after massive loss of blood manifested as hollow pulse which is forceless and empty when pressed by fingers.

Preparation and administration: The drugs are boiled in water for an oral decoction.

Dieda Wan—Bolus for Traumatic Injury (Original name *Junzhong Dieda Wan*—Bolus for Traumatic Injury of Armymen) (A proved recipe from *Dispensary of Traditional Chinese Drugs and Chinese Patent Medicine*)

Ingredients:

Chinese angelica root (*Radix Angelicae Sinensis*)	1 portion
ground beetle (*Eupolyphaga seu Steleophaga*)	1 portion
chuanxiong rhizome	
(*Rhizoma Ligustici Chuanxiong*)	1 portion
dragon's blood (*Resina Draconis*)	1 portion
myrrh (*Myrrha*)	1 portion
ephedra (*Herba Ephedrae*)	2 portions
pyrite (*Pyritum*)	2 portions
frankincense (*Resina Olibani*)	2 portions

Efficacy and indications: Promoting blood circulation to remove blood stasis and accelerating reunion of bones and muscles; used for traumatic injuries with complicated fracture and involvement of the heart due to blood stasis.

Preparation and administration: Pulverize all the drugs together into fine powder which is mixed with boiled honey to prepare boluses, 5g each; take 1—2 bolus(es) each time, 1—2 times a day.

Dieda Wanhua You—Oil From Innumerable Flowers for Traumatic Injury (also known simply as *Wanhua You*—Oil from Innumerable Flowers) (A proprietary)

Ingredients: Omitted.

Efficacy and indications: Inducing detumescense to relieve pain and removing toxic substances to relieve inflammation; used for traumatic injury with swelling and pain, burns, etc.

Preparation and administration: For external application; fill in a sterile container with the oil and then soak antiseptic gauze in the oil for a short while to apply directly to the affected site. If the gauze is applied on a wound, it should be changed daily and if on an injury without open wound, 1—3 days. When the gauze is applied on an unstable fracture fixed with small splints on top, it is unnecessary to unfasten the splints only for the sake of dressing change. The oil can be filled into the gap between splints to be absorbed by the gauze.

As liniment; rub the oil directly onto the affected part. It can also be used during massage.

Dieda Yangying Tang — Nutrition-increasing Decoction for Traumatic Injuries (from *Lin Rugao's Clinical Experience of Bone Setting*)

Ingredients:

 root of American ginseng (*Radix Panacis Quinquefolii*) 3g
 Or substituted with; dangshen
   (*Radix Codonopsis Pilosulae*)   15g
 astragalus root (*Radix Astragali seu Hedysari*)   9g
 Chinese angelica root (*Radix Angelicae Sinensis*)   6g
 chuanxiong rhizome (*Rhizoma Ligustici Chuanxiong*) 4.5g
 rehmannia root (*Radix Rehmanniae*)   (prepared) 15g
 white peony root (*Radix Paeoniae Alba*)   9g
 wolfberry fruit (*Fructus Lycii*)   15g
 Chinese yam (*Rhizoma Dioscoreae*)   15g
 teasel root (*Radix Dipsaci*)   9g
 amomum fruit (*Fructus Amomi*)   3g
 notoginseng (*Radix Notoginseng*)   4.5g
 malaytea scurfpea (*Fructus Psoraleae*)   9g
 drynaria rhizome (*Rhizoma Drynariae*)   9g
 chaenomeles fruit (*Fructus Chaenomelis*)   9g
 licorice root (*Radix Glycyrrhizae*)   3g

Efficacy and indications: Replenishing *qi* and blood, tonifying the liver and kidney and strengthening muscles and bones; used at the middle and late stages of bone fractures.

Preparation and administration: Boil the drugs in water for an oral decoction.

Ding Gui San — Clove and Cinnamon Powder (A proved recipe from *Textbook on Traumatology in Traditional Chinese Medicine*)

Ingredients:
    clove (*Flos Caryophylli*)
    cinnamon bark (*Cortex Cinnamomi*)

                             In equal amounts

Efficacy and indications: Expelling wind and cold and promoting the flow of *qi* by warming the channels; used for relieving pain of swelling and pyogenic sores of *yin* nature.

Preparation and administration: Both drugs are ground together into fine powder which is spread on a medicated plaster to be warmed with fire and applied on the affected spot.

Dingtong Gao — Pain-killing Ointment (from *Standards of Sore Medicine*)

Ingredients:

cottonrose hibiscus leaf (*Folium Hibisci*)	4 portions
Chinese redbud bark (*Cortex Cercis Chinesis*)	1 portion
pubescent angelica root	
(*Radix Angelicae Pubescentis*)	1 portion
arisaema tuber (*Rhizoma Arisaematis*)	1 portion
dahurian angelica root	
(*Radix Angelicae Dahuricae*)	1 portion

Efficacy and indications: Dispelling wind and subduing swelling to relieve pain; used to relieve swelling pain of traumatic injuries and of sores at early stage.

Preparation and administration: The drugs are ground together into fine powder which is mixed with ginger juice, water and rice wine. The mixture is boiled hot for external application. The powder can also be mixed and boiled together with vaseline into an ointment for external application.

292

Dingtong Hexue Tang—Decoction for Regulating Blood Flow and Killing Pain (from *Supplement to Traumatology*)
Ingredients:
  peach kernel (*Semen Persicae*)
  safflower (*Flos Carthami*)
  frankincense (*Resina Olibani*)
  myrrh (*Myrrha*)
  Chinese angelica root (*Radix Angelicae Sinensis*)
  large-leaf gentian root (*Radix Gentianae Macrophyllae*)
  teasel root (*Radix Dipsaci*)
  cat-tail pollen (*Pollen Typhae*)
  trogopterus dung (*Faeces Trogopterorum*)
Efficacy and indications: Regulating and tonifying blood to kill pain; used for injuries in any part with blood stasis and pain.
Preparation and administration: The drugs are boiled in the mixture of water and rice wine in equal amount for an oral dose.

Dushen Tang—Decoction of Ginseng Alone (from *Jingyue's Complete Works*)
Ingredients:
  ginseng (*Radix Ginseng*)   10—20g
Efficacy and indications: Replenishing *qi*, keeping the blood flowing within the vessels and rescuing patient from collapse; used for critical emergent condition marked by restlessness of deficiency type, thirst and collapse due to severe deficiency and exhaustion of *qi*, blood and *yang* as a result of hemorrhage.
Preparation and administration: Boil ginseng in water with slow fire for an oral decoction. In recent years, injection prepared from it is available.

Erhao Xiyao—No. 2 Lotion Recipe (A proved recipe)
Ingredients:
  sichuan aconite root (*Radix Aconiti*)
  wild aconite root (*Radix Aconiti kusnazoffii*)

293

peppertree pricklyash peel (*Pericarpium Zanthoxyli*)
argyi leaf (*Folium Artemisiae Argyi*)
atractylodes rhizome (*Rhizoma Atractylodis*)
pubescent angelica root (*Radix Angelicae Pubescentis*)
cinnamon twig (*Ramulus Cinnamomi*)
ledebouriella root (*Radix Ledebouriellae*)
safflower (*Flos Carthami*)
Chinese siphonostegia (*Herba Siphonostegiae*)
tuberculate speranskia (*Herba Speranskiae Tuberculatae*)
buck grass (*Herba Lycopodii*)

Each of the above drugs 9g

Efficacy and indications: Warming the channels to expel pathogenic cold, relieving rigidity of the muscles, removing obstruction in the collaterals and promoting blood circulation to relieve pain; used at the late stage of a traumatic injury.

Preparation and administration: All the drugs are boiled for a hot lotion used to bathe the injured part.

Fuyuan Huoxue Tang — Decoction for Recovery and Activating Blood Circulation (from *Medical Inventions*)

Ingredients:

bupleurum root (*Radix Bupleuri*)	15g
trichosanthes root (*Radix Trichosanthis*)	10g
Chinese angelica root (*Radix Angelicae Sinensis*)	10g
safflower (*Flos Carthami*)	6g
pangolin scales (*Aquama Manitis*)	10g
rhubarb (*Radix et Rhizoma Rhei*)	

(cured with rice wine) 30g

peach kernel (*Semen persicae*) (cured with rice wine) 12g

Efficacy and indications: Promoting blood circulation to remove blood stasis, and subduing swelling to relieve pain; used for traumatic injury marked by stagnation and accumulation of blood in the hypochondria with unbearable swelling pains.

Preparation and administration: Boil the drugs in water for a decoction which should be taken orally in two times. After the first intake, if the patient has loosed his bowels with his discomforts and pain alleviated, save the remaining decoction, otherwise, he should take the second portion six hours after the first intake.

Gexia Zhuyu Tang—Decoction for Dissipating Blood Stasis Under Diaphragm (from *Correction on the Errors of Medical Works*)
Ingredients:

Chinese angelica root (*Radix Angelicae Sinensis*)	9g
chuanxiong rhizome (*Rhizoma Ligustici Chuanxiong*)	6g
red peony root (*Radix Paeoniae Rubra*)	9g
peach kernel (*Semen Persicae*)	9g
safflower (*Flos Carthami*)	6g
bitter orange (*Fructus Aurantii*)	5g
moutan bark (*Cortex Moutan Radicis*)	9g
cyperus tuber (*Rhizoma Cyperi*)	9g
corydalis tuber (*Rhizoma Corydalis*)	12g
lindera root (*Radix Linderae*)	9g
trogopterus dung (*Faeces Trogopterorum*)	9g
licorice root (*Radix Glycyrrhizae*)	5g

Efficacy and indications: Promoting blood circulation to remove blood stasis; used in the treatment of abdominal injury with accumulation of stagnant blood and pain. Preparation and administration: Boil the drugs in water for an oral dose.

Goupi Gao—Dog-hide Plaster (A proprietary)
Ingredients: Omitted.
Efficacy and indications: Dispelling pathogenic cold to relieve pain, relaxing muscles and tendons and activating the flow of *qi* in the collaterals; used for traumatic injury and arthralgia due to pathogenic wind-cold-dampness.
Preparation and administration: Heat the plaster and apply it on the affected site.

Guipi Tang—Decoction for Invigorating the Spleen and Nourishing the Heart (from *Recipes for Succouring the Sick*)

Ingredients:

white atractylodes rhizome
      (*Rhizoma Atractylodis Macrocephalae*)   10g
Chinese angelica root (*Radix Angelicae sinensis*)   3g
dangshen (*Radix Codonopsis Pilosulae*)   3g
astragalus root (*Radix Astragali seu Hedysari*)   10g
wild jujube seed (*Semen Ziziphi Spinosae*)   10g
costus root (*Radix Aucklandiae*)   1.5g
polygala root (*Radix Polygalae*)   3g
licorice root (*Radix Glycyrrhizae*)   (prepared) 4.5g
longan aril(*Arillus Longan*)   4.5g
poria (*Poria*)   10g

Efficacy and indications: Nourishing the heart, strengthening the spleen and replenishing *qi* and blood; used in the treatment of deficiency of *qi* and blood at the late stage of a bone fracture, neurasthenia, chronic ulcer, etc.

Preparation and administration: Decoct the drugs in water for oral use, a dose a day. Boluses may also be prepared from the drugs for oral use.

Guishe San—Powder of Cinnamon and Musk (from *Revealation of Medical Secrets*)

Ingredients:

ephedra (*Herba Ephedrae*)   15g
asarum herb (*Herba Asari*)   15g
cinnamon bark (*Cortex Cinnamomi*)   30g
abnormal fruit of Chinese honeylocust
      (*Fructus Gleditsiae Abnormalis*)   10g
pinellia tuber (*Rhizoma pinelliae*)   25g
cloves (*Flos Caryophylli*)   30g
arisaema tuber (*Rhizoma Arisaematis*)   25g
musk (*Moschus*)   1.8g
borneol (*Borneolum*)   1.2g

Efficacy and indications: Warming and resolving phlegm and dampness, and subduing swelling to alleviate pain; used to treat

296

unruptured sores of *yin* type.

Preparation and administration: All the drugs are ground into fine powder which is spread on a hot plaster to be applied on the affected site.

Guke Waixi Erfang — No. 2 Lotion Recipe for Bone Injury (A proved recipe from *Traumatology*)

Ingredients:

cinnamon twig (*Ramulus Cinnamomi*)	15g
clematis root (*Radix Clematidis*)	15g
ledebouriella root (*Radix Ledebouriellae*)	15g
acanthopanax bark (*Cortex Acanthopanacis*)	15g
asarum herb (*Herba Asari*)	10g
schizonepeta (*Herba Schizonepetae*)	10g
myrrh (*Myrrha*)	10g

Efficacy and indications: Promoting blood circulation to remove obstruction in the channels and collaterals and expelling wind to relieve pain; used to relieve cold-pain and joint dyskinesia of the limbs at the late stage of trauma, and arthralgia syndrome with pain that is aggravated upon cold stimulation but alleviated by warmth.

Preparation and administration: Boil the drugs in water for a lotion to fumigate and bathe the affected parts. Limbs can be immersed in the lotion and the trunk parts can be covered and rubbed with hot towel soaked with the lotion. Care should be taken that the temperature of the lotion should not be too high so as to avoid skin burn.

Gushang Waixi Yifang — No. 1 Lotion Recipe for Bone Injury (A proved recipe from *Traumatology*)

Ingredients:

treebine stem (*Caulis Cissi*)	30g
uncaria stem with hooks	
(*Ramulus Uncariae cum Uncis*)	30g
Honeysuckle stem (*Caulis Lonicerae*)	30g

vaccaria seed (*Semen Vaccariae*)	30g
Chinese siphonostegia (*Herba Siphonostegiae*)	15g
ledebouriella root (*Radix Ledebouriellae*)	15g
rhubarb (*Radix et Rhizoma Rhei*)	15g
schizonepeta (*Herba Schizonepetae*)	10g

Efficacy and indications: Promoting blood circulation to remove obstruction in the channels and relieving rigidity of muscles to ease pain; effective for clonic spasm of muscles, undesirable articular function, aching and numbness resulting from trauma, or pain due to exopathogenic wind-dampness, used at the middle and late stages of a complicated fracture or when the external fixation is removed and the patient can do functional exercises, after an orthopedic operation.

Preparation and administration: Boil the drugs in water for a lotion to be used for fumigating and bathing the diseased part.

Guzhi Zengsheng Wan—Bolus for Hyperosteogeny (from *Traumatology*)

Ingredients:

prepared rehmannia root	
(*Radix Rehmanniae Praeparata*)	60g
spatholobus stem (*Caulis Spatholobi*)	45g
drynaria rhizome (*Rhizoma Drynariae*)	45g
desertliving cistanche (*Herba Cistanchis*)	30g
pyrola herb (*Herba Pyrolae*)	30g
epimedium (*Herba Epimedii*)	30g
radish seed (*Semen Raphani*)	15g

Efficacy and indications: Tonifying blood, relaxing muscles and strengthening bone; used in the treatment of hypertrofic spondylitis, cervical spondylopathy, joint mouse, osseous spur, calcanodynia and constant distress and pain of incompletely restored bone and muscle injury.

Preparation and administration: All the drugs are ground together into fine powder which is mixed with boiled honey to prepare boluses, 9g each. Take 1—2 bolus(es) a time, 2—3 times a day.

Haitongpi Tang—Decoction of Erythrina Bark (from *The Golden Mirror of Medicine*)
Ingredients:

erythrina bark (*Cortex Erythrinae*)	6g
tuberculate speranshia (*Herba Speranshiae Tuberculatae*)	6g
frankincense (*Resina Olibani*)	6g
myrrh (*Myrrha*)	6g
Chinese angelica root (*Radix Angelicae Sinensis*)	5g
peppertree pricklyash peel (*Pericarpium Zanthoxyli*)	10g
chuanxiong rhizome (*Rhizoma ligustici Chuanxiong*)	3g
safflower (*Flos Carthami*)	3g
clematis root (*Radix Clematidis*)	3g
licorice root (*Radix Glycyrrhizae*)	3g
ledebouriella root (*Radix ledebouriellae*)	3g
dahurian angelica root (*Radix Anglicae Dahuricae*)	2g

Efficacy and indications: Activating collaterals to relieve pain; used to ease pain from traumatic injury.

Preparation and administration: All the drugs are ground together into fine powder which is put into a cloth bag and boiled in water for a decoction to be used for fumigation and bathing of the affected site or to be taken orally.

Heying Zhitong Tang—Decoction for Regulating the Nutrient System and Relieving Pain (from *Supplement to Traumatology*)
Ingredients:

red peony root (*Radix Paeoniae Rubra*)	9g
Chinese angelica root (*Radix Angelicae Sinensis*)	9g
chuanxiong rhizome (*Rhizoma Ligustici Chuanxiong*)	6g
sappan wood (*Lignum Sappan*)	6g
teasel root (*Radix Dipsaci*)	12g
lindera root (*Radix Linderae*)	9g
frankincense (*Resina Olibani*)	6g
myrrh (*Myrrha*)	6g

manshurian aristolochia stem

    (*Caulis Aristolochiae Manshuriensis*)   6g

licorice root (*Radix Glycyrrhizae*)   6g

Efficacy and indications: Promoting blood circulation to relieve pain and removing blood stasis to promote granulation; used for swelling, hematoma and pain from injury.

Preparation and administration: Boil the drugs in water for an oral intake.

Honghua Jiu—Safflower Tincture (A proved recipe)

Ingredients:

Chinese angelica root (*Radix Angelicae Sinensis*)   12g

safflower (*Flos Carthami*)   15g

red peony root (*Radix Paeoniae Rubra*)   12g

arnebia or lithosperm root

    (*Radix Arnebiae seu Lithospermi*)   9g

60% alcohol solution   500ml

Efficacy and indications: Clearing and activating the channels and collaterals; used to prevent bed sores.

Preparation and administration: Immerse the drugs in the alcohol solution for 4—5 days. The tincture is used as a liniment for massage.

Hongsheng Dan—Red Sublimate Powder (from *A Golden Mirror of Medicine*)

Ingredients:

realgar (*Realgar*)   15g

cinnabar (*Cinnabaris*)   15g

melanterite (*Melanteritum*)   18g

mercury (*Hydrargyrum*)   30g

alum (*Alumen*)   30g

niter (*Natrii Nitras*)   120g

Efficacy and indications: Promoting the discharge of pus and necrotic tissues; used for ulcerative sores with difficulty in casting the necrotic tissues.

Preparation and administration: After grinding cinnabar, realgar, nitre, alum and melanterite into powder, add in mercury and grind well. Pour the mixture into a cauldron, spread it out evenly, and melt it with slow fire till it becomes a pancake-like layer which sticks to the cauldron. When it is dry and cool, cover the cauldron with a big bowl. The seam at the place where the brim of the bowl meets the wall of the cauldron should be filled in with wet tissue paper and sealed up with the mixture of vinegar and calcined gypsum powder. Fill in the base concave of the bowl with fine sand, place a cotton ball in the sand and lay two pieces of thick bricks on it. Then heat the cauldron with slow, medium and quick fire in turn for 2—3 hours, and keep observation on the color change of the cotton ball. When it turns to yellowish-black, extinguish the fire. After the cauldron becomes cool, remove the bowl to collect the sublimate crystalline substance and grind it into fine powder. Each time a little powder is spread on the surface of the wound.

Huajian Gao — Tissue-softening Plaster (A proved recipe from *Textbook on Traumatology of Traditional Chinese Medicine*)

Ingredients:

white mustard seed (*Semen Sinapis*)	2 portions
kansui root (*Radix Euphorbiae Kansui*)	2 portions
earthworm (*Lumbricus*)	2 portions
clematis root (*Radix Clematidis*)	2.5 portions
garden balsam seed (*Semen Impatientis*)	2.5 portions
tuberculate speranskia	
(*Herba Speranskiae Tuberculatae*)	2 portions
hemp root (*Radix Cinnabis*)	3 portions
asarum herb (*Herba Asari*)	3 portions
black plum (*Fructus Mume*)	4 portions
pangolin scale (*Aquama Manitis*)	4 portions
carbonized hair (*Crinis Carbonisatus*)	1 portion
croton seed (*Fructus Crotonis*)	1 portion
scorpion (*Scorpio*)	1 portion
ledebouriella root (*Radix Ledebouriellae*)	1 portion

wild aconite root (*Radix Aconiti Kusnezoffii*)	1 portion
purplish sal ammoniac	
(*Sal Ammoniaci Purpurati*)	0. 5 portion
sesame oil (*Oleum Sesami*)	80 portions
red lead (*Minium*)	40 portions

Efficacy and indications: Expelling wind and removing blood stasis; used to relieve sclerosis or adhesion of soft tissues at the late stage of a traumatic injury.

Preparation and administration: Boil all the drugs in the sesame oil till the drugs are exhausted, filter to collect the oil, which is then boiled and concentrated till a drop of it can stay on a surface like a bead. Then add in red lead, churn till no smoke, add in purplish sal ammoniac and churn thoroughly.

Hualeishi San—Ophicalcite Powder (from *Formularies of the Bureau of Pharmacy*)

Ingredients:

| ophicalcite (*Ophicalcitum*) | 1 portion |
| sulfur (*Sulfur*) | 2 portions |

Efficacy and indications: Removing blood stasis and inducing hemo-stasis; used to arrest traumatic hemorrhage.

Preparation and administration: Calcine the drugs together in an earthen pot and then grind them into fine powder. When needed the powder is dusted on the wound prior to bandaging.

Huixiang Jiu — Common Fennel Spirit (A proved recipe from *Textbook on Traumatology of Traditional Chinese Medicine*)

Ingredients:

common fennel fruit (*Fructus Foeniculi*)	15g
cloves (*Flos Caryophylli*)	10g
camphor (*Camphora*)	15g
safflower (*Flos Carthami*)	10g
strong spirit	300g

Efficacy and indications: promoting blood circulation and flow of *qi* to relieve pain; used to ease the swelling pain of sprain or contusion.

Preparation and administration: Immerse all the drugs in the liquor for a week and then filter to collect the tincture which is used to rub the affected part. It can also be used during the manipulation of an injury.

Huoxue Jiu — Medicated Spirit for Promoting Blood Circulation (from *A General Introduction to the Clinical Experience of Bonesetting of Traditional Chinese Medicine*)

Ingredients:

powder for promoting blood circulation	15g
spirit	500g

Efficacy and indications: Removing obstruction in channels and promoting blood circulation; used to relieve pains in the lumbar region and lower extremities chiefly due to cold and dampness left over by old sprain and contusion injury.

Preparation and administration: Soak the powder in the liquor for 7—10 days and drink the liquor.

Huoxue Quyu Pian — Tablet for Activating Blood Circulation and Removing Blood Stasis (A proved recipe)

Ingredients:

dragon's blood (*Resina Draconis*)	30g
(If not available, it can be substituted by 45g of Chinese siphonostegia, *Herba Siphonostegiae*)	
Chinese angelica root (*Radix Angelicae Sinensis*)	30g
red peony root (*Radix Paeoniae Rubra*)	30g
peach kernel (*Semen Persicae*)	24g
safflower (*Flos Carthami*)	24g
pangolin scales (*Squama Manitis*)	24g
notopterygium root (*Rhizoma seu Radix Notopterygii*)	30g
pyrolusite (*Pyrolusitum*) (prepared)	60g
costus root (*Radix Aucklandiae*)	24g
clove (*Flos Caryophylli*)	15g
rhubarb (*Radix et Rhizoma Rhei*)	15g

ground beetle (*Eupolyphaga seu Steleophaga*)   24g
Chinese Honeylocust spine (*Spina Gleditsiae*)   24g
Efficacy and indications: Promoting blood circulation to remove obstruction in channels and collaterals and removing blood stasis to subdue swelling.
Preparation and administration: Prepare the drugs into tablets in the conventional way, each tablet weighing 0. 3g; 8—10 tablets a time for oral administration, 2—3 times a day.

Huoxue Quyu Tang — Decoction for Activating Blood Circulation and Removing Blood Stasis (A proved recipe)
Ingredients:
Chinese angelica root (*Radix Angelicae Sinensis*)   15g
safflower (*Flos Carthami*)   6g
ground beetle (*Eupolyphaga seu Steleophaga*)   9g
pyrite (*Pyritum*)   9g
cibot rhizome (*Rhizoma Cibotii*)   9g
drynaria rhizome (*Rhizoma Drynariae*)   15g
myrrh (*Myrrha*)   6g
frankincense (*Resina Olibani*)   6g
notoginseng (*Radix Notoginseng*)   3g
sweetgum fruit (*Fructus Liquidambaris*)   6g
peach kernel (*Semen Persicae*)   9g
Efficacy and indications: Promoting blood circulation to remove blood stasis, removing obstruction of the collaterals to accelerate subsidence of swelling, and promoting reunion of broken bones, muscles and tendons; used at the early stage of a fracture with soft tissue injury.
Preparation and administration: Boil the drugs in water for an oral decoction, a dose a day.

Huoxue San — Powder Promoting Blood Circulation (from *Introduction to Clinical Experience of Bone Setting in Traditional Chinese Medicine*)
Ingredients:

304

frankincense (*Resina Olibani*) 15g
myrrh (*Myrrha*) 15g
dragon's blood (*Resina Draconis*) 15g
fritillary bulb (*Bulbus Fritillariae*) 9g
notopterygium root (*Rhizoma seu Radix Notopterygii*) 15g
costus root (*Radix Aucklandiae*) 6g
magnolia bark (*Cortex Magnoliae Officinalis*) 9g
sichuan aconite root (*Radix Aconiti*)   (prepared) 3g
wild aconite root (*Radix Aconiti Kusnezoffii*)
(prepared) 3g
dahurian angelica root (*Radix Angelicae Dahuricae*) 24g
musk (*Moschus*) 1.5g
Chinese redbud bark (*Cortex Cercis Chinensis*) 24g
cyperus tuber (*Rhizoma Cyperi*) 15g
common fennel fruit (*Fructus Foeniculi*)   (roasted) 9g
pangolin scale (*Aquama Manitis*) 15g
pyrite (*Pyritum*)   (calcined) 15g
pubescent angelica root (*Radix Angelicae Pubescentis*) 15g
teasel root (*Radix Dipsaci*) 15g
tiger bone (*Os Tigris*) 15g
chuanxiong rhizome (*Rhizoma Ligustici Chuanxiong*) 15g
chaenomeles fruit (*Fructus Chaenomelis*) 15g
cinnamon bark (*Cortex Cinnamomi*) 9g
Chinese angelica root (*Radix Angelicae Sinensis*) 24g

Efficacy and indications: promoting blood circulation, relaxing muscles and regulating flow of *qi* to relieve pain; used for traumatic injuries with ecchymoma and pain, or for a prolonged wound resistant to heal.

Preparation and administration: All the drugs are ground together into fine powder which is mixed with boiled water into a paste for external application on the affected site.

Huoxue Shujin Tang — Decoction for Promoting Blood Circulation and Relaxing Muscles (from *Textbook on Traumatology of Traditional Chinese Medicine*)

Ingredients:

Chinese angelica root (*Radix Angelicae Sinensis*)
red peony root (*Radix Paeoniae Rubra*)
turmeria (*Rhizoma Curcumae Wenyjin*)
buck grass (*Herba Lycopodii*)
nedular branch of pine (*Lignum Pini Nodi*)
erythrina bark (*Cortex Erythrinae*)
herb of asiatic pennywort (*Herba Centellae*)
sweetgum fruit (*Fructus Liquidambaris*)
notopterygium root (*Rhizoma seu Radix Notopterygii*)
pubescent angelica root (*Radix Angelicae Pubescentis*)
ledebouriella root (*Radix Ledebouriellae*)
teasel root (*Radix Dipsaci*)
licorice root (*Radix Glycyrrhizae*)

On the basis of the above prescription, following drugs may be added for troubles in the upper limbs:

chuanxiong rhizome (*Rhizoma Ligustici Chuanxiong*)
cinnamon bark (*Cortex Cinnamomi*)

Or the following two drugs for troubles in the lower extremities:

achyranthes root (*Radix Achranthis Bidentatae*)
costus root (*Radix Aucklandiae*)

Or the following drugs for troubles with severe pain:

frankincense (*Resina Olibani*)
myrrh (*Myrrha*)

Efficacy and indications: Promoting blood circulation, removing blood stasis, relaxing muscular tissues and removing obstruction in collaterals; used for injuries of muscles, ligaments and tendons swelling pain in joints and dysfunction of articular motion.

Preparation and administration: Boil the drugs in water for an oral decoction.

Huoxue Tang — Decoction for Activating Blood Circulation (A proved recipe)

Ingredients:

306

bupleurum root (*Radix Bupleuri*)　　　　　　　　6g
Chinese angelica root (*Radix Angelicae Sinensis*)　　9g
red peony root (*Radix Paeoniae Rubra*)　　　　　9g
peach kernel (*Semen Persicae*)　　　　　　　　9g
spatholobus stem (*Caulis Spatholobi*)　　　　　15g
bitter orange (*Fructus Aurantii*)　　　　　　　9g
safflower (*Flos Carthami*)　　　　　　　　　　5g
dragon's blood (*Resina Draconis*)　　　　　　　3g

Efficacy and indications: Promoting blood circulation to remove blood stasis and subduing swelling to alleviate pain; used at the early stage of bone fractures.

Preparation and administration: Boil the drugs in water for an oral dose.

Huoxue Zhitong San—Powder for Promoting Blood Circulation to Relieve Pain (A proved recipe)

Ingredients:

Chinese angelica root (*Radix Angelicae Sinensis*)　　15g
safflower (*Flos Carthami*)　　　　　　　　　　15g
sappan wood (*Lignum Sappan*)　　　　　　　　15g
dahurian angelica root (*Radix Angelicae Dahuricae*)　15g
turmeria (*Rhizoma Curcumae Longae*)　　　　　15g
clematis root (*Radix Clematidis*)　　　　　　　15g
notopterygium root (*Rhizoma seu Radix Notopterygii*) 15g
acanthopanax bark (*Cortex Acanthopanacis*)　　　15g
erythrina bark (*Cortex Erythrinae*)　　　　　　15g
achyranthes root (*Radix Achyranthis Bidentatae*)　15g
Sichuan chinaberry (*Fructus Meliae Toosendan*)　　15g
Rhizome of glabrous greenbrier
　　　(*Rhizoma Smilacis Glabrae*)　　　　　　　15g
frankincense (*Resina Olibani*)　　　　　　　　6g
peppertree pricklyash peel (*Pericarpium Zanthoxyli*)　9g
tuberculate speranskia
　　　(*Herba Speranskiae Tuberculatae*)　　　　30g

Efficacy and indications: Promoting blood stasis, relaxing muscles and removing obstruction in collaterals to relieve pain.

Preparation and administration: Decoct the drugs in water for a lotion to bathe the affected part.

Huoxue Zhitong Tang — Decoction for Promoting Blood Circulation to Relieve Pain (from *A Great Collection on Traumatology*)

Ingredients:

Chinese angelica root (*Radix Angelicae Sinensis*)	12g
chuanxiong rhizome (*Rhizoma Ligustici Chuanxiong*)	6g
frankincense (*Resina Olibani*)	6g
sappan wood (*Lignum Sappan*)	5g
safflower (*Flos Carthami*)	6g
myrrh (*Myrrha*)	6g
ground beetle (*Eupolyphaga seu Steleophaga*)	3g
notoginseng (*Radix Notoginseng*)	3g
red peony root (*Radix Paeoniae Rubra*)	9g
tangerine peel (*Pericarpium Citri Reticulatae*)	5g
Herb of asiatic pennywort (*Herba Centellae*)	6g
Chinese redbud stem (*Lignum Cercis Chinensis*)	9g

Efficacy and indications: Promoting blood circulation to relieve pain; used for traumatic injury with swelling pain.

Preparation and administration: Boil the drugs in water for an oral decoction.

Huoxue Wan — Bolus for Promoting Blood Circulation (A proved recipe)

Ingredients:

ground beetle (*Eupolyphaga seu Steleophaga*)	5 portions
dragon's blood (*Resina Draconis*)	3 portions
saffron (*Stigma Croci*)	1 portion
frankincense (*Resina Olibani*)	3 portions
myrrh (*Myrrha*)	3 portions
achyranthes root (*Radix Achyranthis Bidentatae*)	2 portions
dahurian angelica root	

(*Radix Angelicae Dahuricae*)	2 portions
catechu (*Catechu*)	2 portions
drynaria rhizome (*Rhizoma Drynariae*)	2 portions
eucommia bark (*Cortex Eucommiae*)	3 portions
teasel root (*Radix Dipsaci*)	3 portions
sappan wood (*Lignum Sappan*)	3 portions
dried rehmannia root (*Radix Rehmanniae*)	3 portions
Chinese angelica root	
(*Radix Angelicae Sinensis*)	5 portions
chuanxiong rhizome	
(*Rhizoma Ligustici Chuanxiong*)	2 portions
pyrite (*Pyritum*)	2 portions
peach kernel (*Semen Persicae*)	2 portions
rhubarb (*Radix et Rhizoma Rhei*)	2 portions
nux-vomica seed (*Semen Strychni*)	2 portions
cinnabar (*Cinnabaris*)	1 portion
borneol (*Borneolum*)	2 portions
honey (*Mel*)	proper amount

Efficacy and indications: Promoting blood circulation to remove blood stasis and subduing swelling to relieve pain; effective for traumatic injury with pain caused by ecchymoma, used at the early and middle stages of bone fracture and other traumatic injuries.

Preparation and administration: Prepare all the drugs into fine powder which is mixed with boiled honey to make boluses, 5g each. One bolus a time for oral administration, 2—3 times a day.

Jianbu Huqian Wan — Pill for Restoring Vigorous Steps (from *Supplement to Traumatology*)

Ingredients:

tortoise plastron glue (*Colla Plastri Testudinis*)	2 portions
antler glue (*Colla Cornus Cervi*)	2 portions
fleece-flower root	
(*Radix Polygoni Multiflori*)	2 portions
cyathula root (*Radix Cyathulae*)	2 portions
eucommia bark (*Cortex Eucommiae*)	2 portions

309

cynomorium (*Herba Cynomorii*)	2 portions
Chinese angelica root	
(*Radix Angelicae Sinensis*)	2 portions
rehmannia root (*Radix Rehmanniae*)	
(prepared)	2 portions
phellodendron bark (*Cortex Phellodendri*)	1 portion
ginseng (*Radix Ginseng*)	1 portion
notopterygium root	
(*Rhizoma seu Radix Notopterygii*)	1 portion
white peony root (*Radix Paeoniae Alba*)	1 portion
white atractylodes rhizome	
(*Rhizoma Atractylodis Macrocephalae*)	1 portion
prepared daughter root of common monkshood	
(*Radix Aconiti Preparata*)	1.5 portion
Honey (*Mel*)	proper amount

Efficacy and indications: Invigorating *qi*, tonifying blood and strengthening muscle and bone; used when there is deficiency of *qi* and blood, flaccidity of extremities and difficulty in walking.

Preparation and administration: All the drugs are ground together into fine powder which is mixed with boiled honey to make pills as big as a mung bean. Take 10g of the pills with saline water of low concentration on an empty stomach, 2—3 times a day.

Jianpi Yangwei Tang — Decoction for Invigorating the Spleen and Stomach (from *Supplement to Traumatology*)

Ingredients:

ginseng (*Radix Ginseng*)

white atractylodes rhizome
(*Rhizoma Atractylodis Macrocephalae*)

astragalus root (*Radix Astragali seu Hedysari*)

Chinese angelica root (*Radix Angelicae Sinensis*)

white peony root (*Radix Paeoniae Alba*)

tangerine peel (*Pericarpium Citri Reticulatae*)

common fennel fruit (*Fructus Foeniculi*)

Chinese yam (*Rhizoma Dioscoreae*)

310

poria (*Poria*)

water-plantain rhizome (*Rhizoma Alismatis*)

Efficacy and indications: Invigorating the spleen and stomach; used for abdominal distension and poor appetite due to weakness of the spleen and stomach.

Preparation and administration: Boil the drugs in water for an oral decoction.

Jiawei Guipi Tang — Modified Decoction for Invigorating the Spleen and Nourishing the Heart (from *Classification and Treatment of Traumatic Diseases*)

Ingredients:

white atractylodes rhizome	
(*Rhizoma Atractylodis Macrocephalae*)	3g
Chinese angelica root (*Radix Angelicae Sinensis*)	3g
poria (*Poria*)	3g
astragalus root (*Radix Astragali seu Hedysari*)	3g
longan aril (*Arillus Longan*)	3g
wild jujube seed (*Semen Ziziphi Spinosae*)	3g
polygala root (*Radix Polygalae*)	3g
costus root (*Radix Aucklandiae*)	1.3g
licorice root (*Radix Glycyrrhizae*)	1g
bupleurum root (*Radix Bupleuri*)	3g
capejasmine fruit (*Fructus Gardeniae*)	3g
ginseng (*Radix Ginseng*)	3g

Efficacy and indications: Invigorating the spleen; tranquilizing the mind and relieving the depressed liver to regulate the circulation of *qi*; used for indisposition in the chest and abdomen, anorexia and insomnia due to stagnation of the liver-*qi*.

Preparation and administration: Boil the drugs in water with due amount of ginger and Chinese date for an oral decoction.

Jiedu Xiyao—Antiphlogistic Lotion (A proved recipe)

Ingredients:

dandelion herb (*Herba Taraxaci*)	30g

flavescent sophora root (*Radix Sophorae Flavescentis*) 12g

phellodendron bark (*Cortex Phellodendri*) 12g

forsythia fruit (*Fructus Forcythiae*) 12g

seed of cochinchina momordica (*Semen Momordicae*) 12g

honeysuckle flower (*Flos Lonicerae*) 9g

dahurian angelica root (*Radix Angelicae Dahuricae*) 9g

red peony root (*Radix Paeoniae Rubra*) 9g

moutan bark (*Cortex Moutan Radicis*) 9g

licorice root (*Radix Glycyrrhizae*) 9g

Efficacy and indications: Clearing away noxious heat, promoting blood circulation to subdue swelling and promoting discharge of pus and necrotic tissues.

preparation and administration: Boil the drugs in water for a lotion to fumigate and bathe wound, 1—2 times a day, 30 minutes each time. For ruptured sore or wound, give routine dressing change after fumigation and bathing.

Jiegu Dan—Bone-knitting Pill

Ingredients:

Prescription 1

(Also known as *Shibao San*—Powder of Ten Precious Ingredients, from *Life-saving Manual of Diagnosis and Treatment of External Diseases*)

dragon's blood (*Resina Draconis*) 4. 8g

realgar (*Realgar*) 12g

safflower (*Flos Carthami*) 12g

catechu (*Catechu*) 0. 72g

cinnabar (*Cinnabaris*) 3. 6g

frankincense (*Resina Olibani*) 3. 6g

Chinese angelica root (*Radix Angelicae Sinensis*) 30g

myrrh (*Myrrha*) 4. 2g

musk (*Moschus*) 0. 09g

borneol (*Borneolum*) 0. 36g

Prescription 2

(Also known as *Duoming Jiegu Dan*—Pill for Knitting Broken

312

Bone and Saving Life, from *Textbook on Traumatology in Traditional Chinese Medicine*)

Chinese angelica root (*Radix Angelicae Sinensis*)	12g
frankincense (*Resina Olibani*)	30g
myrrh (*Myrrha*)	30g
pyrite (*Pyritum*)	30g
drynaria rhizome (*Rhizoma Drynariae*)	30g
peach kernel (*Semen Persicae*)	30g
rhubarb (*Radix et Rhizoma Rhei*)	30g
realgar (*Realgar*)	30g
hyacinth bletilla (*Rhizoma Bletillae*)	30g
dragon's blood (*Resina Draconis*)	15g
ground beetle (*Eupolyphaga seu Steleophaga*)	15g
notoginseng (*Radix Notoginseng*)	15g
safflower (*Flos Carthami*)	15g
catechu (*Catechu*)	15g
musk (*Moschus*)	15g
cinnabar (*Cinnabaris*)	6g
borneol (*Borneolum*)	6g

Efficacy and indications: Promoting blood circulation to relieve pain and promoting bone knitting; used for complicated fracture after traumatic injury.

Preparation and administration: Grind all the drugs together into fine powder and take 2—3g a time, 2 times a day.

Jiegu Gao—Bone Knitting Paste (A proved recipe from *Traumatology*)

Ingredients:

acanthopanax bark (*Cortex Acanthopanacis*)	2 portions
earthworm (*Lumbricus*)	2 portions
frankincense (*Resina Olibani*)	1 portion
myrrh (*Myrrha*)	1 portion
ground beetle (*Eupolyphaga seu Steleophaga*)	1 portion
drynaria rhizome (*Rhizoma Drynariae*)	1 portion
hyacinth bletilla (*Rhizoma Bletillae*)	1 portion

313

                    honey (*Mel*)   proper amount
Efficacy and indications: Promoting bone reunion, blood circulation, and hemostasis; used for fracture injury with ecchymoma and pain.

Preparation and administration: Grind all the drugs together into fine powder which is mixed with honey or liquor into a paste for external application. The powder can also be boiled with vaseline into an ointment for external use.

Jiegu Pian—Bone Knitting Tablet (A proved recipe)

Ingredients:

ground beetle (*Eupolyphaga seu Steleophaga*)		60g
pyrite (*Pyritum*)	(prepared)	90g
dragon's blood (*Resina Draconis*)		90g
pangolin scales (*Aquama Manitis*)		60g
earthworm (*Lumbricus*)		90g
chicken bone (*Os Galli domesticus*)		150g
drynaria rhizome (*Rhizoma Drynariae*)		120g
Chinese angelica root (*Radix Angelicae Sinensis*)		90g
ephedra (*Herba Ephedrae*)		30g
nux-vomica seed (*Semen Strychni*)	(prepared)	9g
pyrolusite (*Pyrolusitum*)	(prepared)	120g

Efficacy and indications: Promoting blood circulation to remove blood stasis and accelerating reunion of broken bones and muscles.

Preparation administration: Pulverize all the drugs together into fine powder, which is prepared into tablets conventionally, 0.3g each tablet. Dosage for adult: 5—7 tablets each time, 3 times a day, taken orally; dosage for children: reduce to proper amount; pregnant women should not take the tablets.

Jiegu Wan—Pill Promoting Bone-knitting (from *The Diagnosis and Treatment of Traumatic Diseases*)

Ingredients:

    Chinese angelica root (*Radix Angelicae Sinensis*)
    white peony root (*Radix Paeoniae Alba*)

poria (*Poria*)
lotus seed (*Semen Nelumbinis*)
dragon's blood (*Resina Draconis*)
safflower (*Flos Carthami*)
catechu (*Catechu*)
cloves (*Flos Caryophylli*)
costus root (*Radix Aucklandiae*)
rhubarb (*Radix et Rhizoma Rhei*) (prepared)
moutan bark (*Cortex Moutan Radicis*)
licorice root (*Radix Glycyrrhizae*)
pyrite (*Pyritum*)
ground beetle (*Eupolyphaga seu Steleophaga*)

Efficacy and indications: Promoting hemogenesis, blood circulation, and bone reunion.

Preparation and administration: Pulverize all the drugs together into fine powder, which is to be prepared into honeyed or water-paste pills. Take 4 — 8g of pills a time with boiled water, 2 — 3 times a day.

Jiegu Xujin Gao — Ointment Promoting Reunion of Bone, Muscle and Ligament (from *Textbook on Traumatology in Traditional Chinese Medicine*)

Ingredients:

pyrite (*Pyritum*)	3 portions
schizonepeta (*Herba Schizonepetae*)	3 portions
ledebouriella root (*Radix Ledebouriellae*)	3 portions
acanthopanax bark (*Cortex Acanthopanacis*)	3 portions
fruit of Chinese honeylocust	
(*Fructus Gleditsiae*)	3 portions
madder root (*Radix Bubiae*)	3 portions
teasel root (*Radix Dipsaci*)	3 portions
notopterygium root	
(*Rhizoma seu Radix Notopterygii*)	3 portions
frankincense (*Resina Olibani*)	2 portions
myrrh (*Myrrha*)	2 portions

315

drynaria rhizome (*Rhizoma Drynariae*)	2 portions
twig of williams elder	
(*Ramutus Sambuci Williamsii*)	2 portions
safflower (*Flos Carthami*)	2 portions
red peony root (*Radix Paeoniae Rubra*)	2 portions
ground beetle (*Eupolyphaga seu Steleophaga*)	2 portions
hyacinth bletilla (*Rhizoma Bletillae*)	4 portions
dragon's blood (*Resina Draconis*)	4 portions
borax (*Borax*)	4 portions
crab powder (*Pulvis Eriocheiris Sinensis*)	4 portions
malt extract (*Saccharum Granorum*) or	
honey (*Mel*)	proper amount

Efficacy and indications: Promoting reunion of broken bone, muscles and ligaments; used for fracture and muscular injury.

Preparation and administration: All the drugs are pulverized together into fine powder, which is to be boiled in malt extract or honey to prepare an ointment for external application.

Jiegu Zhijin Dan — Golden Powder for Bone Reunion (from *A Bright Candle to the Causes and Development of Miscellaneous Diseases*)

Ingredients:
ground beetle (*Eupolyphaga seu Steleophaga*)
frankincense (*Resina Olibani*)
myrrh (*Myrrha*)
pyrite (*Pyritum*)
drynaria rhizome (*Rhizoma Drynariae*)
rhubarb (*Radix et Rhizoma Rhei*)
dragon's blood (*Resina Draconis*)
borax (*Borax*)
Chinese angelica root (*Radix Angelicae Sinensis*)

All in equal amounts

Efficacy and indications: Removing blood stasis, benefiting bone reunion and easing pain; used for traumatic injury with bone fracture and blood stasis.

316

Preparation and administration: Grind all the drugs into fine powder, which is to be taken with boiled water or small amount of rice wine, 3—6g each time.

Jingui Shenqi Wan—Golden Chamber Bolus for Tonifying Kidney-*qi* (from *Synopsis of Prescriptions of the Golden Chamber*)
Ingredients:

prepared rehmannia root	
(*Radix Rehmanniae praeparata*)	25g
Chinese yam (*Rhizoma Dioscoreae*)	12g
dogwood fruit (*Fructus Corni*)	12g
water-plantain rhizome (*Rhizoma Alismatis*)	10g
poria (*Poria*)	10g
moutan bark (*Cortex Moutan Radicis*)	10g
cinnamon bark (*Cortex Cinnamomi*)	3g
prepared daughter root of common monkshood	
(*Radix Aconiti Lateralis Praeparata*)	10g

Efficacy and indications: Warming and recuperating the kidney-*yang*; used for insufficiency of the kidney-*yang* after an injury.

Preparation and administration: Boil the drugs in water for an oral dose, or prepare them into boluses and take with saline water of low concentration.

Jinhuang Gao (San)—Golden Paste or Powder (from *The Golden Mirror of Medicine*)
Ingredients:

rhubarb (*Radix et Rhizoma Rhei*)	5 portions
phellodendron bark (*Cortex Phellodendri*)	5 portions
turmeria (*Rhizoma Curcumae Longae*)	5 portions
dahurian angelica root	
(*Radix Angelicae Dahuricae*)	5 portions
arisaema tuber (*Rhizoma Arisaematis*)	
(prepared)	1 portion
tangerine peel (*Pericarpium Citri Reticulatae*)	1 portion
magnolia bark (*Cortex Magnoliae Officinalis*)	1 portion

licorice root (*Radix Glycyrrhizae*) 1 portion
trichosanthes root (*Radix Trichosanthis*) 10 portions

Efficacy and indications: Clearing away heat, removing toxic substances and blood stasis to promote subsidence of swelling; used in the treatment of infection of *yang* syndrome and swelling pain of traumatic injuries.

Preparation and administration: Pulverize all the drugs together into fine powder, which is applied externally after being mixed with rice wine, sesame oil, juice of towel gourd leaves or of scallion, liquid distilled from flowers or lotus leaves, or vaseline in the proportion of 2:8 to obtain a paste.

Jinqiang Tieshan San — Powder for Metal-inflicted Wound (from *Textbook on Traumatology of Traditional Chinese Medicine*)

Ingredients:
frankincense (*Resina Olibani*) 2 portions
myrrh (*Myrrha*) 2 portions
elephant hide (*Corium Elephantis*) 2 portion
rosin (*Colophonium*) 2 portions
alum (*Alumen*) 1 portion
calamine (*Calamina*) 1 portion
dalbergia wood (*Lignum Dalbergiae Odoriferae*) 1 portion
phellodendron bark (*Cortex Phellodendri*) 1 portion
dragon's blood (*Resina Draconis*) 1 portion

Efficacy and indications: Inducing astringency, promoting pus discharge and granulation; used for various kinds of ulcerative wounds.

Preparation and administration: Grind all the drugs together into very fine powder, which is to be spread directly on a wound.

Juanbi Tang-Decoction for Rheumatic or Rheumatoid Arthritis (from *Strictly Selected Prescriptions*)

Ingredients:
notopterygium root (*Rhizoma seu Radix Notopterygii*) 6g
turmeria (*Rhizoma Curcumae Longae*) 6g

318

Chinese angelica root (*Radix Angelicae Sinensis*)   12g
red peony root (*Radix Paeoniae Rubra*)   9g
astragalus root (*Radix Astragali seu Hedysarii*)   12g
ledebouriella root (*Radix Ledebouriellae*)   6g
licorice root (*Radix Glycyrrhizae*)   (stir-fried) 3g
fresh ginger (*Rhizoma Zingiberis Recens*)   5g

Efficacy and Indications: Promoting blood circulation to remove obstruction in the channels and collaterals and dispelling wind and dampness; used to treat troubles caused by invasion of wind and cold into thecollaterals due to weakness of body resistance after an injury.

Preparation and administration: Boil the drugs in water for an oral decoction.

Kanlisha—Medicated Iron Sand (A proprietary)

Ingredients:
ephedra (*Herba Ephedrae*)
Chinese angelica root (*Radix Angelicae Sinensis*)
prepared daughter root of common Monkshood
    (*Radix Aconiti Lateralis Praeparata*)
tuberculate speronskia (*Herba Speranskia Tuberculatae*)
safflower (*Flos Carthami*)
dried ginger (*Rhizoma Zingiberis*)
cinnamon twig (*Ramulus Cinnamomi*)
achyranthes root (*Radix Achyrantis Bidentatae*)
dahurian angelica root (*Radix Angelicae Dahuricae*)
schizonepeta (*Herba Schizonepetae*)
ledebouriella root (*Radix ledebouriellae*)
chaenomeles fruit (*Fructus Chaenomelis*)
argyi leaf (*Folium Artemisiae Argyi*) prepared
notopterygium root (*Rhizoma seu Radix Notopterygii*)
pubescent angelica root (*Radix Angelicae Pubescentis*)

All in equal amounts
vinegar (*Acetum*)   proper amount

Efficacy and indications: Dispelling pathogenic wind and cold to

319

relieve pain; used to relieve pains in the back and lower extremities and rheumatic arthralgia.

Preparation and administration: Boil the above drugs in the mixture of equal amount of water and vinegar to obtain a thick decoction. Roast iron sand to red and mix it with the decoction. When needed, the prepared iron sand is mixed with about 20ml of vinegar and sealed up in a cloth bag which will become hot by itself. Press the bag on the diseased area. If the bag is too hot, it should be moved to and fro.

Kushen Tang — Decoction of Flavescent Sophora (*from Complete Works of Sore Medicine*)
Ingredients:

flavescent sophora root (*Radix Sophorae Flavescentis*)	60g
cnidium fruit (*Fructus Cnidii*)	30g
dahurian angelica root (*Radix Angelicae Dahuricae*)	30g
honeysuckle flower (*Flos Lonicerae*)	30g
wild chrysanthemum flower	
(*Flos Chrysanthemi Indici*)	30g
phellodendron bark (*Cortex Phellodendri*)	30g
broom cypress fruit (*Fructus Kochiae*)	30g
hemp seed (*Fructus Cannabis*)	30g

Efficacy and indications: Expelling wind to arrest itching, clearing away heat and removing toxic substances; indicated for kinds of scabies, tinea, eczema, and syphilitic skin lesions.

Preparation and administration: Boil the drugs in water for a lotion, into which pig's bile (from 4—5 pieces of gall bladders) is added prior to bathing; bathe 2—3 times a day.

Lidong Wan — Lidong Bolus (from *A Golden Mirror of Medicine*)
Ingredients:

cow-bezoar (*Calculus Bovis*)	1 portion
borneol (*Borneolum*)	1 portion
musk (*Moschus*)	1 portion
Chinese asafetida (*Resina Ferulae*)	5 portions

realgar (*Realgar*)	5 portions
rhubarb (*Radix et Rhizoma Rhei*)	10 portions
catechu (*Catechu*)	10 portions
dragon's blood (*Resina Draconis*)	10 portions
frankincense (*Resina Olibani*)	10 portions
myrrh (*Myrrha*)	10 portions
notoginseng (*Radix Notoginseng*)	10 portions
tabasheer (*Concretio Silicea Bambusae*)	10 portions
gamboge (*Resina Garciniae*)	10 portions

(Gamboge should be heated by boiling its container for a dozen of times, after skimming off the floating foam, it is preferably mixed with goat's blood and dried in the sun, or with lamb's blood instead if the former is not available.)

Efficacy and indications: Eliminating blood stasis to promote granulation; used for traumatic injury with severe pain due to blood stasis and stagnation of *qi*, or with unconsciousness due to accumulation of blood stasis in the interior and for nameless inflammatory swelling, etc.

Preparation and administration: Pulverize the drugs together into fine powder except gamboge which is dissolved in water and mixed with the powder of other drugs to make boluses as big as a gordon seed (*Semen Euryales*). Roast the boluses dry, add a little honey to them and then seal each bolus in a waxed cover. Take 1 bolus a time with boiled water or rice wine; for external use, pestle the bolus with tea (liquid) to rub the affected area.

Liqi Zhitong Tang—Decoction for Regulating the Flow of *qi* to Alleviate Pain (A proved recipe)

Ingredients:

red sage root (*Radix Salviae Miltorrhizae*)		9g
costus root (*Radix Aucklandiae*)		3g
green tangerine peel		
(*Pericarpium Citri Reticulatae Viride*)		6g
frankincense (*Resina Olibani*)	(stir-fried)	5g
bitter orange (*Fructus Aurantii*)		6g

321

cyperus tuber (*Rhizoma Cyperi*) (prepared) 9g
sichuan chinaberry (*Fructus Meliae Toosendan*) 9g
corydalis tuber (*Rhizoma Corydalis*) 5g
root of red thorowax (*Radix Bupleuri*) 6g
sweetgum fruit (*Fructus Liquidambaris*) 6g
myrrh (*Myrrha*) 5g

Efficacy and indications: Promoting blood circulation, and regulating the nutrient system and the flow of *qi* to alleviate pain; used for pains caused by blood stasis due to impairment of the *qi* system.

Preparation and administration: Boil all the drugs in water for an oral decoction.

Liuwei Dihuang Tang (Wan) — Decoction or Bolus of Six Drugs Including Rehmannia (from *Key to Therapeutics of Children's Diseases*)

Ingredients:
prepared rehmannia root
  (*Radix Rehmanniae Praeparata*) 25g
Chinese yam (*Rhizoma Dioscoreae*) 12g
poria (*Poria*) 10g
water-plantain rhizome (*Rhizoma Alismatis*) 10g
dogwood fruit (*Fructus Corni*) 12g
moutan bark (*Cortex Moutan Radicis*) 10g

Efficacy and indications: Removing the pathogenic fire by nourishing the kidney; used in the treatment of deficiency of the kidney-*yin* marked by soreness and aches in the back and lower limbs, dizziness, dry throat, tinnitus, tidal fever, night sweating, and very slow reunion of broken bones at the late stage of fractures.

Preparation and administration: The drugs are decocted in water for oral use, a dose a day; or ground into powder, which is to be mixed with properly boiled honey and made into boluses for oral administration, 10g a time, 3 times a day.

Mafei San — Anesthetic Powder (from *The Secret Biography of*

Hua Tuo—A Miracle-working Doctor)
Ingredients:
root of Chinese azalea (*Radix rhododendri Mollis*)   9g
root of arabian jasmine (*Radix Jasmini Sambae*)   3g
Chinese angelica root (*Radix Angelicae Sinensis*)   30g
grassleaved sweetflag rhizome
(*Rhizoma Acori Graminei*)   0. 9g
Efficacy and indications: Inducing anesthesia to stop pain; used as an anesthetic in surgical operations.
Preparation and administration: Boil the drugs in water for an oral decoction taken lukewarm.

Magui Wenjing Tang—Channel-warming Decoction with Ephedra and Cinnamon (from *Supplement to Traumatology*)
Ingredients:
ephedra (*Herba Ephedrae*)
cinnamon twig (*Ramulus Cinnamomi*)
safflower (*Flos Carthami*)
dahurian angelica root (*Radix Angelicae Dahuricae*)
asarum herb (*Herba Asari*)
peach kernel (*Semen Persicae*)
red peony root (*Radix Paeoniae Rubra*)
licorice root (*Radix Glycyrrhizae*)
Efficacy and indications: Clearing and activating the channels and collaterals to remove blood stasis; used to treat arthralgic pain due to affection of pathogenic wind-cold after an injury.
Preparation and administration: The dosage should be fixed accordingto actual condition, and the drugs are boiled in water for an oral decoction.

Qiangjin Wan — Muscle-strengthening Pill (from *Diagnosis and Treatment of Traumatic Diseases*)
Ingredients:
cyperus tuber (*Rhizoma Cyperi*) (*prepared*)
frankincense (*Resina Olibani*)

myrrh (*Myrrha*)
achyranthes root (*Radix Achyranthis Bidentatae*)
teasel root (*Radix Dipsaci*)
licorice root (*Radix Glycyrrhizae*)
polygala root (*Radix Polygalae*)

Efficacy and indications: Promoting *qi* circulation to remove obstruction in the collaterals, promoting blood circulation and strengthening muscles; used to heal old injuries of ligaments and muscles of joints.

Preparation and administration: The drugs are pulverized together into powder, which is mixed with honey to prepare pills. Take 6g each time, 2—3 times a day.

Qili San—Seven-*li* Anti-bruise Powder (from *Collection of Effective Recipes*)

Ingredients:

dragon's blood (*Resina Draconis*)	30g
musk (*Moschus*)	0.36g
borneol (*Borneolum*)	0.36g
frankincense (*Resina Olibani*)	4.5g
myrrh (*Myrrha*)	4.5g
safflower (*Flos Carthami*)	4.5g
cinnabar (*Cinnabaris*)	3.6g
catechu (*Catechu*)	7.2g

Efficacy and indications: Promoting blood circulation to remove blood stasis, relieving pain and stopping bleeding; used for traumatic injuries with pain due to blood stasis, complicated fracture and bleeding.

Preparation and administration: All the drugs are ground together into a very fine powder for oral use, 0.2g (about seven *li*) a time, 1—2 times a day, taken with rice wine; or mixed with rice wine to be applied on the injured part.

Qingshui Yao—A Clear Medical Liquid (from *Standards of Diagnosis and Treatment*)

324

Ingredients:
  Chinese angelica root (*Radix Angelicae Sinensis*)
  moutan bark (*Cortex Moutan Radicis*)
  chuanxiong rhizome (*Rhizoma Ligustici Chuanxiong*)
  red peony root (*Radix Paeoniae Rubra*)
  dried rehmannia root (*Radix Rehmanniae*)
  scutellaria root (*Radix Scutellariae*)
  coptis rhizome (*Rhizoma Coptis*)
  forsythia fruit (*Fructus Forsythiae*)
  capejasmine fruit (*Fructus Gardeniae*)
  peach kernel (*Semen Persicae*)
  licorice root (*Radix Glycyrrhizae*)

Efficacy and indications: Removing blood stasis to induce detumae-cense, clearing away heat and removing toxic substances; used in the treatment of open fracture, dislocation and injury of soft tissues.

Preparation and administration: Boil the drugs in water for an oral decoction.

Quyu Xiaozhong Gao — Ointment for Removing Blood Stasis and Subduing Swelling (A proved recipe)

Ingredients:

dragon's blood (*Resina Draconis*)	9g
catechu (*Catechu*)	6g
myrrh (*Myrrha*)	9g
frankincense (*Resina Olibani*)	9g
corydalis tuber (*Rhizoma Corydalis*)	12g
peppertree pricklyash peel (*Pericarpium Zanthoxyli*)	6g
musk (*Moschus*)	1.5g
borneol (*Borneolum*)	1.5g
redbean (*Semen Phaseoli*)	30g
earthworm (*Lumbricus*)	30g

Efficacy and indications: Promoting blood circulation to remove blood stasis, and promoting subsidence of swelling to relieve pain.

Preparation and administration: All the drugs are pulverized together into fine powder which is mixed with honey or malt sugar for an ointment to be applied on the injury.

Rushen Jindao San—Holly Powder for Cut-wound (from *Orthodox Manual of External Diseases*)
Ingredients:

rosin (*Colophonium*)	5 portions
alum (*Alumen*)	1 portion
calcined alum	1 portion

Efficacy and indications: Inducing hemostasis and excreting dampness; used for cut oozing or running ulcer.
Preparation and administration: Grind the three drugs into a fine powder to be spread on a wound.

Sanleng Heshang Tang—Burreed Tuber Decoction for Trauma (A proved recipe from *Textbook on Traumatology of Traditional Chinese Medicine*)
Ingredients:
green tangerine peel (*Pericarpium Citri Reticulatae Viride*)
burreed tuber (*Rhizoma sparganii*)
zedoary (*Rhizoma Zedoariae*)
tangerine peel (*Pericarpium Citri Reticulatae*)
white atractylodes rhizome
　　(*Rhizoma Atractylodis Macrocephalae*)
bitter orange (*Fructus Aurantii*)
Chinese angelica root (*Radix Angelicae Sinensis*)
white peony root (*Radix Paeoniae Alba*)
dangshen (*Radix Codonopsis Pilosulae*)
frankincense (*Resina Olibani*)
myrrh (*Myrrha*)
licorice root (*Radix Glycyrrhizae*)
Efficacy and indications: Promoting circulation of blood and *qi* to remove blood stasis and relieve pain; used for old injury in the sternocostal region with vague pain.
Preparation and administration: The dosage of each drug in the

326

recipe should be determined on the basis of the condition and the drugs are boiled in water for an oral decoction, a dose a day.

Sanyu Heshang Tang — Decoction for Removing Blood Stasis and Healing Injury (from *A Golden Mirror of Medicine*)

Ingredients:

nux-vomica seed (*Semen Strychni*)	15g
safflower (*Flos Carthami*)	15g
pinellia tuber (*Rhizoma Pinelliae*)	15g
drynaria rhizome (*Rhizoma Drynariae*)	9g
licorice root (*Radix Glycyrrhizae*)	9g
adventitious root of fistular onion	
(*Radix Allii Fistulosi*)	30g
vinegar (*Acetum*)	60g

Efficacy and indications: promoting blood circulation, eliminating blood stasis and relieving pain; used for ecchymoma and swelling pain from injury of soft tissues and clonic spasm and pain of muscles at the late stage of bone fracture or dislocation.

Preparation and administration: Boil the drugs in water and then add in vinegar and boil again for 5—10 minutes to get a lotion for fumigating and bathing the diseased part, 3—4 times a day. Heat the lotion to boil prior to fumigation and bathing every time.

Shang Yougao — Rubbing Cream for Injury (A proved recipe from *Textbook on Traumatology of Traditional Chinese Medicine*)

Ingredients:

dragon's blood (*Resina Draconis*)	60g
safflower (*Flos Carthami*)	6g
frankincense (*Resina Olibani*)	6g
myrrh (*Myrrha*)	6g
amber (*Succinum*)	3g
catechu (*Catechu*)	6g
borneol (*Borneolum*)	6g
sesame oil (*Oleum Sesami*)	1500g
beeswax (*Cera Flava*)	proper amount

Efficacy and indications: Promoting blood circulation to relieve pain; usually used to rub the affected area during manipulation of an injury as both a liniment and a lubricant.

Preparation and administration: Grind all the drugs except borneol, wax and oil into a fine powder, then add in borneol and grind further. Dissolve the powder in the boiled sesame oil and finally add in the wax to make a cream.

Shangzhi Sunshang Xifang—Lotion Recipe for Injuries in the Upper Limbs (A proved recipe from *Textbook on Traumatology of Traditional Chinese Medicine*)

Ingredients:

buck grass (*Herba Lycopodii*)	15g
tuberculate speranskia	
(*Herba Speranskiae Tuberculatae*)	15g
schizonepeta (*Herba Schizonepetae*)	9g
ledebouriella root (*Radix Ledebouriellae*)	9g
safflower (*Flos Cartharmi*)	9g
homalomena rhizoma (*Rhizom Homalomenae*)	12g
Chinese siphonostegia (*Herba Siphonostegiae*)	9g
cinnamon bark (*Cortex Cinnamomi*)	12g
sappan wood (*Lignum Sappan*)	9g
chuanxiong rhizome (*Rhizoma Ligustici Chuanxiong*)	9g
clematis root (*Radix Clematidis*)	9g

Efficacy and indications: Relieving rigidity of muscles by promoting blood circulation; used to treat clonic spasm and aching of muscles after a bone fracture, dislocation or other traumatic injuries of the upper limbs.

Preparation and administration: The drugs are decocted in water for a lotion for fumigating and bathing the affected limb.

Shenfu Tang — Decoction of Ginseng and Prepared Aconite (from *Effetive Formularies Tested by Physicans of Generations*)

Ingredients:

ginseng (*Radix Ginseng*)	12g

prepared danghter root of common monkshood
   (*Radix Aconiti Lateralis Praeparata*)
                        (Baked off the peel)   10g
Efficacy and indications: Recuperating depleted *yang* and rescuing
patient from collapse; used to treat *yang* depletion after injury or
disease manifested as shock, cold limbs, shortness of breath, hic-
cup, dyspnea and chest stuffiness, sweating and weak thready
pulse.
Preparation and administration: Decoct the drugs in water for an
oral dose.

Shengji Babao San (Dan) — Powder of Eight Precious Ingredients
for Promoting Granulation (A proved recipe from *Textbook on
Traumatology of Traditional Chinese Medicine*)
Ingredients:

gypsum (*Gypsum Fibrosum*) (calcined)	3 portions
red halloysite (*Halloysitum Rubrum*)	3 portions
red lead (*minium*)	1 portion
dragon's bone (*Os Draconis Fossilia*)	1 portion
calomel (*Calomelas*)	3 portions
dragon's blood (*Resina Draconis*)	1 portion
frankincense (*Resina Olibani*)	1 portion
myrrh (*Myrrha*)	1 portion

Efficacy and indications: Promoting granulation and healing of
wounds; used for various kinds of wounds.
Preparation and administration: Grind all the drugs together into
a very fine powder to be spread on a wound.

Shengji Yuhong Gao — Red Jade Plaster Promoting Granulation
(from *Orthodox Manual of Exnual of External Diseases*)
Ingredients:

Chinese angelica root	
(*Radix Angelicae Sinensis*)	5 portions
dahurian angelica root	
(*Radix Angelicae Dahuricae*)	1. 2 portions

insect wax (*Cera Chinensis*)	5 portions
calomel (*Calomelas*)	1 portion
licorice root (*Radix Glycyrrhizae*)	3 portions
arnebia or lithosperm root	
(*Radix Arnebiae seu Lithospermi*)	0. 5 portion
dragon's blood (*Resina Draconis*)	1 portion
sesame oil (*Oleum Sesami*)	40 portions

Efficacy and indications: Promoting blood circulation and removal of putrid tissues, removing toxic substances, relieving pain, nourishing skin tissues and promoting granulation; used to heal ulcers which are long retarded in getting rid of the pus and necrotic tissues and in growing out the new.

Preparation and administration: First soak the Chinese angelica, dahurian agelica, arnebia and licorice in the sesame oil for 3 days and boil them in the oil with a slow fire till they are nearly exhausted. Filter to collect the oil and boil it again. Then add in dragon's blood and when it is completely dissolved, add in the insect wax and melt it with slow fire. Finally, lay a bowl on water and fill it with the paste prepared. A little later, add calomel (*Calomelas*) into the bowl and mix well. The final paste is evenly spread out on a piece of gauze and applied on an ulcer. The powder of other drugs which can promote the discharge of pus and putrid tissues may be dusted on the surface of this paste prior to application so that better result can be expected.

Shengmai San—Pulse-activating Powder (from *On Differentiation of Internal and Traumatic Injuries*)

Ingredients:

ginseng (*Radix Cinseng*)	1. 6g
ophiopogon root (*Radix Ophiopogonis*)	1. 6g
schisandra fruit (*Fructus Schisandrae*)	7 pieces

Efficacy and indications: Replenishing *qi* to arrest sweating and nourishing *yin* to promote the production of body fluid; used in the treatment of impairment of *qi* and body fluid or impairment of *qi* and blood, due to pathogenic heat, marked by sweating, shortness of breath, flaccidity, cold limbs, palpitation and weak pulse.

Preparation and administration: Boil the drugs in water for an oral intake, or grind drugs into a powder, which is infused for oral intake, 1 — 4 doses a day or in the light of the patient's condition. Contemporarily, injection made according to the recipe is available for intramuscular or intravenous purposes, or upon emergency, for direct intracardiac injection.

Shengxue Busui Tang—Decoction Promoting Hematopoiesis(from *Supplement to Traumatology*)

Ingredients:

dried rehmannia root (*Radix Rehmanniae*)	12g
chuanxiong rhizome (*Rhizoma Ligustici Chuanxiong*)	6g
astragalus root (*Radix Astragali seu Hedysari*)	9g
eucommia bark (*Cortex Eucommiae*)	9g
acanthopanax bark (*Cortex Acanthopancis*)	9g
achyranthes root (*Radix Achyranthis Bidentatae*)	9g
safflower (*Flos Carthami*)	5g
Chinese angelica root (*Radix Angelicae Sinensis*)	9g
teasel root (*Radix Dipsaci*)	9g

Efficacy and indications: Regulating *qi* and blood, relaxing muscles and tendons and activating collaterals; used to heal sprain or contusion injuries, and treat unhealed wound and pain of joint dislocation and bone fracture at the middle and late stages.

Preparation and administration: Boil the drugs in water for oral intake, a dose a day.

Shenjin Gao—Muscle-relaxing Plaster (A proved recipe)

Ingredients:

nux-vomica seed (*Semen Strychni*)	9g
earthworm (*Lumbricus*)	12g
tuberculate speranskia	
(*Herba Speranskiae Tubercutatae*)	9g
bean blister beetle (*Epicauta Gorhami*)	12g
pangolin scales (*Aquama Manitis*)	9g

batryticated silkworm (*Bombyx Batryticatus*)	12g
tetrandra root (*Radix Stephaniae Tetrandrae*)	9g
clematis root (*Radix Clematidis*)	12g
Chinese angelica root (*Radix Angelicae Sinensis*)	15g
rhubarb (*Radix et Rhizoma Rhei*)	12g
bulgeweed (*Herba Lycopi*)	12g
frankincense (*Resina Olibani*)	9g
myrrh (*Myrrha*)	9g
drynaria rhizome (*Rhizoma Drynariae*)	9g
vaccaria seed (*Semen Vaccariae*)	9g
asarum herb (*Herba Asari*)	9g
acanthopanax bark (*Cortex Acanthopanacis*)	9g
siegesbeckia herb (*Herba Siegesbeckiae*)	9g
mahobnia leaf (*Folium Mahoniae*)	30g
centipede (*Scolopendra*)	4 pieces
luffa (*Retinervus Luffae Fructus*)	12g
ephedra (*Herba Ephedrae*)	12g
ground beetle (*Eupolyphaga seu Steleophaga*)	12g
pubescent angelica root (*Radix Angelicae Pubescentis*)	9g
wild aconite root (*Radix Aconiti Kusnezoffii*)	9g
kansui root (*Radix Euphorbiae Kansui*)	30g
Chinese gall (*Galla Chinensis*)	9g
cinnamon bark (*Cortex Cinnamomi*)	9g
ledebouriella root (*Radix Ledebouriellae*)	12g
immature bitter orange (*Froctus Aurantii*) *Immaturus*)	9g
arctium fruit (*Fructus Arctii*)	9g
carbonized hair (*Crinis Carbonisatus*)	9g

Efficacy and indications: Dispersing blood stasis to relieve pain, relaxing muscles, promoting blood circulation and dispelling wind to remove obstruction in channels and collaterals.

Preparation and administration: Boil 2 000ml of sesame oil, add in the above drugs and deep-fry them to exhaustion. Then filter to collect the oil and concentrate it till a drop of it can stay on a surface like a bead. Add 1 000g of red lead (*minium*) and mix thoroghly. Take proper amount of the paste and spread it out on a piece of cloth to be applied on the affected site.

Shenjin Pian—Muscle-relaxing Tablet (A proved recipe)
Ingredients:

nux-vomica seed (*Semen Strychni*)   21g
earthworm (*Lumbricus*)   30g
frankincense (*Resina Olibani*)   9g
myrrh (*Myrrha*)   9g
ephedra (*Herba Ephedrae*)   9g
hemp root (*Radix Cannabis*)   (carbonized) 9g
acanthopanax bark (*Cortex Acanthopanacis*)   9g
tetrandra root (*Radix Stephaniae Tetrandrae*)   9g
dragon's blood (*Resina Draconis*)   6g
drynaria rhizome (*Rhizoma Drynariae*)   6g

Efficacy and indications: Provoting blood circulation, relaxing muscles and removing obstruction in channels to relieve pain.
Preparation and administration: Grind all drugs into fine powder to prepare tablets as routine, 0. 3g each tablet. Oral administration: 5 tablets a time, 3 times a day.

Shenling Baizhu San — Powder of Ginseng, Poria and White Atractylodes (from *Formularies of the Bureau of Pharmacy*)
Ingredients:

white hyaciath bean (*Semen Dolichoris Album*)   12g
dangshen (*Radix Codonopsis Pilosulae*)   12g
white atractylodes rhizome
    (*Rhizoma Atractylodis Macrocephalae*)   12g
poria (*Poria*)   12g
licorice root (*Radix Glycyrrhizae*) (*stir-fried*)   6g
Chinese yam (*Rhizoma Dioscoreae*)   12g
lotus seed (*Semen Nelumbinis*)   10g
coix seed (*Semen Coicis*)   10g
platycodon root (*Radix Platycodi*)   6g
amomum fruit (*Fructus Amomi*)   5g
Chinese date (*Fructus Ziziphi Jujubae*)   4 pieces

Efficacyt and indications: Replenishing *qi*, invigorating the spleen and excreting dampness; used for dysfunction of the spleen due to consumption of and impairment to the blood and *qi* at the late stage of an injury.

Preparation and administration: Boil the drugs in water for an oral dose, or prepare all the drugs into a powder except Chinese date which should be boiled for a decoction to go with the powder.

Shentong Zhuyu Tang — Decoction for Relieving Pantalgia due to Blood Stasis (from *Correction on Errors of Medical Works*)

Ingredients:

large-leaf gentian root	
(*Radix Gentianae Macrophyllae*)	9g
chuanxiong rhizome (*Rhizoma Ligustici Chuanxiong*)	9g
peach kernel (*Semen Persicae*)	6g
safflower (*Flos Carthami*)	6g
licorice root (*Radix Glycyrrhizae*)	3g
notopterygium root (*Rhizoma seu Radix Notopterygii*)	9g
myrrh (*Myrrha*)	9g
trogopterus dung (*Faeces Trogopterorum*)	9g
cyperus tuber (*Rhizoma Cyperi*)	9g
achyranthes root (*Radix Achyranthis Bidentatae*)	9g
earthworm (*Lumbricus*)	9g
Chinese angelica root (*Radix Angelicae Sinensis*)	15g

Efficacy and indications: Promoting blood circulation and flow of *qi*, removing blood stasis and obstruction in the channels and relieving pain; used to relieve chronic pains in the shoulders, lumbar region, legs, or all over the body due to obstruction of channels by blood stasis and stagnation of *qi*.

Preparation and administration: Boil all the drugs in water for oral intake. Uncooked, cold and greasy food should be avoided during medical treatment. Pregnant women must not take the decoction.

Shiquan Dabu Tang — Decoction of Ten Powerful Tonics (from *Medical Inventions*)

334

Ingredients:

dangshen (*Radix Codonopsis Pilosulae*)	10g
white atractylodes rhizome	
(*Rhizoma Atractylodis Macrocephalae*)	12g
poria (*Poria*)	12g
licorice root (*Radix Glycyrrhizae*) (stir-fried)	5g
Chinese angelica root (*Radix Angelicae Sinensis*)	10g
chuanxiong rhizome (*Rhizoma Ligustici Chuanxiong*)	6g
rehmannia root (*Radix Rehmanniae*) (prepared)	12g
white peony root (*Radix Paeoniae Alba*)	12g
astragalus root (*Radix Astragali seu Hedysari*)	10g
cinnamon bark (*Cortex Cinnamomi*)	
(fully steamed to make an infusion for ral use)	0. 6g

Efficacy and indications: Invigorating *qi* and enriching blood, used at the late stage of a traumatic injury when there is deficiency of *qi* and blood marked by watery and thin pus from the wound, spontaneous sweating, night sweating, yellow complexion, emaciation, anorexia, lassitude and shortness of breath.

Preparation and administration: The drugs are boiled in water for an oral decoction, a dose a day.

Shuangbai San—Powder or Paste of Biota Tops and Phellodendron (from *Textbook on Traumatology of Traditional Chinese Medicine*)

Ingredients:

biota tops (*Cacumen Biotae*)	2 portions
phelodendron bark (*Cortex Phellodendri*)	1 portion
rhubarb (*Radix et Rhizoma Rhei*)	2 portions
peppermint (*Herba Menthae*)	1 portion
bulgeweed (*Herba Lycopi*)	1 portion

Efficacy and indications: Promoting blood circulation, removing toxic substances, and subduing swelling to relieve pain; used for traumatic injuries at the early stage, or sores at onset marked by local redness, swelling and hot pain, or swollen sore prior to ulceration.

Preparation and administation: All the drugs are ground together into fine powder for use. When needed, the powder is boiled in water and honey for a thick paste, which is applied to the affected site. The powder can also be mixed with proper amount of rice wine, or boiled with vaseline into ointment, for external application.

Shufeng Yangxue Tang — Decoction for Expelling Wind and Nourishing Blood (from *Supplement to Trumatology*)

Ingredients:

schizonepeta (*Herba Schizonepetae*)	9g
notopterugium root (*Rhizoma seu Radix Notopterygii*)	6g
ledebouriella root (*Radix Ledebouriellae*)	6g
Chinese angelica root (*Radix Angelicae Sinensis*)	12g
chuanxiong rhizome (*Rhizoma Ligustici Chuanxiong*)	12g
white peony root (*Radix Paeoniae Alba*)	9g
large-leaf gentian root	
(*Radix Gentianae Macrophyllae*)	9g
peppermint (*Herba Menthae*)	4g
safflower (*Flos Carthami*)	6g
trichosanthes root (*Radix Trichosanthis*)	12g

Efficacy and indications: Nourishing blood and expelling pathogenic wind; used for traumatic injury complicated by affection of pathogenic wind-cold.

Preparation and administration: Boil the drugs in water for an oral decoction.

Shujin Huoxue Tang — Decoction for Relaxing Muscles and Promoting Blood Circulation (from *Supplement to Traumatology*)

Ingredients:

notopterygium root (*Rhizoma seu Radix Notopterygii*)	6g
ledebouriella root (*Radix Ledebouriellae*)	9g
schizonepeta (*Herba Schizonepetae*)	6g
pubescent angelica root (*Radix Angelicae Pubescentis*)	9g
Chinese angelica root (*Radix Angelicae Sinensis*)	12g
teasel root (*Radix Dipsaci*)	12g

336

green tangerine peel

      (*Pericarpium Citri Reticulatae Viride*)   5g

achyranthes root (*Radix Achyranthis Bidentatae*)   9g

acanthopanax bark (*Cortex Acanthopanacis*)   9g

eucommia bauk (*Cortex Eucommiae*)   9g

safflower (*Flos Carthami*)   6g

bitter orange (*Fructus Aurantii*)   6g

Efficacy and indications: Relaxing muscles and tendons and activating the flow of *qi* and blood in the channels and collaterals; used to treat clonic spasm of muscles and pain at the late stage of soft tissues injury, bone fracture and dislocation.

Preparation and administration: Boil the drugs in water for an oral decoction.

Shujin Tang—Decoction for Relaxing Muscles (from *Treatment of Bone and Articulation Injuries with Combined Traditional Chinese Medicine and Western Medicine*)

Ingredients:

Chinese angelica root (*Radix Angelicae Sinensis*)   15g

flower of Chinese Azalea (*Flos rhododendri Mollis*)   15g

peppertree pricklyash peel (*Pericarpium Zanthoxyli*) 15g

tuberculate speranskia

      (*Herba Speranskiae Tuberculatae*)   15g

herb of wooly dutchmanspipe

      (*Herba Aristolochiae Mollissimae*)   15g

buck grass (*Herba Lycopodii*)   15g

teasel root (*Radix Dipsaci*)   15g

erythrina bark (*Cortex Erythrinae*)   15g

Efficacy and indications: Relaxing muscles to ease pain; used to treat stiff joints (ankylosis) after a bone or joint injury, or pain of an old injury on a wet day.

Preparation and administration: Boil all the drugs in large quantity of water to get a tub of hot decoction. Lay a bar or a piece of board across on the tub, place the affected limb on the board and cover it with a cotton-padded quilt or a piece of cloth so that the limb can be fumigated with hot steam from the decoction. The fumigation continues till there is sweat on the limb. Then sprinkle the limb with or bathe it in the decoction till the liquid turns lukewarm. Wipe the limb with a piece of dry cloth and take care that the limb be kept from cold. Repeat the treatment 2 — 3 times a day. For a stiff joint, massage and functional exercise can be done after bathing.

Shujin Wan — Bolus for Relaxing Muscels (also known as *Shujin Zhuangli Wan* — *Bolus for Relaxing and Strengthening and Muscles*) (from *Liu Shoushan's Clinical Experience of Bone-setting*)

Ingredients:

ephedra (*Herba Ephedrae*)		2 portions
nux-vomica seed (*Semen Strychni*)	(prepared)	2 portions
frnkincense (*Resina Olibani*)	(prepared)	1 portion
myrrh (*Myrrha*)	(prepared)	1 portion
dragon's blood (*Resina Draconis*)		1 portion
safflower (*Flos Carthami*)		1 portion
pyrite (*Pyritum*)		
(*Calcined and tempered in vinegar*)		1 portion
notopterygium root		
(*Rhizoma seu Radix Noteopterygii*)		1 portion
pubescent angelica root		
(*Radix Angelicae Pubescentis*)		1 portion
ledebouriella root (*Radix Ledebouriellae*)		1 portion
root-bark of Chinese hydrangeavine (*Coretx*		
Schizophragmatis Integrifdii Radicis)		1 portion
eucommia bark (*Cortex Eucommiae*)		1 portion
chaenomeles fruit (*Fructus Chaenomelis*)		1 portion
cinnamon twig (*Ramulus Cinnamomi*)		1 portion
achyranthes root (*Radix Achyranthis Bidentatae*)		1 portion
fritillary bulb (*Bulbus Fritillariae*)		1 portion
licorice root (*Radix Glycyrrhizae*)		1 portion
honey (*Mel*)		proper amount

Efficacy and indications: Dispelling pathogenic wind and cold, re-

338

laxing muscles and tendons and activating the circulation of *qi* and blood in the channels and collaterals; used in the treatment of muscular injuries with cold-type arthralgia.

Preparetion and administration: All the drugs are ground together into fine powder which is mixed with boiled honey to make boluses, 5g each. Take 1 bolus a time, 1—3 times a day.

Shunqi Huoxue Tang—Decoction for Lowering Adverse Flow of Qi and Promoting Blood Circulation (from *A Great Collection on Traumatology*)

Ingredients:

perilla stem (*Caulis Perillae*)
magnolia bark (*Cortex Magnoliae Officinalis*)
bitter orange (*Fructus Aurantii*)
amomum fruit (*Fructus Amomi*)
Chinese angelica root (*Radix Angelicae Sinensis*)
safflower (*Flos Carthami*)
costus root (*Radix Aucklandiae*)
red peony root (*Radix Paeoniae Rubra*)
peach kernel (*Semen Persicae*)
sappan wood (*Lignum Sappan*)
cyperus tuber (*Rhizoma Cyperi*)

Efficacy and indications: Promoting flow of *qi* and blood and removing blood stasis to relieve pain; used for thoracico-abdominal contusion with pain and distension due to stagnation of *qi*.

Preparation and administration: The dosage of the above drugs should be fixed in the light of patient's condition. The drugs are boiled in water for an oral decoction, taken with a small amount of rice wine.

Si Huang Gao (*San*)—Paste or Powder of the Mixture of Coptis, Phellodendron, rhubarb and Scutellaria (from *Standards of Diognosis and Treatment*)

Ingredients:

coptis rhizome (*Rhizoma Coptidis*)　　　　　　　1 portion

phellodendron bark (*Cortex Phellodendri*) 3 portions
rhubarb (*Radix et Rhizoma Rhei*) 3 portions
scutellaria root (*Radix Scutellariae*) 3 portions

Efficacy and indications: Clearing away heat, removing toxic substances and subduing swelling to relieve pain; used to treat infection after injury and carbuncle of *yang* nature with local reddening, swelling and hot pain.

Preparation and administration: All the drugs are ground together into a fine powder which is mixed with water and honey or with vaseline for external application.

Siwu Tang — Decoction of Four Ingredients (from *Secret Recipes of Treating Wound and Bone-setting Taught by Celestials*)
Ingredients:
chuanxiong rhizome (*Rhizoma Ligustici Chuanxiong*) 6g
Chinese angelica root (*Radix Angelicae Sinensis*) 10g
white peony root (*Radix Paeoniae Alba*) 12g
prepared rehmannia root
　　(*Radix Rehmanniae Praeparata*) 12g

Efficacy and indications: Nourishing blood and promoting hematopoiesis; used in the treatment of deficiency of blood after an injury or illness.

Preparation and administration: Boil the drugs in water for an oral decoction, a dose a day.

Siwu Zhitong Tang — Decoction of Four Ingredients for Relieving Pain (A proved recipe)
Ingredients:
Chinese angelica root (*Radix Angelicae Sinensis*) 9g
chuanxiong rhizome (*Rhizoma Ligustici Chuanxiong*) 6g
white peony root (*Radix Paeoniae Alba*) 9g
dried rehmannia root (*Radix Rehmanniae*) 12g
frankincense (*Resina Olibani*) 6g
myrrh (*Myrrha*) 6g

Efficacy and indications: Promoting blood circulation to relieve

340

pain; used to relieve pain due to blood stasis from injuries of any part.

Preparation and administration: Boil the drugs in water for an oral decoction.

Suhexiang Wan—Storax Bolus (from *Formularies of the Bureau of Pharmacy*)

Ingredients:

white atractylodes rhizome	
(*Rhizoma Atractylodis Macrocephalae*)	2 portions
dutchmanspipe root (*Radix Aristolochiae*)	2 portions
powder of black rhinocero's horn	
(*Pulvis Corni Rhinocerotis*)	2 portions
cyperus tuber (*Rhizoma Cyperi*)	2 portions
cinnabar (*Cinnabaris*)2 portions	
myrobalan (*Fructus Chebulae*)	
(Roasted in fresh cinders to rid of the peel)	2 portions
sandalwood (*Lignum santali*)	2 portions
benzoin (*Benzoinum*)	2 portions
eagle wood (*Lignum Aquilariae Resinatum*)	2 portions
musk (*Moschus*)	2 portions
long pepper (*Fructus Piperis Longi*)	2 portions
borneo-camphor (*Borneo-Camphora*)	1 portion
frankincense (*Resina Olibani*)	1 portion
storax (*Styrax Liquidus*)	1 portion
honey (*Mel*)	proper amount

Efficacy and indications: Warming channels and expelling pathogenic cold to induce resuscitation; used for coma due to intracranial injury.

Preparation and administration: Grind the solid drugs separately into powder. The benzoin powder is boiled in 1000ml of limeless wine to get a paste, which is then mixed with the storax. Add to the mixture the powder of other drugs one by one and mix with boiled honey to make boluses, 3g each. Take 1 bolus with lukewarm water each time; half of the dosage for children.

Taiyi Gao—Taiyi Plaster (from *Orthodox Manual of Extenal Diseases*)

Ingredients:

scrophularia root (*Radix Scrophulariae*)	100g
dahurian angelica root (*Radix Angelicae Dahuricae*)	100g
Chinese angelica root (*Radix Agnelicae Sinensis*)	100g
cinnamon bark (*Cortex Cinnamomi*)	100g
rhubarb (*Radix et Rhizoma Rhei*)	100g
red peony root (*Radix Paeoniae Rubra*)	100g
dried rehmannia root (*Radix Rehmanniae*)	100g
cochinchina momordica seed (*Semen Momordicae*)	100g
Chinese asafetida (*Resina Ferulae*)	15g
calomel (*Calomelas*)	20g
willow twig (*Ramulus Salicis*)	100g
carbonized hair (*Crinis Carbonisatus*)	50g
red lead (*Minium*)	2000g
myrrh (*Myrrha*)	15g
framkincense (*Resina Olibani*)	25g
twig of pagoda tree (*Ramulus Sophorae*)	100g
sesame oil (*Oleum Sesami*)	2500g

Efficacy and indications: Clearing away heat, promoting subsidence of swelling, removing toxic substances and promoting generation of new tissues, used for various kinds of sores and traumatic injuries.

Preparation and administration: Boil all drugs except red lead in sesame oil till they are exhausted and filter to collect the oil. Add red lead into the oil (20g to every 500g of oil), boil and mix well into a paste. Boil the paste container in water to soften the paste so that it can be spread out on a piece of paper or cloth to produce plaster for external application.

Taohong Siwu Tang-also known as *Yuanrong Siwu Tang*-Peach kernel and Safflower Decoction Plus Four Ingredients (from *The Goldern Mirror of Medicine*)

Ingredients:
  Chinese angelica root (*Radix Angelicae Sinensis*)
  chuanxiong rhizome (*Rhizoma Ligustici Chuanxiong*)
  white peony root (*Radix Paeoniae Alba*)
  dried rehmannia root (*Radix Rehmanniae*)
  peach kernel (*Semen Persicae*)
  safflower (*Flos Carthami*)

Efficacy and indications: Promoting blood circulation and removing blood stasis; used for blood stasis after injury.

Preparation and administration: Boil the drugs in water for an oral decoction.

Taohua San — Pink Powder (from *Orthodox Manual of External Diseases*)

Ingredients:

lime (*Calx*)	6 portions
rhubarb (*Radix et Rhizoma Rhei*)	1 portion

Efficacy and indications: Arresting hemorrhage; used to check traumatic bleeding.

Preparation and administration: Boil rhubarb in water for a decoction and pour the decoction into the lime. Turn the lime into powder and roast it till it becomes pink. Sieve the powder for use. When needed, the powder is spread on the wound which is then dressed tightly with gauze.

Taoren Chengqi Tang — Purgative Decoction of Peach Kernel (from *Treatise on Pestilence*)

Ingredients:

peach kernel (*Semen Persicae*)	9g
rhubarb (*Radix et Rhizoma Rhei*)	15g
mirabilite (*Natrii Sulfas*)	6g
Chinese angelica root (*Radix Angelicae Sinensis*)	9g
paeony root (*Radix Paeoniae Alba*)	9g
moutan bark (*Cortex Moutan Radicis*)	9g

Efficacy and indications: Promoting blood circulation, removing blood stasis, expelling the pathogenic heat and inducing purgation; used for traumatic injury with pain due to blood stasis, constipation, or accumulation of stagnant blood in the lower abdomen.

Preparation and administration: Boil the drugs in water for an oral decoction.

Taoren Siwu Tang — Peach Kernel Decoction with Four Ingredients (from *A Dictionary of Traditional Chinese Medicine*)

Ingredients:

peach kernel (*Semen Persicae*)	25g
chuanxiong rhizome (*Rhizoma Ligustici Chuanxiong*)	3g
Chinese angelica root (*Radix Angelicae Sinensis*)	3g
red peony root (*Radix Paeoniae Rubra*)	3g
dried rehmannia root (*Radix Rehmanniae*)	2g
safflower (*Flos Carthami*)	2g
moutan bark (*Cortex Moutan Radicis*)	3g
cyperus tuber (*Rhizoma Cyperi*) (prepared)	3g
corydalis tuber (*Rhizoma Corydalis*)	3g

Efficacy and indications: Removing obstruction in the collaterals to promote blood circulation and promoting flow of *qi* to ease pain; used to relieve swelling pain resulting from *qi* stagnation and blood stasis after bone injury.

Preparation and administration: Boil the drugs in water for an oral decoction.

Tongqiao Huoxue Tang — Decoction for Activating Blood Circulation (from *Correction on Errors of Medical Works*)

Ingredients:

red peony root (*Radix Paeoniae Rubra*)	3g
chuanxiong rhizome (*Rhizoma Ligustici Chuanxiong*)	3g
safflower (*Flos Carthami*)	9g
peach kernel (*Semen Persicae*) (mashed)	9g
mature fistular onion (*Herba Allii Fistulosi Matura*) (cut up into small pieces)	3 stalks

344

Chinese date (*Fructus Ziziphi Jujubae*)   (stoned) 7 pieces
musk (*Moschus*)   0. 15g

Efficacy and indications: Promoting blood circulation to induce re-suscitation ; used to check hemorrhage in the head and face, or blood stasis from craniocerebral injury, or dizziness and headache or concussion of brain after head injury.

Preparation and administration: Boil all the drugs except musk in 250g of rice wine for 15 minutes, filter out the dregs, add in musk and heat the decoction to two boils. Take the decoction before going to bed.

Tuoseng Gao—Litharge Ointment (from *Supplement to Traumatology*)

Ingredients:

litharge (*Lithargyrum*)	40 portions
red peony root (*Radix Paeoniae Rubra*)	1 portion
Chinese angelica root (*Radix Angelicae Sinesnsis*)	1 portion
frankincense (*Resina Olibani*)	1 portion
myrrh (*Myrrha*)	1 portion
red halloysite (*Halloysitum Rubrum*)	0. 5 portion
plant soot (*Pulvis Fumi Carbonisatus*)	4 portions
flavescent sophora root	
(*Radix Sophorae Flavescentis*)	8 portions
tung oil (*Oleum Aleuritis*)	64 portions
sesame oil (*Oleum Sesami*)	32 portions
dragon's blood (*Resina Draconis*)	1 portion
catechu (*Catechu*)	1 portion
rhubarb (*Radix et Rhizoma Rhei*)	16 portions

Efficacy and indications: Removing toxic substances and producing hemostasis; used for traumatic injuries and pains due to local infection.

Preparation and administration: Grind the litharge into a fine powder, stew other drugs in the sesame oil and filter to collect the oil. Mix the litharge powder with the oil to obtain a paste for external use.

345

Waiyong Jiegu Gao (*Dan*)—Plaster Promoting Bone Knitting
(A proved recipe)
Ingredients:

pyrite (*Pyritum*)	(calcined)	45g
frankincense (*Resina Olibani*)		30g
myrrh (*Myrrha*)		30g
Chinese gall (*Galla Chinensis*)		60g
scale on the wall of a pail for urine (*Urina Humana*)		45g
dragon's blood (*Resina Draconis*)		9g

Efficacy and indications: Promoting blood circulation to remove blood stasis, subduing swelling to relieve pain and promoting reunion of broken bone and injured muscles; used in case of retarded healing of fracture or nonunion of fracture.

Preparartion and administration: The actual amount of drugs can be decided to the proportion of the above recipe according to the area of the injury. The drugs should be ground into fine powder which is then mixed with vinegar of good quality into a paste. After being boiled, the paste is spread out on a piece of cloth and applied to the injured site after the injury is washed clean. Small splints may be fixed on top of the plaster, if necessary.

Wanling Gao — Panacea Plaster (from *The Colden Mirror of Medicine*)
Ingredients:

buck grass (*Herba Lycopodii*)	30g
tuberculate speranskia (*Herba Speranskiae Tuberculatae*)	30g
lilac root (*Radix Syringae Oblatae*)	30g
Chinese angelica root (*Radix Angelicae Sinensis*)	30g
pyrite (*Pyritum*)	30g
myrrh (*Myrrha*)	30g
dragon's blood (*Resina Draconis*)	30g
chuanxiong rhizome (*Rhizoma Ligustici Chuanxiong*)	25g
ancient copper coin	

(about 16g; tempered in vinegar) 1 piece

safflower (*Flos Carthami*)   30g

cyathula root (*Radix Cyathulae*)   15g

acanthopanax bark (*Cortex Acanthopanacis*)   15g

grassleaved sweetflag rhizome
(*Rhizoma Acori Graminei*)   15g

atractylodes rhizome (*Rhizoma Atractylodis*)   15g

costus root (*Radix Aucklandiae*)   10g

large-leaf gentian root
(*Radix Gentianae Macrophyllae*)   10g

cnidium fruit (*Fructus Cnidii*)   10g

cinnamon bark (*Cortex Cinnamomi*)   10g

prepared daughter root of common monkshood
(*Radix Aconiti Praeparata*)   10g

pinellia tuber (*Rhizoma Pinelliae*)   10g

dendrobium (*Herba Dendrobii*)   10g

hypoglauca yam (*Rhizoma Dioscoreae Hypoglaucae*)   10g

hairy antler (*Cornu Cervi Pantotrichum*)   10g

tiger's tibia (*Os Tigris*)   two whole pieces

musk (*Moschus*)   6g

sesame oil (*Oleum Sesami*)   5000g

red lead (*minium*)   2500g

Efficacy and indications: Removing blood stasis and toxic substances, relaxing muscles, promoting blood circulation and reunion of broken bones and relieving pain; used to heal a traumatic injury with fracture at the late stage or to relieve local numbness and pain due to pathogenic cold and dampness.

Preparation and administration: The dragon's blood, myrrh and musk are ground into fine powders separately and wrapped for use; other drugs are stewed in sesame oil on a slow fire for three days and then boiled till black; the decoction is filtered to rid of the dregs and collect the oil. After red lead (*Minium*) is added, the oil is decocted again till a drop of the oil mixture can stay on a surface like a bead. When the creamy substance is cooled to warm, it is well mixed with the powders of dragon's blood, myrrh

347

and musk to get a paste, which, when properly cooled, is prepared into plaster. When needed, it is applied on the affected part after being warmed over a fire.

Wanyin Gao—Cure-all Plaster (A proprietary)
Ingredients: Omitted.
Efficacy and indications: Promoting blood circulation to remove blood stasis and warming the channels to promote the flow of *qi*; used in the treatment of traumatic injuries, pains and aching in the muscles and bones due to pathogenic wind, cold and dampness, and pain in the chest and abdomen due to stagnation of *qi* there.
Preparation and administration: Heat the plaster and apply it on the affected site.

Wenjing Tongluo Gao—Ointment Warming the Channels to Promote the Flow of *Qi* (A proved recipe from *Textbook on Traumatology in Traditional Chinese Medicine*)
Ingredients:
    frankincense (*Resina Olibani*)
    myrrh (*Myrrha*)
    ephedra (*Herba Ephedrae*)
    nux-vomica seed (*Semen Strychni*)
                                        All in equal amount
    malt extract (*Saccharum Granorum*)
        or honey (*Mel*)   proper amount
Efficacy and indications: Expelling wind to relieve pain; used for relieving tumescense and pain due to injury of joints and soft tissues, or local arthralgia due to affection by wind, cold and dampness.
Preparation and administration: Grind all the drugs into fine powder, which is mixed with malt extract or honey or is boiled with vaseline for an ointment for external application on the diseased part.

Wujiapi Tang—Decoction of Acanthopanax Bark (from *The Gold-*

en Mirror of Medicine)

Ingredients:

Chinese angelica root (*Radix Angelicae Sinensis*)

(washed with liquor) 10g

myrrh (*Myrrha*)   10g

acanthpopanax bar (*Cortex Acanthopanacis*)   10g

impure mirabilite (*Mirabilitum Impuritum*)   10g

green tangerine peel

(*Pericarpium Citri Reticulatae Viride*)   10g

peppertree pricklyash peel (*Pericarpium Zanthoxyli*) 10g

cyperus tuber (*Rhizoma Cyperi*)   10g

wolfberry bark (*Cortex Lycii Radicis*)   3g

moutan bark (*Cortex Moutan Radicis*)   6g

stalk of fully grown fistular onion

(*Rhizoma Allii Fistulosa*)   3 pieces

musk (*Moschus*)   0.3g

Efficacy and indications: Regulating blood, killing pain and relaxing muscles; used in the late stage of injuries.

Preparation and administration: Boil all the drugs except musk in water to get a lotion for external bathing.

Wuling San—Powder of Five Drugs Including Poria (from *Treatise on Febrile Diseases*)

Ingredients:

umbellate pore-fungus (*Polyporus Umbellatus*)   9g

water-plantain rhizome (*Rhizoma Alismatis*)   9g

white atractylodes rhizome

(*Rhizoma Atractylodis Macrocephalae*)   9g

Poria (*Poria*)   15g

cinnamon bark (*Cortex cinnamomi*)   6g

Efficacy and indications: Regulating the function of *qi* to induce diuresis; used to treat dribbling urination or retention of urine due to dysfunction of the bladder after injury in the back and loin with involvement of the *Du* Channel.

Preparation and administration: The drugs are decocted in water for oral intake, a dose a day; or ground together into a powder which is to be taken orally, 2—3 times a day.

Wulong Gao—Black Dragon Ointment
Ingredients:
  Prescription 1 (from *Supplement to Traumatology*)

plant soot (*Pulvis Fumi Carbonisatus*)	10g
hycinth bletilla (*Rhizoma Bletillae*)	15g
ampelopsis root (*Radix Ampelopsis*)	10g
lily bulb (*Bulbus Lilii*)	15g
stoemona root (*Radix Stemonae*)	10g
frankincense (*Resina Olibani*)	10g
myrrh (*Myrrha*)	15g
musk (*Moschus*)	0.3g
polished glutionous rice (*Oryza Glutinosa*) (parched)	30g
wheat starch (The old is better,parched)	120g
vinegar (*Acetum*)	proper amount

  Prescription 2 (A proved recipe)

buffalo horn (*Cornu Bubali*)	(carbonized)	500g
carbonized hair (*Crinis Carbonisatus*)		500g
carbonized piemarker herb		
(*Herba Abutili Carbonisatus*)		50g
dragon's bone (*Os Draconis Fossilia*)	(calcined)	100g
powder of decomposed lead		
(*Pulvis Plumbi Decompositus*)		5 000g
wheat starch (The old is better)		1 500g
mature vinegar (*Acetum Maturum*)	proper amount	

Efficacy and indications: Promoting blood circulation and reunion of broken bone and subduing swelling to relieve pain.
Preparation and administration:
  Prescription 1: All the drugs are pulverized together into a fine powder which is boiled with vinegar to produce a paste for external application.

Prescription 2 : The buffalo horn is whittled into small shreds and sealed up in an earthen container to be toasted into a tawny charcoal. The hair, after removal of impurities, is also sealed tightly in an earthen container to be baked into a black lustrous charcoal. The piemarker herb is sealed in an earthenware. When it is parched dry, open the container, light it with a fire and immediately seal the container tightly for an hour. Grind these three carbonized drugs into fine powders and mix them with those of decomposed lead and dragon's bone and starch for use. When the plaster is needed, pour mature vinegar into a china container to boil it (if there is no mature vinegar, ordinary vinegar can be used instead by concentrating it into half of the original amount). When the vinegar is heated to boil, add in the powder prepared. Stir the mixture while adding in the powder till the mixture becomes a paste, which is to be stewed further for half an hour. Spread out the paste about 0.3cm thick on a piece of cloth while it is hot. The plaster is applied externally on the affected part and changed every other day, or once a week for mild swelling.

Wuwei Xiaodu Yin—Antiphlogistic Decoction of Five Drugs(from *The Colden Mirror of Medicine*)
Ingredients:

honeysuckle flower (*Flos Lonicerae*)	15g
wild chrysanthemum flower	
(*Flos Chrysanthemi Indici*)	15g
dandelion herb (*Herba Taraxaci*)	15g
viola herb (*Herba Violae*)	15g
root of muskroot-like semiaquilegia	
(*Radix Semiaquilegiae*)	10g

Efficacy and indications: Clearing away heat and removing the poisonous quality of any substances; used in the treatment of pyogenic infection of bone at onset, and early infection of an open injury.
Preparation and administration: The drugs are decocted in water for oral intake, 1—3 doses a day.

Xiangpi Gao—Elephant-hide Paste (from *Supplement to Traumatology*)

Ingredients:

Group 1:

rhubarb (*Radix et Rhizoma Rhei*)	10 portions
chuanxiong rhizome (*Rhizoma Ligustici Chuanxiong*)	5 portions
Chinese angelica root (*Radix Angelicae Sinensis*)	5 portions
dried rehmannia root (*Radix Rehmanniae*)	5 portions
safflower (*Flos Carthami*)	1.5 shares
coptis rhizome (*Rhizoma Coptis*)	1.5 portions
licorice root (*Radix Glycyrrhizae*)	2.5 portions
schizonepeta (*Herba Schizonepetae*)	1.5 portions
cinnamon bark (*Cortex Cinnamomi*)	1.5 portions
sesame oil (*Oleum Sesami*)	85 portions

Group 2:

yellowish beeswax (*Cera Flava Lutea*)	25 portions
purified beeswax (*Cera Flava Alba*)	25 portions

Group 3:

elephant hide (*Corium Elephatis*)	2.5 portions
dragon's blood (*Resina Draconis*)	2.5 portions
frankincense (*Resina Olibani*)	2.5 portions
myrrh (*Myrrha*)	2.5 portions
pearl (*Margarita*)	1 portion
ginseng (*Radix Ginseng*)	1 portion
borneol (*Borneolum*)	0.5 portion
ground beetle (*Eupdyphaga seu Steleophaga*)	5 portions
hyacinth bletilla (*Rhizoma Bletillae*)	1.5 portions
swallowwort root (*Radix Cynanchi Atrati*)	1.5 portions
dragon's bone (*Os Draconis Fossilia*)	1.5 portions
cuttle-bone (*Os Sepiella seu Sepiae*)	1.5 portions
plant soot (*Pulvis Fumi Carbonisatus*)	proper amount

Efficacy and indications: Promoting blood circulation, muscular granulation and reunion of bone and muscle; used for open injury and various ulcers which have cast the necrotic tissues, whose infection is under control without obvious pussy secretion, and which are expected to grow new tissues and heal.

Preparation and administration: The first group of drugs are deep-fried in the sesame oil till they grow exhausted. Filter to discard the dregs and collect the oil. Add the second group of drugs into the oil and boil them to get a paste. Then grind the drugs of the third group (except plant soot) separately into fine powders, mix them together, add them into the paste and churn well. Finally proper amount of plant soot is added to the paste to adjust the consistency. The final paste should be kept in a tight container for use. When needed, proper amount of the paste is spread out on the dressing material for external application. In recent years, the drugs are sometimes pulverized individually into fine powders and are then mixed together and boiled with vaseline for a paste in which gauze is soaked for external application.

Xiangsha Liujunzi Tang — Decoction of Cyperus and Amomum with Six Noble Ingredients (from *Classification and Treatment of Traumatic Diseases*)

Ingredients:
  ginseng (*Radix Ginseng*)
  white atractylodes rhizome
        (*Rhizoma Atactylodis Macrocephalae*)
  poria (*Poria*)
  licorice root (*Radix Glycyrrhizae*)
  tangerine peel (*Pericarpium Citri Reticulatae*)
  pinellia tuber (*Rhizoma Pinelliae*)
  cyperus tuber (*Rhizoma Cyperi*)
  amomum fruit (*Froctus Amomi*)
  agastache (*Herba Agastachis*)

Efficacy and indications: Invigorating *qi* to strengthen and harmonize the spleen and stomach; used to relieve persistent distending pain due to deficiency of promordial *qi*, or distending pain in the epigastria and stomach due to deficiency of *qi* and retention of dampness in the middle-*jiao*.

Preparation and administration: Boil the drugs in water for an oral dose.

Xiao Huoluo Dan — Minor Bolus for Activating Energy Flow in Channels and Collaterals (from *Formularies of the Bureau of Pharmacy*)

Ingredients:

arisaema with bile (*Arisaemacum Bile*)	3 portions
sichuan aconite root (*Radix Aconiti*)	3 portions
wild-aconite root (*Radix Aconiti Kusnezoffii*) (prepared)	3 portions
earthworm (*Lumbricus*)	3 portions
frankincense (*Resina Olibani*)	1 portion
myrrh (*Myrrha*)	1 portion
honey (*Mel*)	proper amount

Efficacy and indications: Warming the channels and collaterals to dispel the pathogenic cold and promoting circulation of blood to remove obstruction in channels; used for chronic pain, numbness of the body and extremities and inability of flexion and extension of limbs due to obstruction of the channels and collaterals by blood stasis after traumatic injury or due to affection of the channels and collaterals by pathogenic wind, cold or dampness.

Preparation and administration: All the drugs are ground together into a fine powder, which is mixed with processed honey to make boluses, 3g each. Take 1 bolus a time, 1—3 times a day.

Xiaoyao San — Ease Powder (from *Formularies of the Bureau of Pharmacy*)

Ingredients:

bupleurum root (*Radix Bupleuri*)	30g
Chinese angelica root (*Radix Angelicae Sinensis*)	30g
white peony root (*Radix Paeoniae Alba*)	30g
white atractylodes rhizome	

(*Rhizoma Atractylodis Macrocephalae*) 30g
poria (*Poria*) 30g
licorice root (*Radix Glycyrrhizae*) 15g

Efficacy and indications: Soothing the liver to regulate the flow of *qi* and invigorating the spleen to tonify blood; used for stagnation of the liver-*qi* and hyperactive liver-*qi* attacking the stomach after an injury manifested as distending pain in the chest and hypochondria, headache, dizziness, thirst, dry throat, listlessness, poor appetite, or alternate spells of fever and chill.

Preparation and administration: All the drugs are ground together into fine powder, 6—9g of which is infused with the decoction prepared from a little fresh ginger and peppermint and taken orally, 3 times a day. The drugs can also be boiled in water for an oral decoction but the dosage of each drug should be reduced in proportion to that in the recipe.

Xiaoyu Gao — Cream for Eliminating Blood Stasis (A proved recipe)

Ingredients:
rhubarb (*Radix et Rhizoma Rhei*) 1 portion
capejasmine fruit (*Froctus Gardeniae*) 2 portions
chaenomeles fruit (*Froctus Chaenomelis*) 4 portions
dandelion herb (*Harba Taraxaci*) 4 portions
turmeria (*Rhizoma Curcumae Longae*) 4 portions
phellodendron bark (*Cortex Phellodendri*) 6 portions
honey (*Mel*) proper amount

Efficacy and indications: Eliminating blood stasis, inducing subsidence of swelling and relieving pain; used for pains caused by ecchymoma after an injury.

Preparation and administration: Grind all the drugs into fine powder, which is mixed with water and honey of equal amount to prepare a cream for external application.

Xiaozhong Zhitong Gao — Repellent and Analgesic Ointment (A proved recipe from Traumatology)

Ingredients:
turmeria (*Rhizoma Curcumae Longae*)
notopterygium root (*Rhizoma seu Radix Notopterygii*)
dried ginger (*Rhizoma Zingiberis*)
capejasmine fruit (*Fructus Gardeniae*)
frankincense (*Resina Olibani*)
myrrh (*Myrrha*)

Efficacy and indications: Removing blood stasis, promoting subsidence of swelling and easing pain; used for ecchymoma and pain at the early stage of trauma.

Preparation and administration: Grind all the drugs together into a fine powder which is mixed with vaseline to prepare an ointment (6 portions of drug powder : 4 portions of vaseline) to be applied on the affected part.

Xiazhi Sunshang Xifang — Lotion for Injury of Lower Limbs (A proved Recipe from *Textbook on Traumatology of Traditional Chinese Medicine*)

Ingredients:

buck grass (*Herba Lycopodii*)	15g
tuberculate speranskia	
(*Herba Speranskiae Tuberculatae*)	15g
acanthopanax bark (*Cortex Acanthopanzcis*)	12g
burreed tuber (*Rhizoma Sparganii*)	12g
zedoary (*Rhizoma Zedoariae*)	12g
large-leaf gentian root	
(*Radix Gentianae Macrophyllae*)	12g
erythina bark (*Cortex Erythrinae*)	12g
achyranthes root (*Radix Achyranthis Bidentatae*)	10g
chaenomeles fruit (*Fructus Chaenomelis*)	10g
safflower (*Flos Carthami*)	10g
sappan wood (*Lignum Sappan*)	10g

Efficacy and indications: Promoting blood circulation to relieve rigidity of muscles; used to relieve muscular spasm and aches of the injured lower limb.

Preparation and administration: The drugs are decocted in water for a lotion for fumigating and bathing the affected limb.

Xinshang Xuduan Tang — Decoction Promoting Reunion of Fresh Bone Injury (A proved recipe from *Textbook on Traumatology in Traditional Chinese Medicine*)

Ingredients:

Chinese angelica root (*Radix Angelicae Sininsis*)	12g
ground beetle (*Eupolyphaga seu Steleophaga*)	6g
frankincense (*Resina Olibani*)	3g
myrrh (*Myrrha*)	3g
red sage root (*Radix Salviae Miltorrhizae*)	6g
pyrite (*Pyritum*) (*calcined and tempered in vinegar*)	12g
drynaria rhizome (*Rhizoma Drynariae*)	12g
bulgeweed (*Folium Lycopi*)	6g
corydalis tuber (*Rhizoma Corydalis*)	6g
sappan wood (*Lignum Sappan*)	10g
teasel root (*Radix Dipsaci*)	10g
mulberry twigs (*Ramulus Mori*)	12g
peach kernel (*Semen Persicae*)	10g

Efficacy and indications: Promoting blood circulation, removing blood stasis, easing pain and accelerating bone reunion; used to heal bone injury at the early and middle stages.

Preparation and administration: Boil the drugs in water for an oral decoction.

Xuefu Zhuyu Tang — Decoction for Removing Blood Stasis in the Chest (from *Correction on the Errors of Medical Works*)

Ingredients:

Chinese angelica root (*Radix Angelicae Sinensis*)	10g
dried rehmannia root (*Radix Rehmanniae*)	10g
peach kernel (*Semen Persicae*)	12g
safflower (*Flos Carthami*)	10g
bitter orange (*Fructus Aurantii*)	6g
red peony root (*Radix Paeoniae Rubra*)	6g

bupleurum root (*Radix Bupleuri*)   3g
licorice root (*Radix Glycyrrhizae*)   3g
platycodon root (*Radix Platycodi*)   4. 5g
achyranthes root (*Radix Achyranthis Bidentatae*)   10g

Efficacy and indications: Promoting blood circulation and removing blood stasis and obstruction in the channels and collaterals to relieve pain due to accumulation of blood stasis, unsmooth blood circulation and obstruction of channels.

Preparation and administration: Boil all the drugs in water for an oral decoction, a dose a day.

Xugu Huoxue Tang—Decoction Promoting Blood Circulation and Bone Reunion (A proved recipe from *Textbook on Traumatoloy in Traditional Chinese Medicine*)

Ingredients:
Chinese angelica root (*Radix Angelicae Sinensis*)   12g
red peony root (*Radix Paeoniae Rubra*)   10g
white peony root (*Radix Paeoniae Alba*)   10g
dried rehmannia root (*Radix Rehmanniae*)   15g
safflower (*Flos Carthami*)   6g
ground beetle (*Eupolyphaga seu Steleophaga*)   6g
drynaria rhizome (*Rhizoma Drynariae*)   12g
pyrite (*Pyritum*)   (calcined) 10g
teasel root (*Radix Dipsaci*)   12g
herb of asiatic pennywort (*Herba Centellae*)   10g
myrrh (*Myrrha*)   6g
frankincense (*Resina Olibani*)   6g

Efficacy and indications: Removing blood stasis, checking hemorrhage, promoting blood circulation and bone reunion; used to heal bone fracture and injury of soft tissues.

Preparation and administration: Boil the drugs in water for an oral dose.

Yangxue Zhitong Wan—Pill Tonifying Blood to Relieve Pain (from *A Concise Manual for Bone Setting*)

358

Ingredients:

white peony root (*Radix Paeoniae Alba*)	21g
red sage root (*Radix Salviae Miltorrhizae*)	21g
spatholobus stem (*Caulis Spatholobi*)	30g
large-leaf gentian root	
(*Radix Gentianae Macrophyllae*)	12g
cinnamon twig (*Ramulus Cinnamomi*)	9g
dried rehmannia root (*Radix Rehmanniae*)	18g
clematis root (*Radix Clematidis*)	24g
cyperus tuber (*Rhizoma Cyperi*)	12g
lindera root (*Radix Linderae*)	9g
cyathula root (*Radix Cyathulae*)	15g
licorice root (*Radix Glycyrrhizae*)	6g

Efficacy and indications: Tonifying blood, promoting blood circulation and easing the movement of joints; used for blood stasis due to deficiency of blood at the late stage of an injury with such signs and symptoms as myophagism, myosclerosis and dysfunction of the injured limb.

Preparation and administration: All the drugs are ground together into fine powder which is mixed with water to make pills. Take the pills with boiled water, 6g a time, 2 times a day.

Yougui Wan—Bolus Reinforcing the Kidney-*yang* (from *Jingyue's Complete Works*)

Ingredients:

prepared rehmannia root	
(*Radix Rehmanniae Praeparata*)	4 portions
Chinese yam (*Rhizoma Dioscoreae*)	2 portions
dogwood fruit (*Fructus Corni*)	2 portions
wolfberry fruit (*Fructus Lycii*)	2 portions
dodder seed (*Semen Cuscutae*)	2 portions
eucommia bark (*Cortex Eucommiae*)	2 portions
antler glue (*Colla Cornus Cervi*)	2 portions
Chinese angelica root	
(*Radix Angelicae Sinensis*)	1.5 portions

prepared daughter root of common monkshood
    (*Radix Aconiti Lateralis Praeparata*)   1 portion
cinnamon bark (*Cortex Cinnamomi*)   1 portion
honey (*Mel*)   proper amount

Efficacy and indications: Reinforcing the kidney-*yang*; used for mental fatigue and fright due to deficiency of *qi*, or palpitation and uneasiness, or cold limbs with flaccidity, resulting from insufficiency of the liver and kidney and deficiency and impairment of the blood and essence at the late stage of injury of bone and soft tissues.

Preparation and administration: Grind all the drugs together into fine powder which is then mixed with honey to produce pills. Take 10g each time 1—2 times a day.

Yunnan Baiyao—Yunnan White Drug-powder (A proprietary)
Ingredients: omitted.

Efficacy and indications: Promoting blood circulation, inducing hemostasis, removing blood stasis and relieving pain; used in the treatment of swelling pain due to blood stasis after injury, traumatic bleeding and pains of bone troubles.

Preparation and administration: For oral use: 0. 5g each time, once every 4 hours; for traumatic bleeding: dusted directly on the wound which is bound up afterwards; it can also be mixed with a liquid for external application.

Zhenggu Zijin Dan—Precious Bolus for Traumatic Injuries (from *The Golden Mirror of Medicine*)
Ingredients:
   clove (*Flos Caryophylli*)   1 portion
   costus root (*Radix Aucklandiae*)   1 portion
   dragon's blood (*Resina Draconis*)   1 portion
   catechu (*Catechu*)   1 portion
   prepared rhubarb
      (*Radix et Rhizoma Rhei Praeparata*)   1 portion
   safflower (*Flos Carthami*)   1 portion

moutan bark (*Cortex Moutan Radicis*)	1/2 portion
licorice root (*Radix Glycyrrhizae*)	1/3 portion

Efficacy and indications: Promoting blood circulation and the flow of *qi* to remove blood stasis and relieve pain; used for all kinds of traumatic injuries with pain, blood stasis or hematoma.

Preparation and administration: All the drugs are ground together into a fine powder, which is mixed with processed honey to form boluses. 10g of the bolus is taken orally with rice wine each time.

Zhenjiang Gao — Zhenjiang Plaster (A proprietary)

Ingredients: omitted.

Efficacy and indications: Expelling wind to relieve pain, dissolving mass in the abdomen, removing blood stasis, relaxing muscles, promoting blood circulation and regulating the flow of *qi*; used for pain of the muscles and bones, traumatic injury, internal injury from overstrain, hemiplegia, numbness of the limbs, arthritis, etc.

Preparation and administration: Heat the plaster and apply it on the diseased part. It should be avoided by those liable to skin allergies or those with skin diseases.

Zhibao Dan — Bolus Equaling a Priceless Treasure (from *Formularies of the Bureau of Pharmacy*)

Ingredients:

rhinocero's horn (*Cornu Rhinocerotis*)	100 portions
hawks bill shell (*Carapax Eretmochelydis*)	100 portions
amber (*Succinum*)	100 portions
cinnabar (*Cinnabaris*)	100 portions
realgar (*Realgar*)	100 portions
borneo-camphor (*Borneo-camphora*)	1 portion
musk (*Moschus*)	1 portion
cow bezoar (*Calculus Bovis*)	50 portions
benzoin (*Benzoinum*)	150 portions

Efficacy and indications: Inducing resuscitation, tranquilizing the mind, clearing away pathogenic heat and removing toxic substances; used for concussion of brain with coma from intracerebral injury, and high fever with convulsion caused by wound infection.

Preparation and administration: Grind all the drugs into a fine powder to make boluses, 3g each; take 1 bolus each time; proper dosage for children.

Zhuangjin Xugu Dan — Pellets Strengthening Muscles and Promoting Reunion of Fracture (from *A Great Collection on Traumatology*)

Ingredients:

Chinese Angelica root (*Radix Angelicae Sinensis*)	60g
chuanxiong rhizome (*Rhizoma Ligustici Chuanxiong*)	30g
white peony root (*Radix Paeoniae Alba*)	30g
prepared rehmannia root	
(*Radix Rehmanniae Praeparata*)	120g
eucommia bark (*Cortex Eucommiae*)	30g
teasel root (*Radix Dipsari*)	45g
acanthopanax bark (*Cortex Acanthopanacis*)	45g
drynaria rhizome (*Rhizoma Drynariae*)	90g
cinnamon twig (*Ramulus Cinnamomi*)	30g
notoginseng (*Radix Notoginseng*)	30g
astragalus root (*Radix Astragali seu Hedysari*)	90g
tiger bone (*Os Tigris*)	30g
malaytea scurfpea (*Fructus Psoraleae*)	60g
dodder seed (*Semen Cuscutae*)	60g
dangshen (*Radix Codonopsis Pilosulae*)	60g
chaenomeles fruit (*Fructus Chaenomelis*)	30g
Chinese siphonostegia (*Herba Siphonostegiae*)	60g
ground beetle (*Eupolyphaga seu Steleophaga*)	90g

Efficacy and indications: Strengthening muscles and promoting reunion of boken bones; used at the middle and late stages of bone fractures, dislocation and injury of muscles and ligaments.

Preparation and administration: Grind all the drugs into a fine powder, mix the powder with syrup to make small pellets, which are taken with warm rice wine, 12g. each time.

Zhuangyao Jianshen Tang (*Wan*) — Decoction for Strengthening the Kidney and Back (A proved recipe)

Ingredients:

prepared rehmannia root (*Radix Rehmanniae Praeparata*)
eucommia bark (*Cortex Eucommiae*)
dogwood fruit (*Fructus Corni*)
wolfberry fruit (*Fructus Lycii*)
malaytea scurfpea (*Fructus Psoraleae*)
safflower (*Flos Carthami*)
notopterygium root (*Radix seu Rhizoma Notopterygii*)
pubescent angelica root (*Radix Angelicae Pubescentis*)
desertliving cistanche (*Herba Cistanchis*)
dodder seed (*Semen Cuscutae*)
Chinese angelica root (*Radix Angelicae Sinensis*)

10g of each of the above drugs

Efficacy and indications: Strengthening the liver, kidney, muscles and bones; used to heal bone fractures and soft tissue injury with insufficiency of the liver and kidney.

Preparation and administration: Boil all the drugs for an oral decoction.

Zijin Jiu — Precious Purple Medicated Wine (from *Treatment of Bone and Articulation Injury by Traditional Chinese Medicine Combined with Western Medicine*)

Ingredients:

dragon's blood (*Resina Draconis*)	60g
safflower (*Flos Carthami*)	60g
camphor (*Camphora*)	30g
galangal rhizome (*Rhizoma Alpiniae Officinarum*)	120g
long peper (*Fructus Piperis Longi*)	90g
asarum herb (*Herba Asari*)	60g
white mustard seed (*Semen Sinapis Albae*)	60g
borneol (*Borneolum*)	30g
dried rehmannia root (*Radix Rehmanniae*)	60g

herb of small centipeda (*Herba Centipedae*)	90g
frankincense (*Resina Olibani*)	45g
myrrh (*Myrrha*)	45g

Efficacy and indications: Subduing swelling to ease pain and promoting blood circulation to remove blood stasis; used in the treatment of traumatic, injury with traumatic edema, cyanosis, pain and complicated fracture.

Preparation and administration: Steep all the drugs in 5kg of spirit and seal the container airtight. After 10 days, the medicated spirit is ready for use. Dip the absorbent cotton into the spirit and rub the injury dozens of times with the affected area feeling from cool at first to hot later on. It can also be used during massage.

Zixue Dan — Purple Snow Powder (from *Formularies of the Bureau of Pharmacy*)

Ingredients:

gypsum (*Gypsum Fibrosum*)

calcite (*Calcitum*)

tale (*Talcum*)

magnetite (*Magnetitum*)

scrophularia root (*Radix Scrophulariae*)

cimicifuga rhizome (*Rhizoma Cimicifugae*)

licorice root (*Radix Glycyrrhizae*)

mirabilite (*Natrii Sulphas*)

niter (*Nitrum*)

cloves (*Flos Caryophylli*)

cinnabar (*Cinnabaris*)

costus root (*Radix Aucklandiae*)

musk (*Moschus*)

rhinoceros horn (*Cornu Rhinocerotis*)

antelope's horn (*Cornu Saigae Tataricae*)

gold (*Aurum*)

eagle wood (*Lignum Aquilariae Resinatum*)

Efficacy and indications: Clearing away heat, removing toxic substances, inducing resuscitation and relieving convulsion; used in the treatment of high fever, dysphoria, unconsciousness, delirium, skin eruptions, jaundice, secondary infection of the inner tissues by sores, carbuncle complicated by septicemia, and dermatitis medicamentosa, or high fever and coma after craniocerebral injury.

Preparation and administration: The dosage of each drug and preparation of the powder are described in detail in *Collection of Prescriptions with Exposition*. Take 1—2g of the powder orally a time, or 3g for severe cases, 1—3 times a day.

Zuogui Wan — Bolus Reinforcing the Kidney-*yin* (from *Jingyue's Complete Works*)

Ingredients:

prepared rehmannia root (*Radix Rehmanniae Praeparata*)	4 portions
Chinese yam (*Rhizoma Dioscoreae*)	2 portions
dogwood fruit (*Fructus Corni*)	2 portions
wolfberry fruit (*Fructus Lycii*)	2 portions
dodder seed (*Semen Cuscutae*)	2 portions
eucommia bark (*Cortex Eucommiae*)	2 portions
antler glue (*Colla Cornus Cervi*)	2 portions
tortoise plastron (*Plastrum Testudinis*)	2 portions
cyathula root (*Radix Cyathulae*)	1.5 portions
honey (*Mel*)	proper amount

Efficacy and indications: Reinforcing the kidney-*yin*; used for lassitude in loin and legs, dizziness, blurred vision, fever of deficiency type, spontaneous sweating, night sweating, etc. due to insufficiency of kidney-*yin* and deficiency of essence after long internal injury or bone troubles.

Preparation and administration: All the drugs are ground together into a fine powder, which is mixed with boiled honey to make boluses. Take 2—3g a time with warm boiled water.

中医正骨医术

张志刚　编著

王宝勤　张玉玺

梁淑谦　赵华英　译

*

山东科学技术出版社出版

（中国济南玉函路 16 号　邮政编码 250002）

山东新华印刷厂德州厂印刷

中国国际图书贸易总公司发行

（中国北京车公庄西路 35 号　邮政编码 100044）

北京邮政信箱第.399 号

1996 年 8 月第 1 版第 1 次印刷

ISBN7－5331－1797－2/R · 518

05550

14－E－2850P